INFECTION CONTROL – UPDATES

Edited by **Christopher Sudhakar**

Infection Control – Updates
Edited by Christopher Sudhakar

Published by InTech
Janeza Trdine 9, 51000 Rijeka, Croatia

Publishing Process Manager Adriana Pecar

Technical Editor Teodora Smiljanic

Cover Designer InTech Design Team

Additional hard copies can be obtained from orders@intechopen.com

Infection Control – Updates, Edited by Christopher Sudhakar
p. cm.
ISBN 978-953-51-0055-3

For EU product safety concerns:
IN TECH d.o.o., Prolaz Marije Krucifikse Kozulić 3, 51000 Rijeka, Croatia,
info@intechopen.com or visit our website at intechopen.com.

Meet the editor

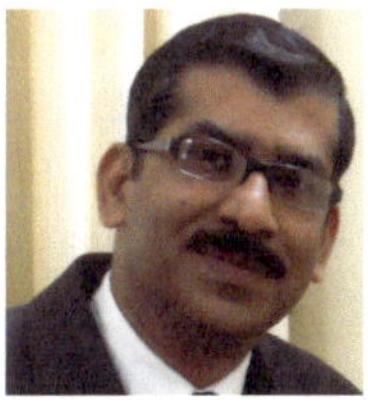

Dr Sudhakar has extensive work experience in Health care associated infection control especially in practice improvement. He is also involved in infection control policy development and developing low cost devices specifically for use in developing countries. He has authored a number of books and chapters and his work has been published within several national and international journals. In addition, he is an editorial board member of national Journal of Nursing science - Rajiv Gandhi University of Health sciences and review panel member of NITTE University journal. His special interests are training and simulation based learning. He is a research guide for PhD, MPhil, Masters and Degree programs and has taught at MPhil, MSc and Bachelor degree level in nursing. BOS and Academic Senate member of many Universities in south India. Dr Sudhakar is a frequent speaker on the subject and has presented at a number of national and international conferences. He has experience as a quality management representative, ISO auditor and assessor for the National Accreditation Board for Hospitals and Health care Providers (NABH), India. Whilst a life member of Hospital Infection Society of India, Academy of Hospital Administration and CMAI and NRSI, he currently works as Dean and professor in MCON, Mangalore, and Manipal University India.

Contents

Preface

Health care associated infection is coupled with significant morbidity and mortality. Prevention and control of infection is indispensable part of health care delivery system. Knowledge of Preventing HAI can help health care providers to make informed and therapeutic decisions thereby prevent or reduce these infections.

Infection control is continuously evolving science that is constantly being updated and enhanced. This book is arranged in various sections like facets of infection control, preventive strategies, practice improvement and emerging trends. The authors have paid particular attention in their field of expertise.

I am confident that this book will be very useful for all health care professionals to combat with health care associated infections. My sincere thanks to all expert contributors from different specialties around the world.

Christopher Sudhakar, Ph.D.
Manipal University
India

Part 1

Facets of Infection Control

1

Healthcare Associated Infections: Nuisance in the Modern Medical Epoch

Aamer Ikram[1] and Luqman Satti[2]
[1]*Department of Pathology, Quetta Institute of Medical Sciences*
[2]*Combined Military Hospital, DI Khan*
Pakistan

1. Introduction

Rapid advancements in the medical sciences have changed the understanding of the diseases down to the molecular level and in turn revolutionized the diagnostics and therapeutics. Similarly, architectural and engineering progression has reshaped the outlooks of the hospitals with the aim of comforting the patients. Despite all that, hospital environments remain a source of infection for the already ailing clientele. The scare of 'super bugs' has further aggravated the situation requiring more consolidated efforts for protection of admitted patients.

Healthcare associated infections (HAIs) are major cause of increased morbidity and mortality (World Health Organization [WHO], 2009). Statistics of various surveys show that 1 out of 10 patients admitted in hospital invariably acquire HAI (Emmerson, 1995). Data from developing countries is sparse, the situation otherwise seems to be much higher as compared to the developed world (Allegranzi et al., 2011). Worldwide around 1.4 million people are affected by HAIs at any given instance (Pittet & Donaldson, 2005). HAIs account for 99,000 deaths in American hospitals according to the Centres for Disease Control & Prevention (CDC) estimates (Klevens et al., 2007), and 37,000 deaths in Europe (WHO, 2011).

HAI or nosocomial infection is defined as localized or systemic infection which reveals itself in patient either during stay in hospital or after discharge, and was not incubating at the time of admission (WHO, 2002). Hospital infection control (HIC) refers to combination of various guidelines, policies and modalities implemented to minimize the risk of spreading infections in a health care facility. In the past, HAIs were restricted only to the hospital environments but in the recent years, various healthcare settings such as ambulatory care, home care have also been included in this category. This chapter essentially focuses on the prime aspects of HAIs especially lately documented.

These unanticipated but otherwise preventable infections have many distressing consequences such as increased mortality, prolonging morbidity and hospital stay, additional diagnostic and therapeutic interventions adding financial burden not only for the patient but also significant economic consequences on the entire healthcare organization. HAIs thus have a negative impact on the patients and their families and in turn the system. The financial effect is humongous as it has been estimated to reach £ 1,000 million each year in the UK (National Audit Office [NAO], 2000), € 7 billion in Europe (WHO, 2011) and $ 6.65 billion in the US in 2007 (Scott, 2009).

In the recent years, duration of patients' hospital stay has decreased but paradoxically, HAIs are increasing at alarming rates (Burke, 2003; Stone et al., 2002). Unfortunately, exact incidence of HAIs is not known or undervalued as many patients develop symptoms after discharge from the hospitals especially post-surgical infectious cases. Intensive care units (ICUs) and surgical units are the main reservoirs for HAIs especially in resource poor countries; reason being that most of the patients, especially in ICUs, have meager immunity or are critically ill (Ikram et al., 2010). However, the main reason for HAIs remains poor adherence to 'standard infection control guidelines' and 'additional precautions' (Siegel, 2007). Any breach in the infection control practices augments the transmission of microorganisms. It is, therefore, obligatory for everyone including doctors, nurses, paramedics, patients and even visitors to strictly follow the standard infection control guidelines.

The sites involved and the sources could be multiple. Surgical site infections comprise 20% of HAIs and around 5% of operated patients develop these infections (de Lissovoy et al., 2009; Gottrup, 2000). Neonatal nosocomial infection doubles the mortality risk and can only be improved by paying comprehensive attention to all aspects of neonatal intensive care (Gill et al., 2011).

Invasive fungal infections in hospitalized patients increase morbidity and mortality. *Candida* spp. is responsible for 15% of HAIs and 72% of nosocomial fungal infections, and invasive candidiasis has mortality rate up to 40-50% in hospitalized patients (Gudlaugsson et al., 2003). Water in the dental units may be contaminated with a variety of organisms which may in turn cause infection during dental procedures (Kumar et al., 2011).

2. Responsibility of infection control team

Infection control in a health care setting requires a multifaceted approach (CDC, 2007) and is responsibility of everyone coming in contact with the patient. The pivotal role is performed by a committed Infection Control Team usually comprising:

- Infection control practitioner or doctor.
- Administrator.
- Infection control nurse.

Infection Control Team is responsible for establishing infection control policies and procedures, providing advice and guidance regarding infection control matters, regular audits and surveillance, identification and investigation of outbreaks, awareness and education of staff (Ayliffe et al., 2000). The team works under Infection Control Committee which chiefly carries the responsibilities of making major decisions, problem discussion with the team, departmental coordination, educational activities, policy modification and recommendations.

3. Factors implicated in healthcare associated infections

Factors predisposing a hospitalized patient to HAI are related to organisms, host and environments.

3.1 Organism-related factors

Practically any microorganism in the vicinity can cause HAI; varying for different settings, populations and countries (WHO, 2002). The organisms may be endogenous causing auto-infection or self-infection, or exogenous. The exogenous organisms are usually transferred through airborne, percutaneous or direct contact transmission. 'Cross-infection' is transmission of organism from one person to another. Organisms commonly responsible for major HAIs are listed in table 1.

Type of Infection	Common organisms involved
Surgical site infections (SSIs)	*S. aureus*, *Enterococcus* spp, *S. pyogenes*, *E. coli*, *Pseudomonas aeruginosa*, *Proteus* spp and anaerobes
Blood stream infections (BSIs)	*S. aureus* including methicillin resistant *S. aureus* (MRSA), coagulase negative staphylococci and *Enterococcus* spp
Urinary tract infections (UTIs)	*E. coli*, *Proteus* spp, *Klebsiella* spp, *Pseudomonas aeruginosa*, *Serratia* spp, *Enterococcus* spp and less commonly *C. albicans*
Ventilator associated pneumonia (VAP)	*Acinetobacter baumannii*, *Pseudomonas aeruginosa*, *S. aureus*, and Enterobacteriaceae

Table 1. Common organisms involved in healthcare associated infections.

Serratia marcescens has been associated with nosocomial outbreaks mostly with contaminated fluids and injections. Recently there has been an outbreak among newborns due to usage of contaminated baby shampoo (Madani et al., 2011). *Clostridium difficile* associated diarrhoea (CDAD) is associated with high mortality rate in hospitalized patients particularly elderly with multiple co-morbidities (White and Wiselka, 2011). *Acinetobacter baumannii* has rapidly emerged as a nosocomial pathogen and that too with acquisition of multidrug resistance. Anti-pseudomonal carbapenems have been utilized against this resistant species, however, one-half to two-third of the isolates have been reported as resistant to this group as well (Tsakris et al., 2006).

Viral infections can be transmitted through different routes in the healthcare settings; airborne viruses such as influenza virus, respiratory syncytial virus, adenovirus, rhinovirus, coronavirus, measles, rubella virus, mumps virus and parvovirus B19 can spread through droplets or indirectly by settling on surfaces; faecal-oral route such as norovirus, rotavirus and human adenovirus 40 and 41 (Lopman et al., 2004); and blood-borne like hepatitis B and C viruses and human immunodeficiency virus (Davanzo et al., 2008).

3.2 Host-related factors

The host could either be a patient or staff. There are numerous risk factors which predispose a host to acquire HAIs including:

- Low body resistance as in infancy and old age.
- Underlying illness gravity - patients with severe diseases / debilitated conditions.
- Prolonged hospitalization.

- Delayed hospital discharge has been associated with increased HAI prevalence. The reason for delayed discharge include long term bed care, pending equipment required at home or access to other services (McNicholas et al., 2011).
- Immunosuppression, malignancy, pregnancy.
- Reduced local tissue resistance.
- Use of medical devices such as I/V cannula, catheters, shunts and procedures such as bronchoscopy, cystoscopy etc.

3.3 Environment-related factors

Environment has a very significant impact on the chances of acquiring HAI and it varies for different places within a hospital. Clean and healthy environments in wards and sterile conditions especially in ICUs, nurseries and operation theatres minimize the risk of HAIs.

Routine cleaning and disinfection is not sufficient in hospitals with continuous flow of patients, healthcare workers (HCWs) and visitors, and more efficient methods may have to be adopted to maintain the requisite standards (Wang et al., 2010).

4. Mode of transmission of microorganisms

It is important to understand the mode of transmission of microorganisms for putting barricades in the chain at healthcare settings. These include (CDC, 1998; 2007):

4.1 Droplet transmission

Droplet particles, produced by coughing, sneezing and even talking, can settle either on surrounding surfaces or on the body mucosa which can be transferred to others. Examples include meningitis and pneumonia.

4.2 Airborne transmission

Particles less than 5 micrometers remain suspended in air and may be inhaled causing infection in a susceptible host. Examples are tubercle bacilli and varicella virus.

4.3 Contact transmission

This is the most common mode of transmission of organisms which can be direct or indirect. In direct transmission, organisms are transferred from an infected or colonized person to another susceptible host by direct skin contact. In indirect transmission, organisms are first transferred from an infected person to a normal host such as a HCW and then to another. Most common example of contact transmission seen in surgical settings is the transfer of *S. aureus* from an infected wound or boils.

4.4 Vector-borne transmission

This mode is unusual in developed countries but it is not so uncommon in resource poor healthcare settings. Organisms are spread by vectors such as flies, mosquitoes and fleas. A common example is spread of dysentery caused by *Shigella* spp. through flies.

4.5 Other modes

There are sometimes incidences where the source of infection in hospital setting is common and many persons get infected through the same source like use of contaminated food, drinking water, ointments, topical solutions and instruments. This can lead to outbreak in hospital setting.

5. Principles for hospital infection control

In general, infection control measures particularly revolve around the following:

- Policies and procedures taken within hospital in different settings such as ICUs, operation theatres, other high risk areas, wards, etc.
- Dedicated infection control teams.
- Maintaining hospital hygiene.
- Effective sterilization and disinfection techniques.
- Proper management of hospital waste.
- Continuous surveillance.
- Outbreak investigation and management in hospital.
- Clinical auditing.

5.1 Measures taken in hospital

These include standard infection control measures and transmission based precautions (CDC, 2007). Standard infection control measures are universally accepted and followed in most healthcare facilities.

5.1.1 Hand washing and hand hygiene

Hand hygiene is one of the key measures for preventing HAIs (Pittet & Boyce, 2001). Hand washing between patient contact and after surgical/invasive procedures is the most simple, economical and easy to perform measure significantly reducing infection transmission. However, its practice and compliance has been the core issue worldwide especially in the developing countries (Collins, 2008). Poor hand hygiene practices in hospital has led to number of outbreaks and adverse outcomes (Jarvis, 2001; Stanton and Rutherford, 2004; Hugonnet et al., 2004). It has been well established that simple hand washing with soap and water can prevent majority of childhood illnesses causing high mortality (Luby et al., 2005). Provision of sinks at various places in hospitals, monitoring of hand hygiene and continued education of staff in hospital can increase the level of patient safety. Hand washing and hand hygiene practices can be improved and monitored by using guidelines, '*How-to-Guide: Improving Hand Hygiene*' (Institute for Healthcare Improvement, 2008). A versatile approach involving HCWs in the form of social marketing or especially directed towards barriers to hand hygiene seems to be much more successful (Forrester et al., 2010).

Preoperative hand scrubbing by surgical team is mandatory to prevent surgical site infection along with wearing of gloves, gown, mask and cap. A latest study recommends appropriate disinfectant application to forearms for 10 s as part of preoperative hand disinfection (Hubner et al., 2011). Another study recommends alcohol-based hand rubs for surgical preparation because of prompt antimicrobial action, broad spectrum, lesser side effects and avoiding the risk of contamination by the rinsing water (Widmer et al., 2010).

Importance associated with hand hygiene awareness requires national commitment. It is mandatory part of national infection control programmes in many countries. A baseline survey of activities in improving hand hygiene was conducted by the WHO First Global Patient Safety Challenge in 2007. In 2009, it was repeated to evaluate the latest situation. Promotion of hand hygiene has become an important initiative with most of the countries; however, coordinated efforts are to be strengthened across the world (Mathai et al., 2011). WHO message remains – 'Clean hands are safer hands'.

Wearing wrist watches augments the bacterial contamination of the wrist but until it is manipulated, excess hand contamination does not ensue (Jeans et al., 2010). The wearing of watch over the chest pocket is definitely preferable.

In demanding situations like patient overload or in critical care units, alcohol based hand rub may be a more realistic approach as it acts rapidly, takes less time and less irritable (Pittet & Boyce, 2001). Goroncy-Bermes et al. (2010) recommended 3 mL of alcohol hand rub containing adequate active concentration for contact time of 30 s. In general, sufficient amount should be utilized to cover all the surfaces of both the hands. Increased application of alcohol hand rub has been associated with noteworthy reduction in MRSA rates in hospital settings (Sroka et al., 2010)

Much valuable time of HIC experts has been spent in the development and implementation of audit tools for hand hygiene. Gould et al (2011) recommended a combined approach of routine screening from product uptake and utilization of infection control experts. A promising consideration adjunct to the safety culture is involvement of patients in the design and promotion of hand hygiene at the institutional level (Pittet et al., 2011).

5.1.2 Physical precautions

Personal clothing is changed after arriving in the hospital and varies for different departments and hospitals. The indication for changing clinical attire is not as intense as other infection control measures like hand hygiene but it should be part of measures for controlling infections and the concept of 'bare below elbows' may be preferred (Shelton et al., 2010).

Personal protective equipment (PPE) is used by healthcare workers for protection against infectious organisms as it acts as a barrier between the worker and fluid or material containing infectious agents. PPE may comprise of gloves, mask/respirator such as N-95, gowns/apron, goggles/face shield, shoe and head covers. Some of the important aspects for proper PPE utilization are:

- **Risk assessment** is an important aspect before deciding about the sort of PPE to be utilized. PPE should be selected according to the risks involved in that particular healthcare setting.
- PPE should not be worn outside the restricted area. There should be properly allocated place for every HCW for keeping PPE.
- Each HCW should have his/her own PPE.

- PPE should be changed between patients' contact followed by proper hand washing.
- Used or old PPE should be disposed of properly.
- Double gloving should be done where indicated and punctured gloves should be changed immediately.

Healthcare setting environments can be protected by provision of physical barriers in the form of isolation of infected cases. Isolation policy and guidelines for the infectious cases thus remain pivotal for curtailing pathogen spread and have to be prepared according to requirements considering transmission mode, risk of spread to others, severity of infection, effective treatment available, and impact of isolation on patients (Ayliffe et al., 1999). Cohorting of the patients infected with same pathogen can be done.

5.1.3 Environmental safeguards

Hospital environments hold a diverse group of microorganisms surrounding a patient which generally originates from normal flora of patient, HCW, visitor, or from infected wounds. In the recent years, much debate is going on the role of environmental cleaning in reducing HAIs. The apparent hygiene of hospital cannot be linked with the risk of HAIs. With the emergence of fear and public panic due to 'superbugs' causing serious HAIs, hospital environments have been blamed for such infections. However, the exact role of hospital environment in causing these infections remains unknown (Dancer, 2009). Some of the superbugs such as *Acinetobacter baumannii* and *Pseudomonas aeruginosa*, after gaining access to hospital environment especially in ICUs, are extremely difficult to eradicate even with the advanced disinfection techniques. Hospital room surfaces and inanimate objects such as blood pressure set, stethoscope, utensils, etc can become colonized with resistant microorganisms such as MRSA, VRE and *Clostridium difficile*. Ungloved hands can become 50% more contaminated with low level pathogenic microorganisms (Bhalla et al., 2004).

For prevention of health associated infections particularly in immuno-compromised patients, special attention should be directed to the quality of air circulating in the hospital environments (Leung and Chan, 2006). Total air change rate should be 15 air changes/hr for operation theatres and delivery rooms; 6 air changes/hr for intensive care units, isolation rooms and laboratories; and 4 air changes/hr for patient rooms. Isolation room, equipment sterilization room and laboratory should have negative pressure control while intensive care unit, operation theatre and delivery room should have positive pressure control. The flow of air has to be from clean towards dirty areas. A latest study by Tang et al. (2011) has nicely observed the role of airflow patterns and movement of suspended material in infection control of aerosol and airborne transmitted diseases employing different techniques. This understanding would be very beneficial in understanding aerosol and airborne infection transmission through precise airflow visualization techniques and in turn developing modalities for preventing them.

Among many sources responsible for nosocomial infections, hospital water is a controllable but overlooked source. Many pathogens can survive in hospital water supply, transfer antibiotic resistance and have been implicated in numerous outbreaks (Anaissie et al., 2002). Proper guidelines for the monitoring and prevention of hospital water borne infections are still limited. *Legionella pneumophila*, pathogenic mycobacteria, parasites and viruses have been implicated in hospital water borne diseases. In the recent years, pathogenic fungi and molds have been increasingly reported (Falvey & Streifel, 2007; Garner & Machin, 2008) thus mounting the need to formulate guidelines for the monitoring of hospital water sources (Hayette et al., 2010). Avoidance of hospital tap water, routine and targeted surveillance cultures of water sources, and hospital staff and patients education are major measures to control water associated nosocomial infections. Marchesi et al. (2011) employed hyperchlorination, thermal shock, chlorine dioxide, monochloramine, boilers and point-of-use filters to control *Legionella* spp. in hospital water supply.

The make of surfaces of hospital items does affect the contamination chances. Copper-containing items tend to reduce the number of microbial surface contamination in hospital environments (Casey et al., 2010). The antimicrobial activity of copper-containing surfaces has been demonstrated to be far more effectual as it decreases the biodurden to a far greater amount as compared to the standard materials (Marias et al., 2010). The routine cleaning of these surfaces, however, is mandatory and the make of surfaces act as additional factors against HAIs.

Central venous catheters are justifiably used in the ICUs whereas reverse is true for non-ICU settings and even for prolonged periods facilitating infections. There is a dire need to prevent infections associated with CVCs and short-term indwelling catheters. Measures should be targeted at insertion time with judicious usage of CVCs in these settings as part of strategy to reduce HAIs (Zingg et al., 2011).

5.1.4 Control of multidrug resistant organism

Multidrug resistant (MDR) organisms in hospital settings add further impetus to the status of HAIs. Empirical use of costly and broad spectrum antibiotics against these organisms further augments their resistance potential. For example, it is much more difficult to treat ventilator associated pneumonia due to MDR *Acinetobacter baumannii* in an ICU than a sensitive strain. A multicentric study showed that bacteremia caused by MRSA strain is associated with higher mortality and prolong hospital stay than caused by methicillin sensitive strain (Cosgrove et al., 2003).

During the past decade, MDR organisms have emerged at an alarming level especially in intensive care units. In these settings, MRSA infections have been dominant with 60% of all the staphylococcal infections followed by VRE, 20% of all the enterococcal infections; while 31% of the enterobacter infections were caused by third generation cephalosporin resistant strains (CDC, 2004). Surveillance data in the USA showed that MRSA accounts for 64% of the invasive nosocomial infections due to *S. aureus*. Various studies have shown that the data of frequency of MDR organisms outside the ICUs is almost similar (Loeb et al., 2003; Trick et al., 2001). Matenez-Capolino et al. (2010) showed that active surveillance cultures with contact precautions augmenting the standard measures could help reducing nosocomial MRSA in healthcare settings.

Strict implementation of HIC guidelines is recommended to prevent the transmission of MDR organisms in hospital environments including:

- Contact precautions, isolation of infected/colonized patients and use of PPE.
- Active surveillance cultures to identify the persons colonized with resistant organisms including HCWs.

- Stringently following standard precautions and hand hygiene.
- Cohorting of patients infected or colonized with MDR organisms.

Nasal carriage of MRSA by the patients as well as staff remains an important source for infection. Many remedies have been tested for nasal elimination of MRSA including local 2% mupirocin application which has lead to emergence of resistant strains. Polyhexanide, a widely used antiseptic, has been shown to be an effective alternate to mupirocin in elimination of nasal MRSA especially mupirocin-resistant strains (Madeo, 2010).

5.1.5 Surveillance

Surveillance comprises continuing systematic collection, analysis, interpretation and dissemination of data pertaining to health related events to be utilized for improving the health system (CDC, 2001). It is a vital component in HIC chain for avoidance and early detection of outbreaks and in turn prompt response as well as determining the need and measuring outcome of actions already adopted (NAO, 2000). Surveillance can be localized or targeted such as to see ventilator associated pneumonia in an ICU or generalized such as to measure infection rate in a hospital. Financial restraints of a hospital are very important to determine the type of surveillance performed. With transformation in healthcare delivery system and advancement in more friendly electronic tools, surveillance methods will continue progression and facilitate effective infection control measures (CDC, 2007).

Staff working in hospital environments has to be protected from catching infections from patients. There should be a regular health surveillance system, ideally part of occupational health services within the setup. The department should address the needs of HCWs especially regarding relevant vaccination status and any accidental exposure, maintaining proper and timely health records, and requisite guidance and training.

5.1.6 Hospital antibiotic policy

Injudicious use of antibiotics especially in hospital settings is a major factor in the development of drug resistant organisms. Each hospital must have its own antibiotic policy based upon the culture and sensitivity results that should be regularly reviewed. Overuse and misuse of antibiotics exerts a selective pressure on bacteria thus resulting in emergence of drug resistance. If possible, usage of newer and costly antibiotics should be restricted to minimum and prescribed only for serious conditions or non-availability of alternate choice in order to prevent the emergence of resistance (Ferguson, 2004). In the recent years, attention has been directed to a greater extent towards prevention through immunization and HIC steps as substitute to reduce the prescription of antibiotics.

Many studies have shown that rational use of antibiotics alone can significantly reduce emergence of drug resistance (Landman et al., 1999; McNulty et al., 1997; Quale et al., 1996; Saurina et al., 2000). In order to reduce emergence of MDR organisms, certain measures should be considered while prescribing antibiotics such as:

- Clinical condition of the patient should be carefully assessed before prescribing any antibiotic.
- Requisite culture and sensitivity results for targeted therapy except in serious infections.

- Substandard drugs, frequent problem in developing countries, should be prohibited.
- Truly infecting organisms should be treated, not colonizers or contaminants.
- Empirical therapy must be advised in the light of existing local susceptibility pattern.
- Combination therapy should be considered in indicated cases.
- Appropriate antibiotic, preferably narrow spectrum, should be advised in precise dose for proper duration.
- Measures must be instilled for ensuring awareness regarding hospital antibiotic policy.

5.1.7 Sterilization and disinfection practices

Hospital sterilization and disinfection policy is crucial and basic component of infection control system. All invasive procedures require direct contact between patient's skin or mucous membrane and medical devices thus carrying a risk of direct transfer of pathogenic organisms. Various steps required to reduce infection rate in hospitals by effective sterilization and disinfection policy include an efficient and dependable team, assessment and implementation of ongoing disinfection policies, adequate staff training and regular audits (Coates and Hutchinson, 1994).

The level of sterilization and disinfection depends on the risk assessment: critical items such as surgical instruments for direct tissue contact require sterilization while semi critical items such as colonoscope with mucous membrane contact and non critical items such as stethoscope with intact skin contact require high level and low level disinfection respectively (Dancer, 2009). Failure to strictly comply with these policies can lead to outbreaks and transmission of pathogenic organisms such as *Mycobacterium tuberculosis* from one person to another through medical or surgical devices such as contaminated endoscopes (CDC, 1998; Garner and Favero, 1986; Uttley and Simpson, 1994).

Spaulding's devised compact and effective scheme for sterilization and disinfection is still in practice with certain modifications (Weber et al., 2002). Critical items can be purchased as sterile or disposable or treated with steam. Heat sensitive instruments can be sterilized by ethylene oxide, hydrogen peroxide gas plasma sterilization or by liquid sterilents if other methods are not appropriate. One of the disadvantages of liquid sterilents is that the devices cannot be wrapped during processing leading to difficulty in maintaining sterilization after processing and during storage.

In case of semi critical items such as endoscope, colonoscope, respiratory therapy equipment, devices should be free of all the pathogenic organisms with exception of small numbers of bacterial spores. These items require high level disinfection with chemical disinfectants such as glutaraldehyde, hydrogen peroxide, ortho-phthalaldehyde, peracetic acid with hydrogen peroxide, and chlorine. After disinfection, these items should be thoroughly rinsed with sterile water and allowed to dry thus reducing the chances of contamination by eliminating the wet environment favourable for bacterial growth (Garner and Favero, 1986; Spaulding, 1968). Non critical items such as stethoscope, bedpans, bed rails, blood pressure cuff, furniture and floors do not require sterilization or high level disinfection as they come in contact with the intact skin. They do not require separate processing unit and can be disinfected at the same place. There is no documented report of a non critical item causing direct transmission of an infectious agent to patients (CDC, 2003). However, they can contribute to secondary transmission mode by contaminating the hands of HCWs and subsequently to the patients. Quaternary ammonium compounds, chlorine based compounds and phenols are some of the commonly used low level disinfectants.

As skin antiseptics prior to venous puncture, alcoholic products appear to be better than non-alcoholic solutions (Caldeira et al., 2011). Spores of *C. difficile* can contaminate the healthcare settings and require use of appropriate disinfectant. Many available disinfectants like alcohol-containing gels, detergents and quaternary ammonium compounds are ineffective against *C. difficile* spores. Chlorine releasing agents are reliable for its control but with limitations under dirty conditions (Fraise, 2011).

The importance of sporicidal disinfectants can never be undervalued especially under the present circumstances. Commercially available sporicides have to be evaluated through testing standards. Although a number of such standards are available in Europe, these have limitations such as prolonged application time and do not involve surface contamination. Organization for Economic Cooperation & Development is presently preparing a more realistic set of standards (Humphreys, 2011).

5.1.8 Hospital waste management

Proper disposal of hospital waste is the last requisite in the chain of an effective HIC system. The hospital waste is a threat not only for the patients and the concerned staff but also to public health and environment (Singh & Sharma, 1996). It is a bit neglected part in the developing countries leading to spread of infectious diseases like hepatitis B, hepatitis C.

Hospital waste includes all types of waste generated in a healthcare facility including laboratories. The infectious waste comprises pathological, isolation, laboratory, surgical, autopsy and animal waste, human blood and blood products and contaminated sharps. Others include chemical, genotoxic and radioactive waste. Sharps contaminated with blood are the major risk factors for infection transmission (WHO, 2002).

Calculation of infectious waste output is obligatory for each healthcare setting so as to streamline the final disposal. Studies have shown that in the US, the rate of average waste production is 5.9 to 10.4 kg/bed/day while in Western Europe it is around 3-6 kg/bed/day (Brunner, 1986; Halbawach, 1994). Disposal of this infectious waste remains intricate and expensive with special concerns like environmental hazards related to incineration. As such, infectious waste reduction leads to cost reduction (Daschner, 1991).

Various components of hospital waste management include: collection of waste by defined persons, segregation/sorting of waste, transportation, storage and disposal.

5.1.8.1 Principles of waste management

- Dedicated hospital waste management committee is a prerequisite.
- Suitable waste management plan based on risks and types of waste generated.
- **Waste minimization** is an imperative aspect to be highlighted to HCWs.
- Color coded bags must be utilized according to the type of waste.
- Waste to be transported in trolleys or carts and stored at specified restricted places.
- Sharps should be stored in proper boxes with biohazard sign.

- Sharps should be first autoclaved and then buried in a secured area after compaction. Animal carcasses and anatomical waste should be incinerated while radioactive waste should be dealt according to the national laws.

5.1.9 Education and training

Awareness of the HCWs has to be ensured and updated in the form of regular educative and training activities. Not only that, patients and their relatives have also to be imparted awareness regarding infection control measures in order to break the transmission chain. Healthcare infection control should be a mandatory component of training at postgraduate and undergraduate level for HCWs and also imparted to all others coming in contact with patients or medical equipment (CDC, 2007).

6. International efforts

Determined efforts and concern for HAI control at the international level especially by the WHO have to be acknowledged. The material available at the WHO website provides plenty of guidance in this respect. The material can easily be downloaded and utilized in preparing local policies. The global involvement in raising awareness about hand hygiene has been commendable. Similarly, assistance can be sought through abundant valuable information provided by the CDC website. These are truly helpful for the developing world.

Regular live and archived lectures are available through courtesy of Webber Training Inc (www.webbertraining.com). These have ample latest information that can provide guidance to the HCWs especially concerned with infection control.

7. References

Allegranzi, B., Nejad, S.B., Combescure, C., Graafmans, W., Attar, H., Donaldson, L., & Pittet, D. (2011). Burden of endemic healthcare-associated infection in developing countries: systematic review and meta-analysis. *Lancet*, Vol. 377, pp. 228-241.

Anaissie, E.J., Penzak, S.R., & Dignani, M.C. (2002). The hospital water supply as a source of nosocomial infections: a plea for action. *Arch Intern Med*, Vol. 162, No. 13, pp. 1483-1492.

Ayliffe, G.A.J., Babb, J.R., & Taylor, L.J. (Eds.). (1999). *Hospital-acquired infection. Principles and Practice*, (3rd Edition), Butterworth and Heinemann, ISBN 0192620339, Oxford.

Ayliffe, G.A.J., Fraise, A.P., Geddes, A.M., & Mitchell, K. (Eds.). (2000). *Control of Hospital Infection*, (4th Edition), Arnold, ISBN 0340759119, London.

Bhalla, A., Pultz, N.J., Gries, D.M., Ray, A.J., Eckstein, E.C., Aron, D.C., & Donskey, C.J. (2004). Acquisition of nosocomial pathogens on hands after contact with environmental surfaces near hospitalized patients. *Infect Control Hosp Epidemiol*, Vol. 25, No. 2, pp. 164-167.

Brunner, C.R. (1986). *Hazardous air emission from incineration*. (2nd Edition), Champman & Hall New York, NY.

Burke, J.P. (2003). Infection control—a problem for patient safety. *N Engl J Med*. Vol. 25, No. 348, pp. 651-656.

Caldeira, D., David, C., & Sampaio, C. (2011). Skin antiseptics in venous puncture-site disinfection for prevention of blood culture contamination: systematic review with meta-analysis. *J Hosp Infect*, Vol. 77, pp. 223-232.

Casey, A.L., Adams, D., Karpanen, T.J., Lambert, P.A., Cookson, B.D., Nightingale, P., Miruszenko, L., Shillam, R., & Christian, P. (2010). Role of copper in reducing hospital environment contamination. *J Hosp Infect*, Vol. 74, pp. 72-77.

Centers for Disease Control & Prevention. (1996). Guidelines for isolation precautions in hospitals. Hospital Infection Advisory Committee. Accessed on 15 July 2011. Available from: <http://wonder.cdc.gov/wonder/prevguid/p0000419.asp>

Centers for Disease Control & Prevention. (1998). Ambulatory and inpatient procedures in the United States, 1996. Atlanta, GA, pp. 1-39.

Centers for Disease Control & Prevention. (2001). Updated Guidelines for Evaluating Public Health Surveillance Systems. Recommendations from the Guidelines Working Group. MMWR Recomm Rep, 50(RR-13), pp. 1-35.

Centers for Disease Control. (2003) Guidelines for Environmental Infection Control in Health-Care Facilities, 2003. MMWR, Vol. 52 (No. RR-10), pp. 1-44.

Centers for Disease Control & Prevention. (2004). National nosocomial infections surveillance (NNIS) system report, data summary from January 1992 through June 2004, issued October 2004. *Am J Infect Control*, Vol. 32, pp. 470–85.

Centers for Disease Control & Prevention. (2007). Guidelines for isolation preventions: preventing transmission of infectious agents in healthcare settings. Accessed on 16 July 2011. Available from:
<http://www.cdc.gov/hipac/pdf/isolation/isoaltion2007.pdf>

Coates, D., & Hutchinson, D.N. (1994). How to produce a hospital disinfection policy. *J Hosp Infect*, Vol. 26, No. 1, pp. 57-68.

Collins, A.S. (2008). Preventing Health Care-Associated Infections. In: *Patient Safety and Quality: An Evidence-Based Handbook for Nurses.* Hughes, R.G. Rockville. Rockville, Agency for Healthcare Research and Quality, US. Accessed on 12 July 2011. Available from: <http://www.ncbi.nlm.nih.gov/books/NBK2683/>

Cosgrove, S.E., Sakoulas, G., Perencevich, E.N., Shwaber, M.J., Karchmer, A.W., & Carmeli, Y. (2003). Comparison of mortality associated with methicillin-resistant and methicillin-susceptible *Staphylococcus aureus* bacteremia: a meta-analysis. *Clin Infect Dis*, Vol. 36, pp. 53–55.

Dancer, S.J. (2009). The role of environmental cleaning in the control of hospital-acquired infection. *J Hosp Infect*, Vol. 73, No. 4, pp. 378-85. Epub 2009 Sep 1.

Daschner, F. (1991). Unnecessary and ecological cost of hospital infection. *J Hosp Infect*, Vol. 18, pp. 73-78.

Davanzo, E., Frasson, C., Morandin, M., & Trevisan, A. (2008). Occupational blood and body fluid exposure of university health care workers. *Am J Infect Control*, Vol. 36, pp. 753-756.

de Lissovoy, G., Fraeman, K., Hutchins, V., Murphy, D., Song, D., & Vaughn, B.B. (2009). Surgical site infection: incidence and impact on utilization and treatment costs. *Am J Infect Control*, Vol. 37, pp. 387-397.

Emmerson, A.M. The impact of surveys on hospital infection. (1995) *J Hosp Infect*, Vol. 30, pp. 421-40.

Falvey, D.G., & Streifel, A.J. (2007). Ten-year air sample analysis of *Aspergillus* prevalence in a university hospital. *J Hosp Infect*, Vol. 67, No. 1, pp. 35-41.

Ferguson, J. (2004). Antibiotic prescribing: how can emergence of antibiotic resistance be delayed? *Aust Prescr*, Vol. 27, pp. 39-42.

Forrester, L.A., Bryce, E.A., & Mediaa, A.K. (2010). Clean Hands for Life™: results of a large, multicentre, multifaceted, social marketing hand-hygiene campaign. *J hosp Infect*, Vol. 74, pp. 225-231.

Fraise, A. (2011). Currently available sporicides for use in healthcare, and their limitations. *J Hosp Infect*, Vol. 77, pp. 210-212.

Garner, D., & Machin, K. (2008). Investigation and management of an outbreak of mucromycosis in a paediatric oncology unit. *J Hosp Infect*, Vol. 70, No. 1, pp. 53-59.

Garner, J.S., & Favero, M.S. (1986). CDC Guideline for handwashing and hospital environmental control, 1985. *Infect Control*, Vol. 7, pp. 231-243.

Garner, J.S., & Favero, M.S. (1986). CDC guidelines for the prevention and control of nosocomial infections. Guideline for handwashing and hospital environmental control, 1985. Supersedes guideline for hospital environmental control published in 1981. *Am J Infect Control*, Vol. 14, pp.110-29.

Gill, A.W., Keil, A.D., Jones, C., Aydon, L., & Biggs, S. (2011). Tracking neonatal nosocomial infection: the continuous quality improvement cycle. *J Hosp Infect*, Vol. 78, pp. 20-25.

Goroncy-Bermes, P., Koburger, T., & Meyer, B. (2010). Impact of amount of hand rub applied in hygienic hand disinfection on the reduction of microbial counts on hands. *J Hosp Infect*, Vol. 74, pp. 212-218.

Gottrup, F. (2003). Prevention of surgical wound infections. *N Eng J Med*, Vol. 342, pp. 202-204.

Gould, D.J., Drey, N.S., & Creedon, S. (2011). Routine hand hygiene by direct observation: has nemesis arrived. *J Hosp Infect*, Vol. 77, pp. 290-293.

Gudlaugsson, O., Gillispie, S., Lee, K., Vande Berg, J., Hu J., Messer, S., Herwaldt, L., Pfaller, M., & Diekema, D. (2003). Attributable mortality of nosocomial candidemia, revisited. *Clin Infect Dis*, Vol. 37, pp. 1172-1177.

Halbawach, H. (1994). Solid waste disposal in District health facilities, Geneva. World Health Forum, Vol. 15, No. 4, pp. 363-367.

Hubner, N.O., Kellner, N.B., Partecke, L.I., Koburger, T., Heidecke, C.D., Kohlmann, T., & Kramer, A. (2011). Determination of antiseptic efficacy of rubs on the forearm and consequences for surgical hand disinfection. *J Hosp Infect*, Vol. 78, pp. 11-15.

Hayette, M.P., Christiaens, G., Mutsers, J., Barbier, C., Huynen, P., Melin, P., & de Mol, P. (2010). Filamentous fungi recovered from the water distribution system of a Belgian university hospital. *Med Mycol*, Vol. 48, No. 7, pp. 969-974.

Hugonnet, S., Harbarth, S., Sax, H., Duncan, R.A., & Pittet, D. (2004). Nursing resources: a major determinant of nosocomial infection? *Curr Opin Infect Dis*, Vol. 17, No. 4, pp. 329-333.

Humphreys, P.N. (2011). Testing standards for sporicides. *J Hosp Infect*, Vol. 77, pp. 193-198.

Ikram, A., Shah S.I.H., Naseem, S., Absar, S.F., Ullah, S., Ambreen, T., Sabeeh, S.M., & Niazi, S.K. (2010). Status of hospital infection control measures at seven major tertiary care hospitals of northern Punjab. *J Coll Physicians Surg Pak*, Vol. 20, No. 4, pp. 266-70.

Institute for Healthcare Improvement. How-to guide: improving hand hygiene. A guide for improving practices among health care workers. Accessed 23 July 2011. Available from: <http://www.ihi.org/knowledge/Pages/Tools/HowtoGuideImprovingHandHygiene.aspx>

Jarvis, W.R. (2001). Infection control and changing health-care delivery systems. *Emerg Infect Dis*, Vol. 7, No. 2, pp. 170-173.

Jeans, A.R., Moore, J., Nicol, C., Bates, C., & Read, R.C. (2010). Wristwatch use and hospital-acquired infection. *J Hosp Control*, Vol. 74, pp. 16-21.

Klevens., M.R., Edwards, J.R., Richards, J.C.L., Horan, T.C., Gaynes, R.P., Pollock D.A., & Cardo D.M. (2007). Estimating health care-associated infections and deaths in U.S. hospitals, 2002. *Public Health Rep*, Vol. 122, pp. 160-166.

Kumar, S., Atray, D., Paiwal, D., Balasubramanyam, G., Duraiswamy, P., & Kulkarni, S. (2011). Dental unit waterlines: source of contamination and cross-infection. *J Hosp Infect*, Vol. 74, pp. 99-111.

Landman, D., Chockalingam, M., & Quale, J.M. (1999). Reduction in the incidence of methicillin-resistant *Staphylococcus aureus* and ceftazidime-resistant *Klebsiella pneumoniae* following changes in a hospital antibiotic formulary. *Clin Infect Dis,* Vol. 28, pp. 1062-1066.

Leung, M., & Chan, A.H. (2006). Control and management of hospital indoor air quality. *Med Sci Monit*, Vol. 12, No. 3, pp. SR17-23. Epub 2006 Feb 23.

Loeb, M.B., Craven, S., McGeer, A.J., Simor, A.E., Bradley, S.F., Low, D.E., Armstrong-Evans, M., Moss, L.A., & Walter, S.D. (2003). Risk factors for resistance to antimicrobial agents among nursing home residents. *Am J Epidemiol*, Vol. 157, pp. 40–47.

Lopman, B.A., Reacher, M.H., Vipond, I.B., Hill, D., Perry, C., Halladay, T., Brown, D.W., Edmunds, W.J., & Sarangi, J. (2004). Epidemiology and cost of nosocomial gastroenteritis, Avon, England, 2002-2003. *Emerg Infect Dis*, Vol. 10, pp. 1827-1834.

Luby, S.P., Agboatwalla, M., Feikin, D.R., Painter, J., Billhimer, W., Altaf, A., & Hoekstra, R.M. (2005). Effect of handwashing on child health: a randomised controlled trial. *Lancet*, Vol. 366, No. 9481, pp. 225-33.

Madani, T.A., Alsaedi, S., James, L., Eldeek, B.S., Jiman-Fatani, A.A., Alawi, M.M., Marwan, D., Cudal, M., Macapagal, M., Bahlas, R., & Farouq, M. (2011). *Serratia marcescens*-contaminated baby shampoo causing an outbreak among newborns at King Abdulaziz University Hospital, Jeddah, Saudi Arabia. *J Hosp Infect*, Vol. 78, pp. 16-19.

Madeo, M. (2010). Efficacy of a novel antimicrobial solution (Prontoderm) in decolonizing MRSA nasal carriage. *J Hosp Infect*, Vol. 74, pp. 290-291.

Marchesi, I., Marchegiano, P., Bargellini, A., Cencetti, S., Frezza, G., Miselli, M., & Borella, P. (2011). Effectiveness of different methods to control *Legionella* in the water supply: ten-year experience in an Italian university hospital. *J Hosp Infect*, Vol. 77, pp. 47-51.

Marias, F., Mehtar, S., & Chalkley, L. (2010). Antimicrobial efficacy of copper touch surfaces in reducing environmental bioburden in a South African healthcare facility. *J Hosp Infect*, Vol. 74, pp. 80-81.

Martinez-Capolino, C., Reyes, K., Johnson, L., Sullivan, J., Samuel, L., DiGiovine, B., Eichenhorn, M., Horst, H.M., Varelas, P., Mickey, M.A., Washburn R., & Zervos, M. (2010). Impact of active surveillance on methicillin-resistant *Staphylococcus aureus* transmission and hospital resource utilization. *J Hosp Infect*, Vol. 74, pp. 232-237.

Mathai, E., Allegranzi, B., Kilpatrick, C., Nejad, S.B., Graafmans, W., & Pittet, D. (2011). Promoting hand hygiene in healthcare through national/subnational campaigns. *J Hosp Infect*, Vol. 77, pp. 294-298.

McNicholas, S., Andrews, C., Boland, K., Shields, M., Doherty, G.A., Murray, F.E., Smith, E.G., Humphreys, H., & Fitzpatrick, F. (2011). Delayed acute hospital discharge and healthcare-associated infections: the forgotten risk factors. *J Hosp Infect*, Vol. 78, pp. 157-158.

McNulty, C., Logan, M., Donald, I.P., Ennis, D., Taylor, D., Baldwin, R.N., Bannerjee, M., & Cartwright, K.A. (1997). Successful control of *Clostridium difficile* infection in an elderly care unit through use of a restrictive antibiotic policy. *J Antimicrob Chemother*, Vol. 40, pp. 707-711.

National Audit Office. (2000). The management and control of hospital acquired infections in acute NHS Trust in England. Report by the Comptroller and Auditor General, HC 230, Session 1999-00.

Pittet, D., & Boyce, J.M. (2001). Hand hygiene and patient care: pursuing the Semmelweis legacy. *Lancet Infect Dis*, April, pp. 9-20.

Pittet, D., & Donaldson, I. (2005). Clean Care is Safer Care: a worldwide priority. *Lancet*, Vol. 366, pp. 1246-1247.

Pittet, D., Panesar, S.S., Wilson, K., Longtin, Y., Morris, T., Allan, V., Storr, J., Cleary, K., & Donaldson, L. (2011). Involving the patient to ask about hospital hand hygiene: a National Patient Safety Agency feasibility study. *J Hosp Infect*, Vol. 77, pp. 299-303.

Quale, J., Landman, D., Saurina, G., Atwood, E., DiTore, V., & Patel, K. (1996). Manipulation of a hospital antimicrobial formulary to control an outbreak of vancomycin-resistant enterococci. *Clin Infect Dis*, Vol. 23, pp. 1020-1025.

Rutala, W.A., & Weber, D.J. Disinfection and sterilization in health care facilities: what clinicians need to know. *Clin Infect Dis*, Vol. 39, No. 5, pp. 702-709. Epub 2004 Aug 12.

Saurina, G., Quale, J.M., Manikal, V.M., Oydna, E., & Landman, D. (2000). Antimicrobial resistance in Enterobacteriaceae in Brooklyn, NY: epidemiology and relation to antibiotic usage patterns. *J Antimicrob Chemother*, Vol. 45, pp. 895-898.

Scott, R.D. (2009). The direct medical cost of healthcare associated infections in U.S. hospitals and the benefits of prevention. Coordinating Center for Infectious Diseases, Centers for Disease Control and Prevention, March 2009. Accessed on 25 July 2011. Available from: <http://www.cdc.gov/ncidod/dhqp/pdf/scott_costpaper.pdf>

Shelton, C.L., Raistrick C., Warburton, K., & Siddiqui, K.H. (2010). Can changes in clinical attire reduce likelihood of cross-infection without jeopardizing the doctor-patient relationship. *J Hosp infect*, Vol. 74, pp. 22-29.

Siegel, J.D., Rhinehart, E., Jackson, M., & Chiarello, L. (2007). Guideline for isolation precautions: preventing transmission of infectious agents in health care settings 2007. *Am J Infect Control*, Vol. 35, pp. S65–164.

Singh, I.B., & Sharma, R.K. (1996). Hospital waste disposal system and technology. *J Acad Hosp Adm*, Vol. 8, No. 2, pp. 44-88.

Spaulding, E.H. (1968). Chemical disinfection of medical and surgical materials. In: *Disinfection, sterilization, and preservation*. Lawrence C., & Block, S.S. pp. 517-531, Lea & Febiger, Philadelphia.

Sroka, S., Gastmeier, P., & Meyer, E. (2010). Impact of alcohol hand-rub on methicillin-resistant *Staphylococcus aureus*: an analysis of the literature. *J Hosp Infect*, Vol. 74, pp. 201-211.

Stanton, M.W., & Rutherford, M.K. (2004). Hospital nurse staffing and quality of care. Rockville, MD: Agency for Healthcare Research and Quality. Research in Action, Issue 14. AHRQ Pub. No. 04–0029.

Stone, P.W., Larson, E., & Kawar, L.N. (2002). A systematic audit of economic evidence linking nosocomial infections and infection control interventions: 1990-2000. *Am J Infect Control*, Vol. 30, No. 3, pp. 145-152.

Tang, J.W., Noakes, C.J., Nielsen, P.V., Eames, I., Nicolle, A., Li, Y., & Settles, G.S. (2011). Observing and quantifying airflows in the infection control of aerosol- and airborne-transmitted diseases: an overview of approaches. *J Hosp Infect*, Vol. 77, No. 3, pp. 213-222.

Trick, W.E., Weinstein, R.A., DeMarais, P.L., Kuehnert, M.J., Tomaska, W., Nathan, C., Rice, T.W., McAllister, S.K., Carson, L.A., & Jarvis, W.R. (2001). Colonization of skilledcare facility residents with antimicrobial-resistant pathogens. *J Am Geriatr Soc*, Vol. 49, pp. 270–276.

Tsakris, A., Ikonomidis, A., Pournaras, S., Tzouvelekis, L.S., Sofianou, D., Legakis, N.J., & Maniatis, A.N. (2006). VIM-1 metallo-beta-lactamase in *Acinetobacter baumannii*. *Emerg Infect Dis*, Vol. 12, pp. 981-983.

Uttley, A.H., & Simpson, R.A. (1994). Audit of bronchoscope disinfection: a survey of procedures in England and Wales and incidents of mycobacterial contamination. *J Hosp Infect*, Vol. 26, pp. 301-308.

Wang, Y.L., Chen, W.C., Chen, C.C., Tseng S.H., Chien, L.J., Wu, H.S., & Chiang, C.S. (2010). Bacterial contamination on surfaces of public areas in hospitals. *J Hosp Infect*, Vol. 74, pp. 195-196.

Weber, D.J., Rutala, W.A., & DiMarino, A.J.Jr. (2002). The prevention of infection following gastrointestinal endoscopy: the importance of prophylaxis and reprocessing. In: *Gastrointestinal diseases: an endoscopic approach*. DiMarino, A.J.Jr, Benjamin, S.B., eds. pp. 87-106. Thorofare, Slack Inc., NJ.

White, H.A., & Wiselka, M.J. (2011). Inpatient mortality and death reporting associated with *Clostridium difficile* infection in a large teaching hospital. *J Hosp Infect*, Vol. 77, pp. 369-370.

Widmer, A.F., Rotter, M., Voss, A., Nthumba, P., Allegranzi, B., Boyce, J., & Pittet, D. (2010). Surgical hand preparation: state-of-the-art. *J Hosp Infect*, Vol. 74, pp. 112-122.

World Health Organization. (2002). Prevention of hospital acquired infections - a practical guide. 2nd ed. Geneva: WHO, 2002. Document no. WHO/CDS/EPH/2002.12.

World Health Organization. (2009). WHO guidelines on hand hygiene in health care. Geneva: WHO, 2009.

World Health Organization. (2011). Report on the burden of endemic health care-associated infections worldwide. WHO Document Production Services, ISBN 9789241501507, Geneva.

Zing, W., Sandoz, L., Inan, C., Cartier, V., Clergue, F., Pittet, D., & Walder, B. (2011). Hospital-wide survey of the use of central venous catheters. *J Hosp Infect*, Vol. 77, pp. 304-308.

2

Health Care Associated Infections: Sources and Routes of Transmission

Hans Jørn Kolmos
Department of Clinical Microbiology, Odense University Hospital
Denmark

1. Introduction

Health care associated infections are infections that patients acquire, while they are in contact with the healthcare system. Contact includes all procedures associated with diagnostics, treatment, care, and rehabilitation. Health care associated infections were formerly called hospital or nosocomial infections. Hospitals still account for the vast majority of cases; however, for practical reasons the concept has been widened to comprise infections in all parts of the health care system, because a growing part of disease management takes place outside hospitals, e.g. in out patient clinics, nursing homes and general practice. The spectrum of health care associated infections ranges from simple common colds to life threatening sepsis with multidrug resistant organisms. With the above definition, around 10 % of patients on average will become infected while they are in contact with the health care system. Health care associated infections also include occupational infectious diseases acquired by health care workers.

Health care associated infections are determined by a number of risk factors related to the patients themselves, the procedures they are exposed to, the organisms that cause disease, and buildings and rooms where treatment takes place (Fig. 1). Patients have an increased susceptibility to infection because they are weakened by disease, and in addition often elderly. Old age weakens the immune system and the function of vital organs. Lifestyle factors such as poor quality food, lack of exercise, and tobacco and alcohol abuse also play a role. Invasive procedures, like surgery and insertion of catheters break down the natural barriers of skin and mucous membranes and thereby predispose for health care associated infections. Cytostatics and other immunosuppressive agents also enhance the risk of infection, and the same applies to broad spectrum antibiotics through their impact on the patients' endogenous microbial flora. Hospital bacteria may have an enhanced potential for producing health care associated infections. A high consumption of broad spectrum antibiotics selects for multi-drug resistant organisms, which spread in hospitals despite infection control measures. Their spread may be favoured by genetic links between antibiotic resistance and virulence factors such as adhesion to cell surfaces (Di Martino et al 1997) and medical devices. Building facilities also play a role. Overcrowding and lack of facilities for isolation of contagious patients predispose for health care associated infections. Reduction of domestic cleaning leads to accumulation of pathogens on contact surfaces, which may subsequently be transmitted to patients.

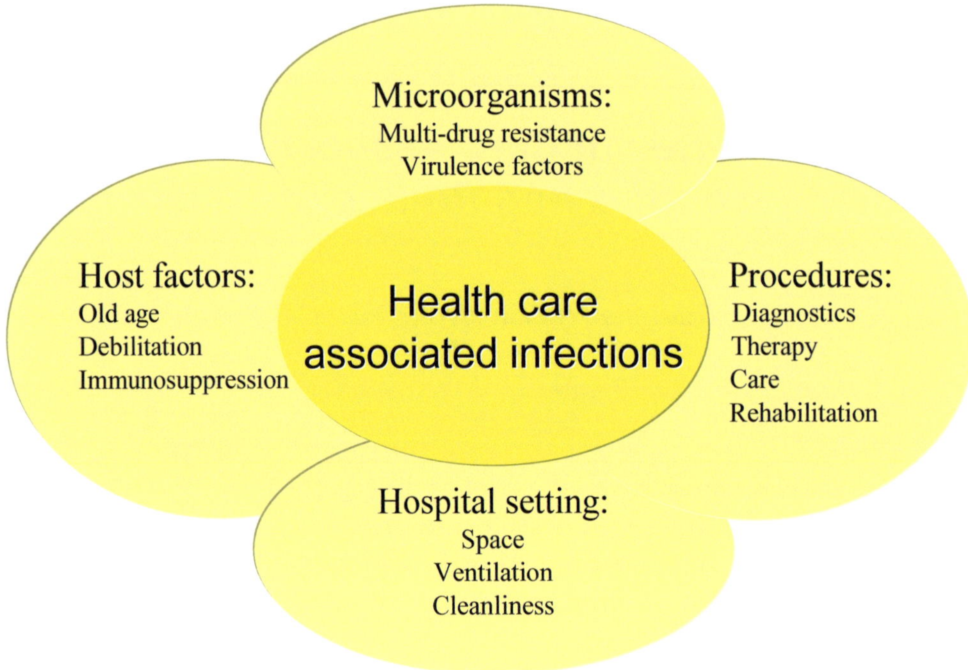

Fig. 1. Factors determining health care associated infections.

This aim of this paper is to give a comprehensive survey of the more important sources of health care associated infections and the way they are spread in the health care setting. The source of infection may be the patient's own microbial flora (self-infection), or organisms from other patients, hospital staff, and the hospital environment (cross-infection). Transmission may take place by direct or indirect contact, by the airborne route, or through a vehicle (e.g. water, food and drugs). Airborne transmission may take place by large particle droplets, by small particle droplets (droplet nuclei), and by dust. Table 1 summarizes the sources and modes of transmission, clarified by examples of risk factors and the types of infections they give rise to. A more detailed description of the single elements is given in the paragraphs below.

2. Self-infection

Patients may acquire health care associated infections from organisms belonging to their own normal flora on skin and mucous membranes. This colonizing flora may become invasive after break-down of natural barriers following surgery and insertion of catheters. The most important organisms are *Staphylococcus aureus* and *Escherichia coli*. Treatment with broad spectrum antibiotics may destroy the susceptible part of the endogenous flora, and instead patients become colonized with more resistant species originating from other patients or from the hospital environment. Examples of such resistant organisms are methicillin-resistant coagulase-negative staphylococci, ampicillin-resistant enterococci, *Klebsiella pneumoniae*, *Pseudomonas aeruginosa* and *Stenotrophomonas maltophilia*. This new colonizing flora may eventually give rise to infection.

Sources of infection	Modes of transmission	Examples of risk factors	Examples of infections
Self-infection	Break of natural barriers (skin and mucous membranes)	Surgery. Insertion of peripheral or central line catheters. *Staphylococcus aureus* carriage	Surgical site infections & catheter related infections due to *Staphylococcus aureus.* Urinary tract infections due to *Escherichia coli*
Cross-infection from other patients	Via hands of staff	Failing hand hygiene before and after patient contact	Surgical site infections & catheter related infections due to *Staphylococcus aureus* Respiratory tract infections due to RSV & other respiratory pathogens
	Via instruments & equipment not properly sterilized	Heat-sensitive equipment, e.g. fibre-optic endoscopes	Tuberculosis transmitted by fibre-optic bronchoscope
	Via the environment	Insufficient domestic cleaning leading to accumulation of pathogens on contact surfaces	Diarrhoea due to *Clostridium difficile*
	Via donor blood & drugs	Medication of several patients From the same multi-dose vial	Hepatitis B or C transmitted with drugs from multi-dose vials accidentally contaminated with blood or body fluids
Hospital staff	Hand-borne	MRSA carriage. Insufficient handhygiene in connection with treatment and care of patients	Surgical wound infections. Catheter related infections
	Air-borne during surgery	Carrrier of *Streptococcus pyogenes* in the operating theatre	Puerperal fever & surgical wound infections with *Streptococcus pyogenes*
Hospital environment	Contact with contaminated tap water	Aspiration of oral secretions following ingestion of tap water contaminated with *Legionella*. Immunosuppression	*Legionella* pneumonia
	Inhalation of dust from buildings	Rebuilding of hospitals. Immunosuppression	Lung infection due to *Aspergillus fumigatus*

Table 1. Sources of healthcare associated infections, modes of transmission, and associated risk factors illustrated by examples

2.1 Staphylococcus aureus carriage

About 25 % of the normal population are chronic carriers of *Staphylococcus aureus*, and the carriage rate is even higher - around 50 % - in insulin dependent diabetics, dialysis patients, and intravenous drug addicts (Kluytmans et al 1997). The primary carriage sites are nostrils and throat, from where the organism is spread to the skin. Persons with a high concentration of *Staphylococcus aureus* in their nostrils have a three to six times higher risk of acquiring surgical wound infections, as compared to non carriers or persons with only a low concentration (Bode et al 2010). The same applies to catheter related infections in dialysis patients and patients with long term indwelling intravenous catheters. The pathogenesis is only partly understood, but it probably plays a role that most nasal carriers are at the same time skin carriers. Prospective studies have shown that more than 80 % of all *Staphylococcus aureus* blood stream infections are of endogenous origin (von Eiff et al 2001). As to surgical site infections the origin of *Staphylococcus aureus* is less well described; however, it is estimated that at least 50 % are due to self-infection (Perl et al 2002). The evidence for a causative relationship between *Staphylococcus aureus* carriage and risk of surgical wound infection is proved by the fact that preoperative eradication of *Staphylococcus aureus* carriage leads to a substantial reduction in surgical site infections (Bode et al 2010).

2.2 Gram-negative bacilli

Escherichia coli and other intestinal organisms may give rise to ascending urinary tract infections in patients with indwelling urinary catheters (Tambyah et al 1999) and to wound infections following abdominal surgery. Enterobacteria may also colonize the airways of critically ill patients and give rise to ventilator associated pneumonia. In healthy individuals the throat flora is dominated by Gram-positive bacteria, which adhere to cell surfaces by surface molecules such as fibronectin. However, in critically ill patients throat epithelial cells often lose their fibronectin-binding surface molecules and thereby their capacity to bind Gram-positive bacteria. This paves the road for colonization with enterobacteria and other Gram-negative bacilli (Woods 1987).

Ventilator associated pneumonia is often due to silent aspiration of bacteria-bearing secretions from the upper airways, which leak down along the outer side of the endotracheal tube. The aspirated material may also originate from the stomach, which has been colonized with intestinal flora following prophylactic treatment with antacids (Safdar et al 2005). The role of aspiration in ventilator associated pneumonia is the major rationale for using selective decontamination of the oropharynx and digestive tract to prevent such cases (Van Saene et al 2003)

3. Cross infection

The most important route of transmission of organisms from patient to patient is by indirect contact via staff's hands because hand hygiene is neglected or performed inadequately (Fig. 2). Transmission may also occur by direct contact between patients or by the airborne route, if they are placed on the same ward.

Staff is not the only factor involved in cross transmission. It may also occur via the environment by contact with surfaces that have been contaminated with organisms from other patients (fomites). This will be discussed in a separate paragraph below. Finally, cross transmission may occur via equipment and utensils that have not been decontaminated adequately before being reused, and through drugs and blood products. These aspects will also be covered in separate paragraphs below.

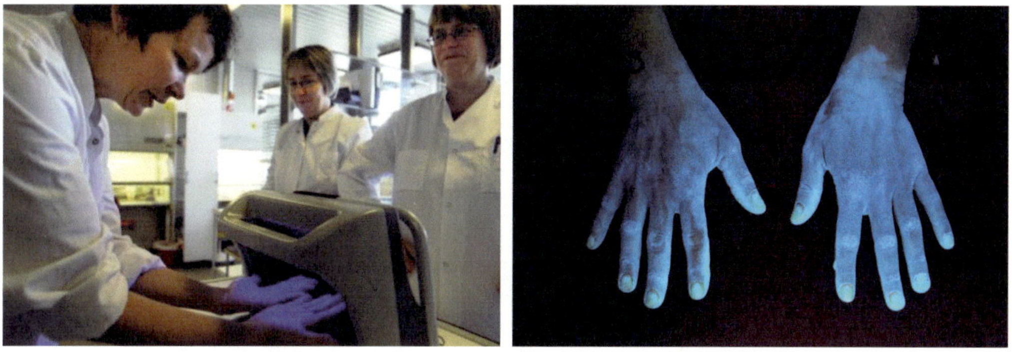

Fig. 2. The quality of hand hygiene may be visualised with fluorescent alcohol in an ultraviolet light box. Studies have shown that even experienced staff may have a low technical performance (Kolmos et al 2006). Right-hand persons often miss the back of their right hand and fingers, as illustrated on the photo to the right (courtesy: Infection Control Team, Odense University Hospital).

3.1 Cross transmission by health care workers' hands

The importance of cross transmission by health care workers' hands has been documented in a large number of studies (Pittet et al 2006). Wearing rings increases the level of skin contamination by a factor ten (Trick et al 2003). Artificial nails are also associated with increased levels of pathogens on hands (McNeil et al 2001). Pathogens are transmitted to health care workers' hands during contact with patients and their body secretions, and during contact with touch sites in the environment that have been contaminated with pathogens released from patients (Fig. 3). Hands become progressively contaminated during patient care: the longer the duration of care, the higher the level of contamination. Skin contact, diaper change, and respiratory care are associated with particularly high levels of transmission (Pessoa-Silva et al 2004). Most pathogens from patients can survive for sufficient time on health care workers' hands to be transmitted to other patients in a busy hospital setting. Organisms tolerant to desiccation form a particular problem. Examples of such agents are *Staphylococcus aureus* and other staphylococci, enterococci, *Clostridium difficile*, *Acinetobacter baumannii* and naked viruses such as noro- and rotavirus. However, organisms adapted to moist environments are also readily transmissible. Examples of such agents are *Escherichia coli*, *Klebsiella pneumoniae*, *Pseudomonas aeruginosa*, and more fragile viruses such as influenza virus and respiratory syncytial virus (RSV). Gloves offer some protection, but do not fully protect health care workers' hands from contamination. Model calculations indicate that they only halve skin contamination in connection with heavily contaminated procedures such as respiratory care and diaper change (Pessoa-Silva et al 2004).

The role of health care workers' hands in cross transmission of organisms is best illustrated by the ability of hand hygiene campaigns to reduce health care associated infections. A striking example is the study by Pittet and coworkers, where a hospital-wide hygiene campaign with emphasis on alcoholic hand rub led to a sustained increase in hand hygiene compliance and a reduction in hospital acquired infections by more than 40 %. Transmission of MRSA was reduced by more than 50 % (Pittet et al 2000).

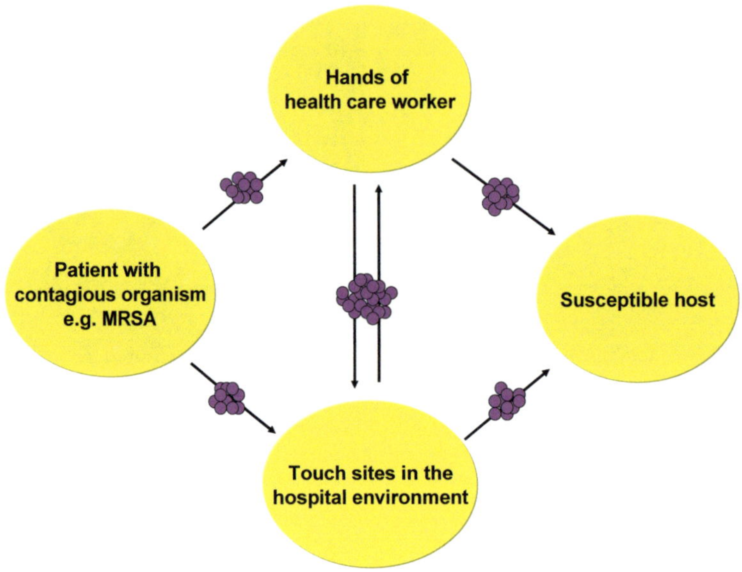

Fig. 3. Interactions between health care workers' hands and touch sites in the hospital environment on transmission of pathogens from one patient to another.

3.2 The role of airborne transmission

Many respiratory pathogens are transmitted from patient to patient by the airborne route. The large majority are carried by large droplets. This applies particularly to RSV, influenza and common cold viruses, and to bacteria like pneumococci, meningococci and haemolytic streptococci. Large droplets settle rapidly, and these organisms are therefore only directly transmissible within a distance of 1 or 2 metres from the infected patient. However, more importantly these organisms can also be transmitted by indirect contact, particularly with staff's hands, if hand hygiene is neglected between patient contacts. Transmission may also take place after contact with contaminated surfaces close to an infected patient (fomites). This has been clearly documented with RSV (Hall 2000), but probably also applies to the other respiratory pathogens mentioned above. Measles, rubella and varicella-zoster virus are mainly spread by droplet nuclei, which can keep airborne for long time and therefore be transmitted over long distances (Tang et al 2006, Roy & Milton 2004).

Laboratory studies indicate that *Mycobacterium tuberculosis* can be transmitted by droplet nuclei; however the clinical significance of this remains controversial (Fennelly et al 2004, Nardell 2004). Transmission by large droplets plays a much larger role. Furthermore, *Mycobacterium tuberculosis* can survive for long time in dust and dried up secretions, which implies that it also has a potential for transmission by fomites.

The mode of transmission of influenza virus is still controversial. Most clinical studies point to transmission by contact and airborne transmission by large droplets; however, airborne transmission by droplet nuclei also seems to play a role. This is particularly the case with influenza pneumonitis, which is associated with the generation of droplet nuclei (Brankston et al 2007, Tellier 2006). Tracheal suctions and endotracheal intubation give rise the formation of aerosols, which may pose a risk to health care workers involved with these procedures.

4. Health care workers as a source of health care associated infections

As illustrated above health care workers play a key role in transmitting organisms from one patient to another. However, they may also be a source of infection themselves, if they are colonized or infected with pathogens which they pass on to patients. This applies particularly to *Staphylococcus aureus*, including MRSA, haemolytic streptococci (*Streptococcus pyogenes*), and to influenza A and hepatitis B viruses.

4.1 Staphylococcus aureus

At least 25 % of all staff are permanent carriers of *Staphylococcus aureus* in their nostrils. From here the organism is spread to skin and hands. Special attention has been paid to carriers of MRSA, however, ordinary susceptible staphylococci are equally transmissible. As a rule the risk of transmitting *Staphylococcus aureus* from asymptomatic nasal carriers is low, provided that they perform proper hand hygiene before contact with patients. However, the risk may rise dramatically with sneezing, if they catch a common cold or suffer from a burst of hay fever. Rhinorrhoea and sneezing transforms a staphylococcal carrier into a staphylococcal disperser (Sherertz et al 2001, Bassetti et al 2005, Bischoff et al 2006). It is often referred to as the cloud phenomenon, indicating that the carrier is virtually surrounded by a cloud of staphylococci, when sneezing. Bacteria expelled by sneezing are usually carried on large droplets that will settle within a distance of 1-2 metres. Thus staphylococci from a carrier will not spread airborne over long distances; however, the organisms may settle on surfaces and act as fomites, which can be transmitted to patients by contact, if surfaces are not properly cleaned (Kramer et al 2006). Staphylococcal carriers with scaling skin diseases may also shed large amounts of organisms to the environment.

4.2 Streptococcus pyogenes

Haemolytic streptococci (*Streptococcus pyogenes*) can be contagious with an extremely low inoculum. Surgical staff and staff attending wounds may be a source of severe surgical wound infections and puerperal fever, if they are carriers of *Streptococcus pyogenes* . Several outbreaks have been reported that could be traced to a carrier (Kolmos et al 1997). Approximately 5 % of the normal population are healthy throat carriers. This may involve a risk of transmission, particularly in relation to a common cold (cloud phenomenon, see above). However, more remarkably vaginal and anal carriage also seems to involve a high risk during surgery. Anal carriage may be seen in relation to minor disorders such as haemorrhoids and fissures; vaginal carriage is probably secondary to anal carriage. The mode of transmission from anal and vaginal carriers during surgery is not fully understood; however, the fact that carriers have given rise to outbreaks even without being close to patients in the operating theatre suggests that airborne transmission plays a role. Two cases of surgical wound sepsis due to *Streptococcus pyogenes* arising close to each other shortly after surgery is an alarm signal that should lead to considerations about a carrier among the surgical staff.

4.3 Influenza and other respiratory tract infections

Health care workers are considered the main source of nosocomial influenza (Salgado et al 2002). The primary reason is that they meet on work with symptoms that are interpreted as a common cold, but are in fact influenza. Half of all cases of influenza A virus infection do not give rise to classical flu symptoms, but are subclinical or present with ordinary cold symptoms. The role of staff in the transmission of nosocomial influenza was highlighted in a Scottish study where vaccination of the staff led to a substantial decrease in mortality among residents in long-term care facilities over a winter season (Carman et al 2000). Staff in pediatric units may also transmit *Bordetella pertussis* (whooping cough) and RSV, which frequently give rise to re-infections with uncharacteristic cold symptoms in adulthood (Sherertz et al 2001, Singh & Lingappan 2006, Hall et al 2001).

4.4 Blood borne viruses

Transmission of hepatitis B virus (HBV) to patients by infected surgeons has been reported in several studies. Transmission presumably takes place during surgery where the operating field is exposed to blood from the surgeon in connection with needle sticks and other skin injuries. Clusters of cases have primarily been seen with surgeons, whose serum contained hepatitis B e antigen (HBeAg), which is associated with particularly high concentrations of circulating virus and therefore great infectivity; however, HBeAg negative surgeons have also infected patients (The Incident Investigation Teams and Others 1997). Surgeons may also transmit hepatitis C virus and HIV (Heptonstall 2000).

5. Cross transmission by medical devices

Instruments and utensils may transmit pathogens if they are not decontaminated properly after patient use. The transmitted pathogens may originate from other patients, or from sources in the hospital environment. Overall, these problems have been declining over the past decades due to the introduction of more single-use equipment and safer and more efficient disinfecting techniques for multiple-use equipment. One of the more important improvements is the introduction of ward based automatic washing machines with heat disinfection programmes, which have replaced older and less safe techniques based on the use of chemical disinfectants. However, in recent years new challenges have arisen with the introduction of fragile and sophisticated equipment, which cannot be heat sterilized.

5.1 Fibre-optic endoscopes

Fibre-optic endoscopes are an example of such heat sensitive equipment. Decontamination takes place by a combination of mechanical cleansing with an enzymatic cleaner and chemical disinfection with a high level disinfectant, such as peracetic acid or glutaraldehyde (Rutala & Weber 2004). The process may be performed manually, but usually takes place in an automatic disinfector (Fig. 4). Bronchoscopes are the medical devices that most commonly give rise to hygienic problems. Numerous outbreaks and pseudo-outbreaks due to the use of contaminated bronchoscopes have been reported, both with person-to-person transmission of pathogens (e.g. *Mycobacterium tuberculosis*), and transmission of pathogens from the environment (e.g. *Mycobacterium chelonae* and *Pseudomonas aeruginosa*). Contamination has been associated with breaches in technique both in the bronchoscopes and the disinfecting machines used for reprocessing (Weber & Rutala 2001, Srinivasan et al 2003). By contrast, transmission of infection has only been recognized in very few cases with endoscopes used in gastrointestinal endoscopy (Nelson & Muscarella 2006).

The sterility safety of surgical instruments is extremely high, given that they are reprocessed and sterilized under well controlled conditions in an autoclave. However, one matter of concern is the emergence new prion-related disorders, like variant Creutzfeldt-Jakob disease (CJD), since this type of prion protein is not fully inactivated by traditional autoclaving. Instruments that have been in contact with brain, spinal cord, eye tissues, lymph nodes, spleen, and terminal ileum pose a special risk for transmitting variant CJD (Sutton et al 2006).

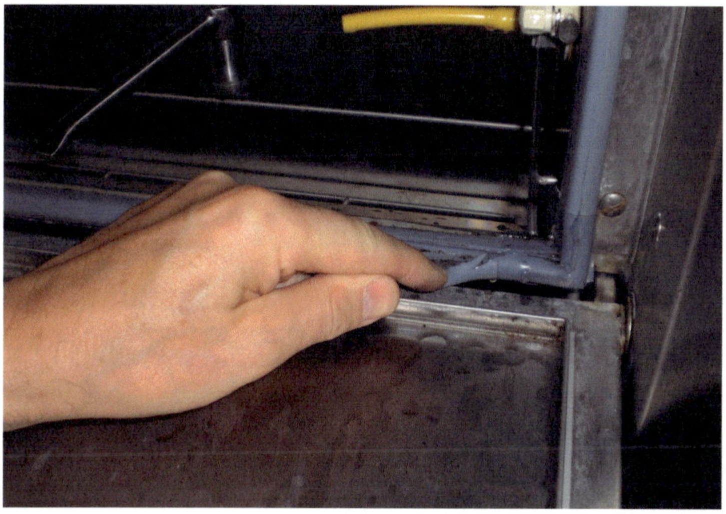

Fig. 4. Damaged rubber gasket in a poorly maintained disinfector used for reprocessing endoscopes. Formation of biofilm in the disinfector resulted in a pseudo-outbreak of *Mycobacterium gordonae* among patients undergoing bronchoscopy with bronchoscopes reprocessed in the disinfector (Courtesy: Infection Control Team, Odense University Hospital).

6. Infections transmitted through a vehicle

Transmission of organisms from other patients or from the environment may take place through a vehicle, e.g. water, food, drugs, and donor blood.

6.1 Tap water

Tap water in most hospitals is colonized with *Legionella pneumophila*, which may give rise to pneumonia and other severe manifestations in immunocompromised patients, such as organ transplant recipients. Patients with impaired throat reflexes and intubated patients are other important risk groups. The most important mode of transmission is by silent aspiration of contaminated secretions from the oral cavity (Sabria & Yu 2002). Contamination of the oral cavity may occur with drinks or ice cubes made from tap water, or with tap water used for oral hygiene. Thus, transmission of *Legionella* in hospitals differs significantly from transmission outside the health care setting, where transmission usually takes place through inhalation of aerosols from contaminated air condition facilities. It is often assumed that showering plays a role in transmission of *Legionella* in hospitals, but there is little evidence that this is actually the case (Sabria & Yu 2002).

Contaminated tap water may give rise to wound infections, if used for cleansing wounds. This was for instance the case in an outbreak of *Pseudomonas aeruginosa* infections in a burns unit, where tap water was used for irrigation of burns as part of the first aid treatment, which patients received when entering the hospital. Contamination was restricted to the showers and plastic tubing, which were permanently connected to the taps. This led to stagnant water inside the tubings and heavy contamination due to biofilm formation. Water sampled directly from the taps of the metal pipes was not contaminated, and the outbreak stopped, when plastic tubings and showers were dismantled and disinfected (Kolmos et al 1993).

6.2 Food

Virtually any food pathogen that occurs in the community can give rise to food borne infections in the health care setting. Much attention is being paid to zoonotic *Salmonella enterica*, which despite enhanced surveillance strategies still gives rise hospital outbreaks (Sion et al 2000, Guallar et al 2004). Outbreaks due to *Listeria monocytogenes* have also been reported (Johnsen et al 2010). A characteristic feature of food borne outbreaks due to these organisms is that they predominantly hit debilitated patients, who have a much higher attack rate than other patients. A major reason for this is that they develop infection with a lower inoculum than other exposed patients, who often stay asymptomatic and therefore go unnoticed. Debilitated patients may therefore be regarded as a sentinel population for recognition of food borne outbreaks, with symptomatic cases representing only the tip of the iceberg.

Norovirus is another important pathogen, which may give rise to food borne outbreaks in the health care setting, affecting both patients and staff. The virus is extremely contagious, which implies that secondary cases often occur (Stevenson et al 1994). A food borne outbreak is therefore often a mix of food transmitted cases and secondary cases acquired by patient to patient transmission, which makes source identification more difficult.

Buffets carry a risk of cross transmission, particularly if food is handled by self-service (Fone et al 1999). The same applies to ice produced by ward based ice machines (Ravn et al 1991).

6.3 Intravenous drugs

Despite efforts to improve safety, transmission of blood borne viruses through intravenous drugs is an ongoing problem.

In recent years there have been reports on transmission of both hepatitis B and C viruses, as well as HIV (Fisker et al 2006, Wenzel & Edmond 2005, Katzenstein et al 1999). In the majority of cases the sources of infection were capped multi-dose vials used for medication of a series of patients. Virus may be spread to the vials by accidental reuse of hypodermic needles and syringes contaminated with virus after medication of infected patients. Alternatively, the rubber membrane of vials may become contaminated with blood aerosols if blood specimens are handled close by, and virus may be introduced by subsequent needle perforations, if the membrane is not disinfected properly. This was probably the case in a recent outbreak of hepatitis B virus infection in a paediatric oncology ward (Fig. 5). Due to crowding and lack of proper room facilities the ward's preparation room was used for collecting blood samples, drying bone marrow smears and occasionally for blood sampling and transfusions, and multi-dose vials in use were placed next to the disposal pot for used hypodermic needles and syringes (Fisker et al 2006). Similarly, a large outbreak of hepatitis C virus infection among haematology/oncology patients visiting an outpatient clinic could be traced back to shared saline bags. Contamination of the saline bags probably occurred because the syringe used for collection of blood specimens from the patient was reused to withdraw saline to flush the catheter after blood sampling (Macedo de Oliveira et al 2005).

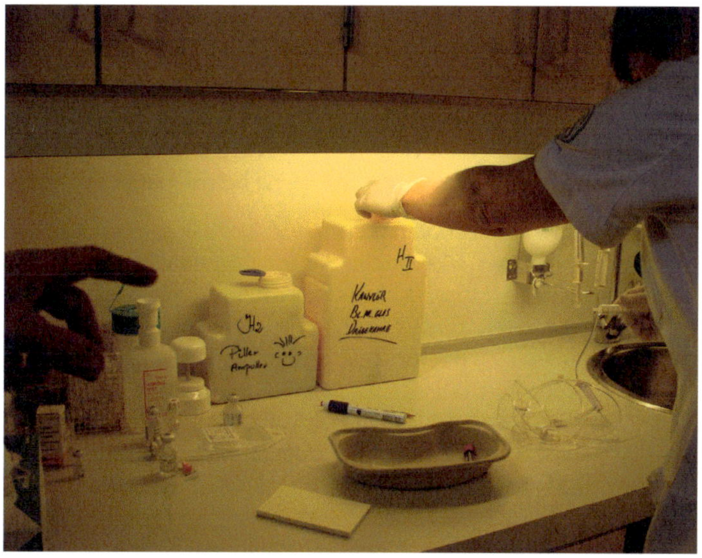

Fig. 5. Snapshot showing the preparation of an infusion with cytostatic agents in the preparation room of a paediatric oncology unit. To the right is the infusion line, rolled up on the table and connected to the infusion bag (hidden behind the nurse). To the left are several multi-dose vials with broken seals, containing drugs for preparation of the infusion. Between the infusion line and multi-dose vials is a bowl with a blood sample from a patient and disposal pots for hypodermic needles, syringes, and vials. This mingling of sterile procedures with handling of blood specimens and disposal of used needles gave rise to a large outbreak of hepatitis B (Fisker et al 2006) (Courtesy: Infection Control Team, Odense University Hospital).

6.4 Donor blood and blood products

Transfusion blood is not a sterile product. Donors may be silent carriers of blood borne viruses, like HBV, HCV, HIV, and HTLV, which may be transmitted to recipients of blood and blood products. Transmission of bacteria like *Yersinia enterocolitica* and protozoa like *Plasmodium falciparum* from apparently healthy donors has also been reported (Leclercq et al 2005, Bihl et al 2007). Rigorous screening of donors and pathogen inactivation in blood components have minimized such cases; however, donor blood may still be contaminated as a result of management errors in the blood bank during collection, preparation, and storage of blood and blood products. Transfusion related bacteraemia may also arise from contaminated blood collection bags. This was the case in a nationwide outbreak of *Serratia marcescens* bacteraemia among transfusion recipients, which could be traced back to commercial blood collection bags contaminated at the production plant. Water used for cooling the bags upon autoclaving was the source of contamination (Heltberg et al 1993).

7. Hospital environment

7.1 Cross infection from contaminated surfaces (fomites)

Cross infection may take place by contact with contaminated surfaces (fomites) in the health care setting. Examples of contact surfaces are door handles, bed tables, chairs, toilet seats, and floors.

Patients discharge large amounts of organisms to the hospital environment, particularly if they suffer from skin, wound, and respiratory tract infections, and from diarrhoea (Fig. 6). The discharged organisms settle with skin scales, droplets, and secretions on contact surfaces and accumulate in dust. From here they may be passed on to other patients, if they touch the contaminated surfaces. Health care workers also play a role in transmission if they touch contaminated surfaces and neglect hand hygiene before patient contact.

Organisms that are tolerant to dessication have a particularly high potential for transmission in the health care setting, because they keep viable for long time in the environment after having been discharged from patients. Such organisms are *Clostridium difficile, Staphylococcus aureus, Acinetobacter baumannii, Enterococcus faecium,* and *Mycobacterium tuberculosis.* Yeasts, and naked viruses like norovirus can also survive for long time outside the human body. Until recently microbial contamination of the hospital environment was considered unimportant in regard to transmission of health care associated infections. However, this has changed with the emergence of new evidence indicating that cross transmission from the environment is in fact a common phenomenon that has to be taken into consideration (Dancer 2008, Dancer 2011).

One way to illustrate a relationship between contamination of the hospital environment and health care associated infections is to study the risk of acquiring a specific pathogen, if a patient is admitted into a room that was previously occupied by a patient colonized or infected with the same pathogen. With this setup an increased risk of acquisition has been shown with *Clostridium difficile*, methicillin resistant *Staphylococcus aureus* (MRSA), vancomycin resistant *Enterococcus* (VRE), and *Acinetobacter baumannii* (Carling & Bartley 2010). The excess risk of acquiring MRSA and VRE was studied in a large multi-centre cohort study comprising more than 10,000 ICU patients, who underwent routine admission and weekly screenings for these two agents. The risk increased by 40 %, if patients were admitted into rooms previously occupied by patients harbouring MRSA or VRE (Huang et al 2006). A subsequent intervention study with focus on adherence to defined cleaning standards, including the use of a quaternary ammonium agent, reduced contamination with both organisms, and more importantly, it eliminated the excess risk of acquiring MRSA, whereas the risk of acquiring VRE remained largely unchanged (Datta et al 2011). This study confirms a previous report, where an outbreak of MRSA in a urological ward was contained successfully after intensifying domestic cleaning with special focus on dust removal and use of alcohol to disinfect contact surfaces (Rampling et al 2001). Similarly, the frequency of *Clostridium difficile* associated diarrhoea was reduced significantly in a number of wards, after the organism had been eliminated from the environment by hydrogen peroxide vapour (Boyce et al 2008).

7.2 Dust from demolition and construction works

Demolition and construction of buildings are ongoing processes in all big hospitals. Dust from building materials contains large amounts of spores of environmental fungi, which may pose a threat to heavily immunocompromised patients. (Hansen et al 2008). There are numerous reports of outbreaks of severe fungal respiratory tract infections among haematology, oncology and organ transplant patients originationg from inhalation of contaminated dust that could be traced back to demolition and renovation works in the hospital setting. The fungi most frequently involved were *Aspergillus fumigatus* and *Aspergillus flavus* (Vonberg & Gastmeier 2006).

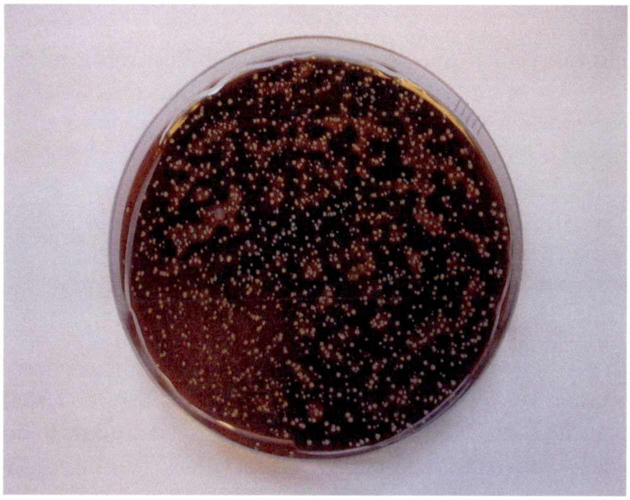

Fig. 6. Methicillin resistant *Staphylococcus aureus* (MRSA) on a sedimentation plate exposed for 12 hours on an overbed table of a dermatitis patient colonized with MRSA (Courtesy: Infection Control Team, Odense University Hospital).

8. Discussion

Sources and transmission routes of health care associated infections are numerous and complex. In many cases they are only partly understood, and the hygienic measures taken to control transmission are not always ideal. In many areas there is a need for more research to clarify the epidemiology and pathogenesis of health care associated infections in order to develop and implement more efficient and targeted interventions. This research should focus not only on technical and biological aspects, but should also involve behavioural sciences, since human behaviour is one of the key factors in transmission of infections in the health care setting.

Failure to perform hand hygiene is probably the single most important factor in transmission of health care associated infections. Taking into account the strength of evidence for the importance of hand hygiene, it is noteworthy that compliance is still so low. Several studies have documented that in daily clinical practice hand hygiene is hardly performed in more than half of the cases where it should, and only one third of those who perform hand hygiene do it correctly (Kolmos et al 2006). A major reason is probably that the complexity of hand hygiene is grossly underestimated. It is often taken for granted that everybody masters the technique; however, to clean hands requires in fact a systematic and elaborate washing technique, which has to be trained. Furthermore, the tools for hand hygiene are far from optimal. A nurse in an intensive care unit with seven patient contacts each hour will for instance have to spend nearly one hour a day washing hands with soap and water, if the recommended procedure is to be followed (Voss & Widmer 1997). Apart from being time consuming, this may give rise to skin problems. Alcoholic hand rub is faster and more gentle to the skin, and even more importantly, much more efficient to kill pathogens. It can replace soap and water in most cases, provided that hands are not visibly dirty (Pittet et al 2000). However, there are important exceptions: spore-forming bacteria, like *Clostridium difficile* and naked viruses, like norovirus (Kampf et al 2005) are not very susceptible to alcohol, which implies that health care workers must stick to soap and water, when dealing with patients suffering from infections due to these pathogens. It appears from this that what at first glance looks simple is in fact a demanding clinical procedure, which requires background knowledge and has to be trained in the same systematic manner as e.g. the skills necessary for insertion of an i.v. line. Essentially, hand hygiene techniques have not changed very much over the past century. With today's knowledge about the lack of compliance and quality with hand hygiene performance and the ability of some organisms to resist alcohol, there is a clear need for development of more efficient hand hygiene techniques that are universally applicable, and at the same time fast and user-friendly.

For many years it has been a matter of discussion, whether transmission of pathogens from the hospital environment plays a significant role in acquisition and spread of health care associated infections. A major reason is lack of well designed studies to document this route of transmission, which may be attributed to the fact that cleaning until recently was not considered an issue worth investigating (Dancer 2008). From the 1970s and until recently cleaning was considered merely an aesthetic issue, and budgets were cut down by hospital management in order to meet the demands for resources in other parts of the health care system. This was endorsed even by infection control practitioners, partly because of the lack of evidence for its importance as an infection control measure, partly because they feared that focus on cleaning would draw attention away from more important measures, like hand hygiene. This attitude has gradually shifted with the emergence of new well designed studies highlighting the role of the environment in transmission of hospital acquired infections and the ability of disinfecting cleaning to reduce such cases (Boyce et al 2008, Dancer 2008, Datta et al 2011).

Accumulating evidence suggests that there is a dynamic interaction between the hands of health care workers and the environment in transmitting organisms from one patient to another (Dancer 2008) (Fig. 3). The question whether focus should be put on hand hygiene or cleaning the hospital environment is no longer meaningful. It is not an either or, rather it is a both and. If cross transmission is to be controlled there is a need to develop new and more efficient methods both for hand hygiene and environmental decontamination. Current cleaning methods used in the health care setting are primarily designed to fulfil aesthetic purposes, and they do not remove organisms from touch sites in the environment to any significant degree (French et al 2004). Cleaning combined with liquid disinfectants, such as hypochlorite and quaternary ammonium agents reduces surface contamination with pathogens, like *Clostridium difficile*, MRSA, and VRE (Wilcox et al 2003, Datta et al 2011). However, occupational hazards and concern for the environment implies that they are not used in daily routine cleaning. Hydrogen peroxide fumigation is an efficient and attractive alternative from an environmental point of view (French et al 2004, Boyce et al 2008). However, it is not suited for daily routine cleaning either. Clearly there is a need for more user-friendly methods that can be used in daily practice to decontaminate touch sites, without posing any risks to humans, materials, and environment. Furthermore, we are in need of universally accepted standards to define and monitor microbial cleanliness of surfaces (Dancer 2011).

Transmission of pathogens by heat sensitive equipment, such as bronchoscopes is still a matter of concern. Problems usually relate to breaches in technique, both in the bronchoscopes and the disinfectors used for reprocessing. Failures in maintenance are one of the major reasons for technical breaches that lead to failing disinfection and eventually to transmission of pathogens to patients undergoing examination (Fig. 4). An important reason for failures is that responsibilities for maintenance are often shared by different parties, and demands are not always clearly defined. Furthermore, when buying this type of equipment there may be a tendency to underestimate working expenses for maintenance, which usually requires paid expertise from an external supplier. In a situation with need for budget cuts, reduction of maintenance may be one way to obtain savings, which may become critical if responsibilities and demands are not clearly defined. A clear definition of responsibilities and documentation of maintenance in accordance with written guidelines are essential measures to secure a satisfactory hygienic standard with this type of fragile equipment. Furthermore, when negotiating with a supplier, purchase and maintenance of equipment should be seen as one combined package, defining a plan for its maintenance in the years ahead. Finally, producers of fibre-optic endoscopes should be encouraged to produce more robust equipment, which can tolerate safer sterilization methods, if possible based on heat.

This review has focused on the sources and routes of transmission seen today and over the past few decades. However, it is important to note that the situation is not static. Growing age and debilitation of patients predispose for more infections. Furthermore, since health care associated infections are in part determined by the procedures used in diagnostics, treatment, care and rehabilitation they change with the development of the health care system. New sources and transmission routes emerge, while others disappear. The risk of new infections can be minimized by making a systematic hygienic risk assessment, when introducing new health care procedures and new technology, and by keeping a sharp eye on unsuspected findings in the microbiology laboratories (Kolmos 2001).

9. References

Bassetti, S.; Bischoff, WE.; Walter, M. et al. (2005). Dispersal of Staphylococcus aureus into the air associated with a rhinovirus infection. *Infect Control Hosp Epidemiol*; 26: 196-203.

Bihl, F.; Castelli, D.; Marincola, F. et al. (2007). Transfusion-transmitted infections. *J Transl Med*; 5: 25

Bischoff, WE.; Wallis, ML.; Tucker, BK. et al. (2006). "Gesundheit!" Sneezing, common colds, allergies and Staphylococcus aureus dispersion. *J Infect Dis*; 194: 1119-26.

Bode, L.; Kluytmans, J.; Wertheim, H. et al. (2010). Preventing surgical-site infections in nasal carriers of Staphylococcus aureus. *N Engl J Med*; 362: 9-17.

Boyce, JM.; Havill NL.; Otter, JA. et al. (2008). Impact of hydrogen peroxide vapor room decontamination on Clostridium difficile environmental contamination and transmission in the health care setting. *Infect Control Hosp Epidemiol*; 29: 723-9.

Brankston, G.; Gitterman, L.; Hirji, Z. et al. (2007). Transmission of influenza A in human beings. *Lancet Infect Dis*; 7: 257-65.

Carling, PC. & Bartley, JM. (2010). Evaluating hygienic cleaning in health care settings: What you do not know can harm your patient. *Am J Infect Control*; 38 (Suppl 1): S41-50.

Carman, WF.; Elder, AG.; Wallace, LA. et al. (2000). Effects of influenza vaccination of health-care workers on mortality of elderly people in long-term care: a randomised controlled trial. *Lancet*; 355: 93-7.

Dancer, SJ. (2008). Importance of the environment in methcillin-resistant Staphylococcus aureus acquisition: the case for hospital cleaning. *Lancet Infect Dis*; 8: 101-13.

Dancer, SJ. (2011). Hospital cleaning in the 21st century. *Eur J Clin Microbiol Infect Dis*; 30: 1473-81.

Datta, R.; Platt, R.; Yokoe, DS. et al. (2011). Environmental cleaning intervention and risk of acquiring multi-drug resistant organisms from prior room occupants. *Arch Intern Med*; 171: 491-4.

Di Martino, P.; Sirot, D; Joly, B et al. (1997). Relationship between adhesion to intestinal caco-2 cells and multidrug resistance in Klebsiella pneumoniae clinical isolates. *J Clin Microbiol*; 35: 1499-1503.

Fennelly, KP.; Martyny, JW.; Fulton, KE. et al. (2004). Cough-generated aerosols of Mycobacterium tuberculosis. A new method to study infectiousness. *Am J Respir Crit Care Med*; 169: 604-9.

Fisker, N.; Carlsen, NL.; Kolmos, HJ. et al. (2006). Identifying a hepatitis B outbreak by molecular surveillance: a case study. *BMJ*; 332: 343-5.

Fone, DL.; Lane, W. & Salmon, RL. (1999). Investigation of an outbreak of gastroenteritis at a hospital for patients with learning difficulties. *Commun Dis Public Health*; 2: 35-8.

French, GL.; Otter, JA.; Shannon, KP. et al. (2004). Tackling contamination of the hospital environment by methicillin-resistant Staphylococcus aureus (MRSA): a comparison between conventional terminal cleaning and hydrogen peroxide vapour decontamination. *J Hosp Infect*; 57: 31-7.

Guallar, C.; Ariza, J.; Dominguez, MA. et al. (2004). An insidious nosocomial outbreak due to Salmonella Enteritidis. *Infect Control Hosp Epidemiol*; 25: 10-5.

Hall, CB.; Long, CE. & Schnabel, KC. (2001). Respiratory syncytial virus infections in previously healthy working adults. *Clin Infect Dis*; 33: 792-6.

Hall, CB. (2000). Nosocomial respiratory syncytial virus infections: the "Cold War"has not ended. *Clin Infect Dis*; 31: 590-6.

Hansen, D.; Blahout, B.; Benner, D. et al. (2008). Environmental sampling of particulate matter and fungal spores during demolition of a building on a hospital area. *J Hosp Infect*; 70: 259-64.

Heltberg, O.; Skov, F.; Gerner-Smidt, P. et al. (1993). Nosocomial epidemic of Serratia marcescens septicemia ascribed to contaminated blood transfusion bags. *Transfusion*; 33: 221-7.

Heptonstall, J. (2000). Surgeons who test positive for hepatitis C should be transferred to low risk duties. *Rev Med Virol*; 10: 75-8.

Huang, SS.; Datta, R. & Platt, R. (2006). Risk of acquiring antibiotic-resistant bacteria from prior room occupants. *Arch Intern Med*; 166: 1945-51.

Johnsen, BO.; Lingaas, E.; Torfoss, D. et al. (2010). A large outbreak of Listeria monocytogenes infection with short incubation period in a tertiary care hospital. *J Infect*; 61: 465-70.

Kallen, AJ.; Wilson, CT. & Larson, RJ. (2005). Perioperative intranasal mupirocin for prevention of surgical-site infections: systematic review of the literature and meta-analysis. *Infect Control Hosp Epidemiol*; 26: 916-22.

Kampf, G.; Grotheer, D. & Steinmann J. (2005). Efficacy of three ethanol-based hand rubs against feline calicivirus, a surrogate virus for Norovirus. *J Hosp Infect*; 60: 144-9.

Katzenstein, T.; Jørgensen, LB.; Permin, H et al. (1999). Nosocomial HIV-transmission in an outpatient clinic detected by epidemiological and phylogenetic analyses. *AIDS*; 13: 1737-44.

Kluytmans, J.; van Belkum, A. & Verbrugh, H. (1997). Nasal carriage of Staphylococcus aureus: Epidemiology, underlying mechanisms, and associated risks. *Clin Microbiol Reviews*; 10: 505-20.

Kolmos, HJ.; Thuesen, B.; Nielsen, SV. et al. (1993). Outbreak of infection in a burns unit due to Pseudomonas aeruginosa originating from contaminated tubing used for irrigation of patients. *J Hosp Infect*; 24: 11-21.

Kolmos, HJ.; Petersen, A.; Hilsberg, P. et al. (2006). Room for improvement: Two third of hospital staff do not use proper hand disinfection technique. *J Hosp Infect*; 64 (suppl 1): S54.

Kolmos, HJ.; Svendsen, RN. & Nielsen SV. (1997). The surgical team as a source of postoperative wound infections caused by Streptococcus pyogenes. *J Hosp Infect*; 35: 207-14.

Kolmos, HJ. (2001). Role of the clinical microbiology laboratory in infection control - a Danish perspective. *J Hosp Infect*; 48 (Suppl A): S50-4.

Kramer, A.; Schwebke, I. & Kampf, G. (2006). How long do nosocomial pathogens persist on inanimate surfaces? A systematic review. *BMC Infect Dis*; 6: 130.

Leclercq, A.; Martin, L.; Vergnes, ML. et al. (2005). Fatal Yersinia enterocolitica biotype 4 serovar O:3 sepsis after red blood cell transfusion. *Transfusion*; 45: 814-8.

Macedo de Oliveira, A.; White, KL; Leschinsky, DP. et al. 2005. An outbreak of hepatitis C virus infections among outpatients in a hematology/oncology clinic. *Ann Intern Med*; 142: 898-902.

McNeil, SA.; Foster, CL.; Hedderwick, SA. Et al. (2001). Effect of hand cleansing with antimicrobial soap or alcohol-based gel on microbial colonization of artificial fingernails worn by health care workers. *Clin Infect Dis*; 32: 367-72.

Nardell, EA. (2004). Catching droplet nuclei. Toward a better understanding of tuberculosis transmission. *Am J Respir Crit Care Med*; 169: 553-4.

Nelson, D. & Muscarella, LF. (2006). Current issues in endoscope reprocessing and infection control during gastrointestinal endoscopy. *World J Gastroenterol*; 12: 3953-64.

Perl, TM.; Cullen, JJ.; Wenzel, RP. et al. (2002). Intranasal mupirocin to prevent postoperative Staphylococcus aureus infections. *N Engl J Med*; 346: 1871-7.

Pessoa-Silva, CL.; Dharan, S.; Hugonnet, S. et al. (2004). Dynamics of Bacterial Hand Contamination during Routine Neonatal Care. *Infect Control Hosp Epidemiol; 25*: 192-7.

Pittet, D.; Allegranzi, B.; Sax, H. et al. (2006). Evidence-based model for hand transmission during patient care and the role of improved practices. *Lancet Infect Dis*; 6: 641-52.

Pittet, D.; Hugonnet, S.; Harbarth, S. et al. (2000). Effectiveness of a hospital-wide programme to improve compliance with hand hygiene. *Lancet*; 356: 1307-12.

Rampling, A.; Wiseman, S.; Davis, L. et al. (2001). Evidence that hospital hygiene is important in the control of methicillin-resistant Staphylococcus aureus. *J Hosp Infect*; 49: 109-16.

Ravn, P.; Lundgren, JD.; Kjaeldgaard, P. et al. (1991). Nosocomial outbreak of cryptosporidiosis in AIDS patients. *BMJ*; 302: 277-80.

Roy, CJ. & Milton, DK. (2004). Airborne transmission of communicable infection - the elusive pathway. *N Engl J Med*; 350: 1710-2.

Rutala, WA. & Weber, DJ. (2004). Disinfection and sterilization in health care facilities: what clinicians need to know. *Clin Infect Dis*; 39: 702-9.

Sabria, M. & Yu, VL. (2002). Hospital-acquired legionellosis: solutions for a preventable infection. *Lancet Infect Dis*; 2: 368-73.

Safdar, N.; Crnich, CJ. & Maki, DG. (2005). The pathogenesis of ventilator-associated pneumonia: Its relevance to developing effective strategies for prevention. *Respir Care*; 50: 725-39.

Salgado, CD.; Farr, BM.; Hall, KK. et al. (2002). Influenza in the acute hospital setting. *Lancet Infect Dis*; 2: 145-55.

Sherertz, RJ.; Bassetti, S.; Bassetti-Wyss, B. (2001). "Cloud" health-care workers. *Emerg Infect Dis*; 7: 241-4.

Singh, M.; Lingappan, K. (2006). Whooping cough. The current scene. *Chest*; 130: 1547-53.

Sion, C.; Garrino, M-G.; Glupczynski, Y. et al. (2000). Nosocomial outbreak of Salmonella enteritidis in a university hospital. *Infect Control Hosp Epidemiol*; 21: 182-3.

Srinivasan, A.; Wolfenden, LL.; Song, X. et al. (2003). An outbreak of Pseudomonas aeruginosa infections associated with flexible bronchoscopes. *N Engl J Med*; 348: 221-7.

Stevenson, P.; McCann, R.; Duthie, R. et al. (1994). A hospital outbreak due to Norwalk virus. *J Hosp Infect*; 26:261-72.

Sutton, JM.; Dickinson, J.; Walker, JT. et al. (2006). Methods to minimize the risk of Creutzfeldt-Jakob disease transmission by surgical procedures: where to set the standard? *Clin Infect Dis*; 43: 757-64.

Tambyah, PA.; Halvorson, KT. & Maki DG. (1999). A prospective study of pathogenesis of catheter-associated urinary tract infection. *Mayo Clin Proc*; 74: 131-6.

Tang, JW.; Li ,Y.; Eames, I. et al. (2006). Factors involved in the aerosol transmission of infection and control of ventilation in health care premises. *J Hosp Infect*; 64: 100-14.

Tellier, R. (2006). Review of aerosol transmission of influenza A virus. *Emerg Infect Dis*; 12: 1657-62.

The Incident Investigation Teams and Others. (1997). Transmission of hepatitis B to patients from four infected surgeons without hepatitis B e antigen. *N Engl J Med*; 336: 178-84.

Trick, WE.; Vernon, MO.; Hayes, RA. et al. (2003). Impact of ring wearing on hand contamination and comparison of hand hygiene agents in a hospital. *Clin Infect Dis*; 36: 1383-90.

Van Saene, HKF.; Petros, AJ.; Ramsay, G. et al. (2003). All great truths are iconoclastic: selective decontamination of the digestive tract moves from heresy to level 1 truth. *Intensive Care Med*; 29: 677-90.

Von Eiff, C.; Becker, K.; Machka, K. et al. (2001). Nasal carriage as a source of Staphylococcus aureus bacteremia. *N Engl J Med*; 344: 11-6.

Vonberg, R-P.; Gastmeier, P. (2006). Nosocomial aspergillosis in outbreak settings. *J Hosp Infect*; 63: 246-54.

Voss, A. & Widmer, AF. (1997). No time for hand washing!? Hand washing versus alcoholic rub: can we afford 100% compliance? *Infect Control Hosp Epidemiol*; 18: 205-8.

Weber, DJ. Rutala, WA. (2001). Lessons from outbreaks associated with bronchoscopy. *Infect Control Hosp Epidemiol*; 22: 403-8.

Wenzel, RP. & Edmond, MB. (2005). Patient-to-patient transmission of hepatitis C virus. *Ann Intern Med*; 142: 940-1.

Wilcox, MH.; Fawley, WN; Wigglesworth, N. et al. (2003). Comparison of the effect of detergent versus hypochlorite cleaning on environmental contamination and incidence of Clostridium difficile infection. *J Hosp Infect*; 54: 109-14.

Woods DE. (1987). Role of fibronectin in the pathogenesis of Gram-negative bacillary pneumonia. *Rev Infect Dis*; 9 (Suppl 4): S386-90.

3

Models of Hospital Acquired Infection

Pietro Coen
University College London Hospitals NHS Trust
United Kingdom

1. Introduction

This chapter will not dwell on how mathematical models are built, better covered elsewhere (Bailey, 1975; Renshaw, 1991; Scott & Smith, 1994; Coen, 2007). It will focus on the impact of mathematical models on the understanding of infections spread in hospitals and their control. Hospital Acquired Infections (HAIs) made their first appearance with the invention of hospitals, mostly associated with surgical operations carried out when germ theory and hand-hygiene were unheard of and post-surgical mortality could be as high as 90% (La Force, 1987). The invention of antibiotics reduced mortality, but subsequently led to the emergence of infections adapted to survival in the antimicrobial-rich hospital environment. An arms race ensued where the bacterium and the pharmacist are to this day fighting to outwit each other (Sneader, 2005). Bacteria like Meticillin-resistant *Staphylococcus aureus* (MRSA) and Vancomycin-resistant Enterococci (VRE) were detected in UK hospitals as early as the 1960s (Stewart & Holt, 1962), but it was not until the mid 1990s that they 'took off' as a significant problem for hospital managers and inpatients (Austin & Anderson, 1999). If only 10% of adult HAI infections could be prevented, £93 million could be saved in England and Wales alone (Plowman et al., 1999).

Hospital inpatients are difficult subjects for study. They are only 'available' for a short time window, measured in days; too debilitated to all cooperate to the same degree; an extremely heterogeneous population; and major ethical issues are met when it comes to experimentation, especially when infection is asymptomatic. Their environment is heterogeneous and constantly changing, as technologies improve medical practice change. Under these circumstances, HAI models have a distinct advantage over uncontrolled observational studies (Cooper et al., 2003). This point is illustrated in section 4.2.

When designing the structure of a model it is necessary to strike a balance between realism and generality (Bonten et al., 2001). A model needs to be complex enough to capture all those essential features of the process under study, ensuring realism and providing sufficient information so that all questions can be addressed using the model framework. Yet models must not be too complex lest conclusions are only generalizable to a small number of situations of little interest for much of the health care public. As complexity increases, providing information for a model may become prohibitive, less tools for analysis may be available for checking errors in formulation, and exact solutions may not exist so that numerical approximations are needed. Nevertheless HAIs are complex things, and modellers are forced to abandon generality; at worst mathematical models may be too simple to be realistic. This chapter explores the nature of this complexity (Section 2), review methods used for fitting models to observational data (Section 3), focus on lessons learnt for some areas of infection control (Section 4). Finally I give an example of a stochastic model of norovirus on a geriatric ward (Section 5).

2. Essential features of HAI

This in part depends on the questions addressed and the biological characteristics of the HAIs modelled. The general idea is that (susceptible) patients spend time on a ward, they have physical contacts with health-care workers ([HCWs] nurses, doctors, cleaners etc.), visitors, other patients and with contaminants in the environment. Such exposure can lead to colonization with infectious organisms that may sooner or later cause debilitating clinical infection. The devil is in the detail.

2.1 Mechanism of infection

Some HAIs manifest themselves soon after colonization, regardless of the kind of healthcare. This is typical of many viruses, such as varicella, measles, norovirus and adenovirus where susceptibles acquire infection and after an incubation period of a few days suffer symptoms of infection coincident with infectiousness to others and subsequently recover or die (section 5). Such aetiologies are typically associated with outbreaks characterized by 'attack rates' and outbreak durations.

In contrast most HAIs are not just about acquiring the organism. Many bacterial infections may be carried for months in the absence of clinical symptoms, such as in the nares (MRSA), the skin (Coagulase-negative Staphylococci [CNS]), the gastrointestinal tract (*Escherichia coli, Clostridium difficile*). This silent infection may last months to years, makes the patient a 'carrier', more or less infectious to others depending on the organism and other circumstances. Only when natural barriers are breached, often as a result of health-care intervention (e.g. surgery, line and catheter insertion), bacteria will invade tissues that are otherwise sterile, they multiply and cause life-threatening clinical illness. An extreme example is *Streptococcus pyogenes* (or Group A Streptococcus [GAS]), an airborne infection that typically causes sore throat, but can be life threatening if allowed to invade subcutaneous tissues (necrotizing fasciitis), such as via a stab wound or burn. Untreated it can result in multiple organ failure and very high fatality rates (Aziz & Kotb, 2008).

Hence the epidemiology of most HAIs is the result of a two-step process: the acquisition of the organism (acting on susceptibles), and the subsequent invasion of sterile tissues (acting on carriers). The slow turn-over of carriage (relative to the average length of stay in hospital) means that these HAIs are typically endemic and their burden measured in terms of prevalence and incidence. The first step is usually modelled with the rate of infection per susceptible-carrier pair, known as the 'transmission coefficient', β (Anderson & May, 1991), sometimes factorized as $\beta = ab$, where a is the contact rate and b is the probability of transmission per contact (Austin et al., 1999a). The second step is modelled as a rate per carrier. For example, Coello et al., (1997) estimate 0.59% daily probability of MRSA carriers developing infection. Cooper and Lipsitch (2004) estimate 35% per day for MRSA in ITU.

Other HAIs present with mixed aetiologies, such as *C difficile,* which in one third of patients causes life threatening infection of the colon on acquisition, while two thirds remain asymptomatic. The latter may yet suffer infection as a result of as poorly understood triggers, such as antimicrobial administration (Johnson et al., 1990). Recent evidence suggests that norovirus is carried asymptomatically by 12% of individuals in the community (Phillips et al., 2010). Such carriers may well become infectious in hospital when diarrhoea sets in, perhaps the result of laxatives and antibiotics.

2.2 Forms of clinical infection

At one end of the clinical spectrum organisms enter the bloodstream through a cut in the skin, are able to multiply and systemically affect the rest of the body (bacteraemia or sepsis). Bacteraemias are relatively rare (1.3% of all HAIs in England; Hospital Infection Society & Infection Control Nurses Association, 2007), are expensive to treat and life threatening. Other infections are more localized in their effects. Surgical wounds may become infected (Surgical Site Infections [SSI]), causing a wide range of problems. Their seriousness depends on whether they are peripheral, deep incisional or whether inner body spaces and organs are affected (Health Protection Agency [HPA], 2011a). These are rarely life threatening, although they make up 16% of all HAIs in England, are expensive to treat (Plowman, 1999), may lead to unpleasant consequences (delayed care) and if inappropriately treated may lead to bacteraemia, amputation and death. A milder form of HAI is the urinary tract infection (UTI) typically caused by insertion of temporary indwelling bladder catheters kept long enough for bacteria to move up the urinary tract and infect normally sterile sites such as the kidneys. UTIs are very common (21% of all HAIs in England), and can lead to pain and distress, general debilitation and occasionally bacteraemia (Bryan et al., 1984).

Many mathematical models distinguish between carriers and clinical infections, but most lump all infections into one homogeneous black box, ignoring heterogeneity in frequency and consequences. Bacteraemias may be expensive to treat and life threatening, but contribute little to infectious spread. SSIs, on the other hand, are not as life-threatening, but are more common and more infectious. Treating SSIs and bacteraemias as a uniform entity may lead to significant discrepancy between model prediction and reality.

2.3 The aetiological agent

Most HAIs are caused by bacteria although viruses and fungi are often involved. Most are resistant to some classes of antibiotic. Examples from the Gram-positive bacteria are MRSA (penicillins and cephalosporins), VRE (some penicillins and glycopeptides), *C difficile* (fluoroquinolones). Many Gram-negative bacteria cause bacteraemias and UTIs, such as *E coli, Pseudomonas aeruginosa, Klebsiellas* spp., *Citrobacter, Enterobacter,* and *Proteus*. Some of these produce enzymes known as extended-spectrum beta-lactamases (ESBL), which confer resistance to many antibiotic classes (penicillins, cephalosporins, fluoroquinolones and aminoglycosides) (Kullik et al., 2010). ESBLs are not a homogeneous group, inheritance may be chromosomal or via plasmid, and several genotypes exist (TEM-10, TEM-26, CTX-M etc.; Livermore 2001). Resistance to carbapenems, one of the last lines of defence against ESBLs, is beginning to emerge (Grundmann et al., 2011). Other bacteria are more sensitive to antibiotics but are common enough to cause significant infection (e.g. Meticillin-susceptible *Staphylococcus aureus* [MSSA]).

The genetic structure of most bacterial populations is clonal (Smith et al., 1993), and antibiotic-resistant HAIs are no exception, so that *de novo* emergence of antibiotic resistance is rare on the hospital-admission time-scale, and resistant variants may be modelled independently of sensitive counterparts. This is the case of MRSA and MSSA (Feil et al., 2003), *E coli* (Milkman & Bridges, 1990), *C difficile* (Griffiths et al., 2010). In contrast, Enterococci (e.g. VRE) and Gram negatives like the *Klebsiella* exhibit considerable inter-strain genomic diversity, mainly linked to the presence of transposable agents such as phages and plasmids - often responsible for the resistance phenotype (van Schaik & Willems, 2010; Zhao et al., 2010). It is then possible for sensitive variants to become resistant in hosts colonized with both variants.

Regardless of the genetics, there may be important differences between HAI genotypes. One example is *C difficile* which has hundreds of different 'ribotypes'. Ribotype 027 can produce 16 to 23-fold higher concentrations of toxin (Warny et al., 2005) and is associated with twice the mortality than other strains (HPA, 2011b). Some *S aureus* variants, known as community-acquired MRSA (CA-MRSA), produce the Panton-Valentine Leukocydin (PVL) toxin, are abundant in the community, are much more sensitive to antibiotics and are more associated with 'soft-skin' infections. But they are also known to cause life-threatening necrotizing pneumonia. CA-MRSA is on the increase in North America and is making its appearance in the hospital (David & Daum, 2010), although relatively unknown in UK hospitals (HPA, 2011c).

Competition for colonization space is an interesting issue when modelling two or more variants. MRSA and MSSA, for example share the same ecologic 'niche' as they both colonize the nares of human beings, as well as many other aspects of infection aetiology and a degree of competition may well exist (Dall'Antonia et al., 2005). The problem is that most mathematical models of antibiotic resistance make implicit assumptions regarding competition with important implications on model dynamics (see section 4.3). These models either include two variants (sensitive and resistant), or only consider the resistant one. One-strain models are consistent with complete coexistence with other variants (e.g. Austin et al., 1999a). Two-strain models are consistent with complete competition whenever the 'co-carrier' state is ignored (i.e. a resistant strain may not colonize a host that is already colonized with the sensitive strain; e.g. Austin et al. 1999b).

2.4 The nature of infectious spread

2.4.1 Transmission routes

Some modellers (Cooper et al., 1999, 2004a; Smith et al., 2004) followed the implicit approach of embedding all possible routes of infection within the value of the transmission coefficient β, which measures the effective transmission rate between any susceptible-infected pair, regardless of the exact route. Bootsma et al. (2007) estimate transmission coefficients for 3rd generation cephalosporin-resistant Enterobacteriaceae (CRE) and consider the addition of the 'endogenous' route, whereby the patient's already present pathogens grow to detectable levels. They find this route to be responsible for more acquisitions than the cross-infection route, which brings into doubt the definition of 'hospital acquired' as infections detected 48 hours after admission for Enterobacteriaceae like *E coli*.

Other modellers are more explicit and usually make the case for the predominance of a single transmission route. Examples are models of VRE and MRSA in ITU where patients are not free to move and transmission takes place via the HCW (Austin et al., 1999a;

Grundmann et al., 2002). Failure of contact precautions is blamed for any transmission. If P is the number of patients and W is the number of HCWs, the total number of infectious contacts per day is C = aPW (*a* as defined in section 2.1). Notice that for a given total number of contacts C, the number of contacts per patient (= aW) may not necessarily equal the number of contacts per HCW (= aP = aP(W/P)). These are only expected to equal when the HCW-patient ratio is 1:1 (as maybe the case on the ITU). This is not realistic when some HCWs visit more patients than others.

In wards where patients are mobile, or where transmission can take the airborne route, more transmission coefficients are needed. The airborne route is especially relevant to the spread of pulmonary tuberculosis (TB), measles and influenza. Models of the airborne route require the measurement of parameters like quantum generation rates (a measure of infectious material in the air), room volume, room ventilation rates, pulmonary ventilation rates (Beggs et al., 2010). It is common practice to isolate patients susceptible to infection (e.g. immunocompromised cases) in isolation rooms with positive pressure (to keep infectious quanta out), and infectious cases with negative pressure (to keep infectious quanta within the confines of the isolation room). The implicit approach may still enable the analysis of the success of isolation, when different transmission coefficients are used, for isolated and non-isolated patients (Forrester et al., 2007).

2.4.2 Quantifying transmission

It is possible to follow a cohort of inpatients and measure the acquisition rate of infection (Jernigan et al., 1996). This is the 'force of infection', λ, and is equivalent to $\beta.I$, where I is the average number of infectious patients per unit time on the ward. It is possible to use this number to calculate β from the expected number of daily visits to infectious patients. Raboud et al. (2005) estimate βs for patient-HCW contact ranging from 0.017% to 6.7%, depending on whether the patient was in isolation and whether HCWs complied with hand-washing. Forrester et al. (2007) estimated 1.03% acquisitions per day (background rate, β_0) and transmission coefficients β_1 = 1.31% (not isolated), and β_2 = 0.45% (isolated). Cooper & Lipsitch (2004) estimate transmission coefficients 33% (MRSA), 26% (VRE) for patients in ITU. Ong et al. (2008) used transmission coefficients for influenza stratified by 5 categories of staff, ambulant and non-ambulant inpatients and visitors.

Other modellers use the "basic case reproduction number", R_0, as a summary measure of infectious spread (Anderson & May, 1991). This is defined as "the average number of secondary infections produced when one infectious individual is introduced into [an infinite] host population in which every host is susceptible". It follows that the infection can persist in the population only when $R_0 > 1$. Real life populations are finite and seldom completely susceptible so that we are more likely to observe *effective* basic case reproduction numbers, $R_e = R_0.s^*$ where R_0 is discounted by the proportion of susceptibles in the population (s^*). Cooper et al. introduced the refinement of having $R_0 = R_A.\xi$, where R_A is the effective basic reproduction number observed within a single admission, and ξ is a constant that accounts for the probability of re-admission while still infectious (Cooper et al., 2004a). The implication is that even when good infection control practice reduces R_A to values less than 1, the infection will establish itself as a result of re-admission if ξ is large enough. Cooper *et al.* chose transmission coefficients for MRSA consistent with R_0 ranging between 1.1 (self-limiting clusters of secondary cases) to 1.3 (endemic pattern).

2.4.3 The role of the environment

The hospital environment, as a source of infection, is an extremely complex entity and difficult to model explicitly. Hospital surfaces can harbour live HAI agents (e.g. Staphylococci, Enterobacteriaceae, C *difficile* spores etc). The problem is that even where it is possible to establish associations between bacterial flora on patients and their immediate environment (Asoh *et al.*, 2005), the direction of the causal arrow is not known. Wards are also extremely heterogeneous places. Bacterial counts sampled from sites most likely associated with direct patient contact (e.g. hand-rails, soap dispensers, bedding, curtains) are much lower than other sites (e.g. floor) (Hamilton et al., 2010), and porous surfaces are more difficult to clean (Oie et al., 2005). To explicitly model these environmental sites it is necessary to choose the appropriate site, sample for organisms at appropriate intervals, and follow up patients for contact rates with the site as well as their carriage status. An alternative is to model the environment as a black box and set its 'colonization' and 'turnover' rates, tweaking them so as to obtain a model output close to observation (Kouyos et al., 2011).

2.5 The patient

Many inpatients have co-morbidities that put them at special risk of infection: HIV cases, diabetics, bone-marrow transplant patients, those on chemotherapy, in elderly care wards, those undergoing surgery, to mention a few. There are behavioural differences: some patients are more likely to be re-hospitalized, and those with a history of hospitalization are more likely to carry HAIs. Cooper et al. (2004a) stratified patients into two categories of re-admission frequency (see section 2.7), while Bootsma et al. (2006) allowed 1% of inpatients colonized with MRSA to be 'super-spreaders' (10 times more infectious than other carriers).

In the UK patients rarely stay on the same ward for the duration of their admission. There are at least two distinct patterns of patient flow (Figure 1): *elective* admissions, planned weeks or

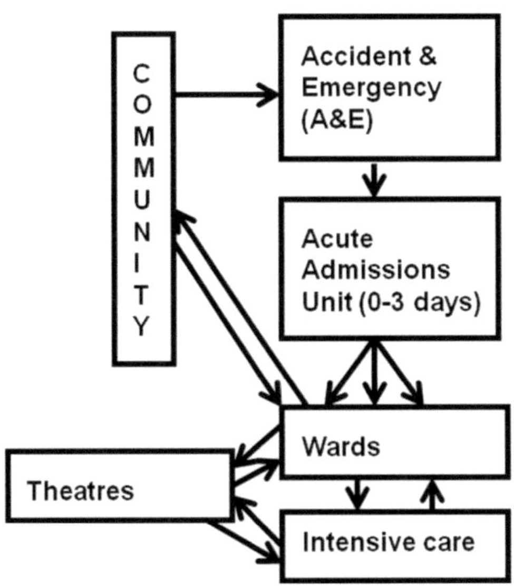

Fig. 1. Schematic description of patient flow in a UK hospital.

months in advance, are usually taken directly to specialist wards. In contrast, *emergency* admissions present to A&E and are subsequently moved to a temporary unit, known in the UK as the Acute Admissions Unit (AAU) and stay there for 1-3 days prior to being admitted to specialist wards. Patients may also be taken to ITU, infectious diseases wards, or may be moved to theatre to undergo surgery, to then recover in a different ward. The role of ITU is thought to be important in the seeding and spread of certain antimicrobial resistant HAIs to other wards (Edgeworth, 2011). Bootsma et al. (2006) and Hubben et al. (2011) modelled patients admitted to one of three hospitals with 36 wards each and 5 ITUs, whose inpatient population had differing lengths of ward stay depending on whether patients were in ITU (mean of 3 days) or other wards (7 days).

2.6 The staff

Some modellers assume all transmission between inpatients to take place via the medium of the ward environment - HCWs being part of it (Cooper et al., 2004a). Others explicitly model HCWs and are seen as the most responsible transmission component (Austin et al., 1999a). Because staff members work on on the ward for much longer than the average patient length of stay, they have a huge potential to spread infection. Hence they cannot play as large a role in transmission as inpatients lest we expect every inpatient to become infected (Beggs et al., 2008). HCWs are a heterogeneous group. Ong et al. (2008) stratified HCWs into cleaners, clerks, doctors, health-attendants, and nurses for an influenza model. Their "Who-Acquires-Infection-From-Whom" (WAIFW) matrix suggest heterogeneous contact rates with patients and each other: cleaners, health-care attendants and clerks mostly contacted nurses; doctors had them mostly with nurses, patients and their visitors; nurses had them mostly with other nurses, patients and visitors. Bootsma et al. (2006) stratified staff into those that have contact with patients on a single ward (1:1 staff patient ratios in ITU, and 5:18 ratios on other wards), and staff with unrestricted contact across wards and hospitals. Some have greater hand-hygiene compliance than others (Pittet et al., 1999). Raboud et al. (2005) stratified them into daytime and night-time staff and went as far as including the detail of staff looking after the patients of other staff during coffee breaks!

2.7 The community

Early HAI models ignored the impact of the population outside hospital walls (the "extramural" population), and patients admitted into hospital were either assumed uncolonized or came with a fixed probability of acquiring infection (Austin et al., 1999a; Lipsitch et al., 2000). Cooper et al. (2004a) broke this tradition and modelled the extramural population, stratifying it into those with a high vs. low rate of readmission (0.57% vs. 0.06% readmissions per day). Hubben et al. (2011) stratify patients by ward within three hospitals and by risk of readmission with 22,000 'high-risk' patients who are 10 times more likely to be readmitted, out of a catchment population of 220,000 - resulting in 50% high risk patients within the hospital population. This kind of HAI model predicts low extramural MRSA prevalence, which matches observation (Lu et al., 2005). Austin & Anderson (1999) modelled the spread of MRSA across 400 NHS hospitals in England and conclude that the largest hospitals are responsible for most 'transmission' events, and make the case in favour of active surveillance.

2.8 Infection control

No hospital applies exactly the same infection control strategy as any another at any one time. Several interventions are invariably applied simultaneously. Many of the decisions taken by hospital managers are based on quasi-experimental and observational data at best. This point is illustrated in the review of the evidence in favour of inpatient isolation for the control of MRSA infection (Cooper et al., 2003; Cooper et al., 2004b). This is an area where mathematical models can contribute. As it is not possible to manipulate the real world of patients in hospitals, we can resort to manipulating a simulated hypothesis of it, and draw some conclusions, aware of all the assumptions made in its design. One approach is to fit the model to infection data and estimate unknown parameters (see section 3), and subsequently to use it to run simulations and test infection control strategies (Section 4).

Some infection control methods are easier to model because they directly affect the transmission cycle: cohorting (Austin et al., 1999a), hand-hygiene (Austin et al., 1999a; Beggs et al., 2008, 2009), isolation (Cooper et al., 1999, 2003). *Cohorting*, the neutralization of transmission routes into 1:1 HCW:patient contacts, is only possible in settings where staff numbers exceed patient numbers, such as on the ITU. On other wards patients can exceed staff numbers by at least 5:1, and only degrees of cohorting are possible, especially when patients are mobile (see section 5; Raboud et al., 2005). *Hand-hygiene*, the cleaning of staff hands before and after patient contact, has two dimensions (Beggs et al., 2008): *compliance* (the proportion of staff that actually clean their hands) and *effectiveness* (the probability of effective removal of contaminants during hand-cleaning). The problem with most hand-hygiene models is their assumption of a linear relationship between hand-washing compliance and the reduction of the transmission coefficient, β - for which there is no evidence. If effectiveness is inversely proportional to compliance non linear effects are expected (Coen, 2007). *Isolation*, the removal of patients into secluded areas so as to prevent contacts with other patients, does not eliminate transmission completely (Forrester et al., 2007; Cepeda et al., 2005), and moving patients to isolation facilities comes with a risk of death on the ITU (section 4.2). Modelling isolation is achieved by adding isolated 'categories' of patients in the model structure (e.g. Cooper *et al.*, 1999). More difficult is to include the realism of true isolation which is the result of competition with a range of other priorities, such as privacy, dignity, avoiding disturbance from difficult patients, and infections caused by other organisms (Jeanes et al., 2011).

Other interventions are the control of hospital demography (closing wards to admissions; sending affected staff home; Section 5), environmental cleaning whose effectiveness is difficult to measure; surveillance and feedback, such as the health-care bundle audits and screening of patients on admission (Raboud et al., 2005; Hubben et al., 2011; section 4.1); antibiotic usage (section 4.3). The practice of training staff to minimize infection risk, such as in the safe taking of blood, the insertion of central lines and catheters, has never been modelled and requires the colonization vs. infection stratification (section 2.1). Rare are the models where several infection control method are compared simultaneously (Austin et al., 1999a; Raboud et al., 2005; Hubben et al., 2011).

2.9 Small population sizes and the role of chance

Even the largest hospitals are broken up into wards which are small enough to make chance events of significant importance. Observing zero cases in a particular month does not mean absence of transmission, and in doing surveillance it is necessary to gather infection data over a wide time period in order to obtain a reliable average incidence rate. For this reason *stochastic* models (which approximate the probability distribution of model behaviour) are preferable to *deterministic* models (which approximate average model behaviour). The advantage of stochastic models - also known as Markov Chain Monte Carlo (MCMC) models - is that they give an indication of the variability in the expected trends (Renshaw, 1991). This variability can be so significant that control measures expected to be successful on average can fail "catastrophically" as a result of chance alone (Cooper et al., 2004a). Their disadvantage is that when parameters are unknown, computer-intensive statistical methods are needed to obtain estimates (section 3). There are many examples of HAI stochastic models: MRSA (Cooper et al., 2004a; Raboud et al., 2005; Hubben et al., 2011), VRE (Austin et al., 1999a), influenza (Ong et al., 2008), Severe Acute Respiratory Syndrome ([SARS]; Fukutome et al., 2007) and norovirus (section 5).

2.10 The finance

Treating infections costs money, so that spending money to implement infection control can save money. Hence, it is important to show that infection control interventions are cost effective. Mathematical models can help provide estimates of the number of cases prevented, N, as a result of intervention. This was done for MRSA screening (Raboud et al., 2005; Hubben et al., 2011). If C_T is the cost of treating one infection, C_I the overall cost of intervention then the cost per case averted (or the 'average Cost Effectiveness Ratio' [aCER]), is C_I / N. The *net benefit* of an intervention is given by (N x C_T) - C_I. The aCER is an indication of the return to the health-care system for each £ spent. A positive net benefit indicates that the intervention will save money. It follows that it does not pay to prevent a rare infection (low N) unless treatment costs are sufficiently high (large C_T), and intervention costs, C_I, are low. Estimates of C_T for MRSA infections are $10,000-$16,000 (Raboud et al., 2005). In the mid 1990s Plowman et al. (1999) estimated C_Ts of £5397 (bloodstream infections), £2398 (lower respiratory tract infections), £1618 (SSIs), £1237 (UTIs) and £9152 (multiple infections). Lopman et al. (2004) estimate costs per norovirus inpatient bed-day of £145 (elderly care ward).

3. Dealing with unknown parameters

The design of a mathematical model should be informed by observation. There are numerous ways to achieve this. Some parameters can be 'fixed' by using estimates from direct measurement possibly from the literature (e.g. the mean duration of infection). WAIFW matrices were estimated from conversations (surrogates of infectious contacts) for varicella (Zagheni et al., 2008), and from direct observations of HCW and patients the wards (Ong et al., 2008). Overlapping stay on the same ward (available from hospital computer records) can be used as surrogate measures of exposure to HAI cases. Alternatively *sensitivity analysis* uses a range of plausible values and the outcomes compared. Examples are screening costs (Hubben et al., 2011), contact rates (Beggs et al., 2008), days from detection of the index case to isolation of SARS cases (Fukutome et al., 2007).

Another approach is to identify the range of parameter values that minimize the discrepancy between model and data. This is usually done via numerical minimization algorithms such as Powell's direction set methods (Press et al., 1994; Chapter 10). *Maximum likelihood* uses the probability of observing some body of data, **y**, when the model **θ** is 'true', and is usually presented as $l = p(\mathbf{y} \mid \boldsymbol{\theta})$, where **y** are the data and **θ** the unknown model parameters (Edwards, 1972). Confidence intervals may be achieved by means of profile likelihood methods (Aitkin, 1998; Press et al., 1994; Chapter 15). This was applied to time-series data of the inpatient 'admission experience' (dates of admission and discharge, swab test dates and results, dates of isolation). The unknown part of the model was kept to a minimum (e.g. transmission coefficients and dates of acquisition of carriage) (Pelupessy et al., 2002; Cooper & Lipsitch, 2004; Bootsma et al., 2007). Cooper and Lipsitch (2004) applied a hidden MCMC model to time-series of MRSA, VRE and resistant Gram-negative rods (R-GNR) clinical infection in order to estimate parameters such as the patient-patient transmission coefficient (β) and the probability of colonization on admission (υ). A 'hidden' MCMC model (based on β and υ) described colonization and a Poisson process of rate λ described infection rates per carrier. Their model gave superior fits to HAI data compared with quality control processes based on the Poisson distribution (Grigg et al., 2003). The latter are nevertheless useful to the local ward manager as null models, the lack of fit indicating the existence of infectious spread (and infection control breakdown), than the estimate of transmission parameters whose confidence intervals may be wide.

Bayesian methods have been applied to iterative MCMC models (Forrester et al., 2007; Kypraios et al., 2010). These are based on sampling algorithms known as the *Gibbs' sampler* and *Hastings-Metropolis*, which are based on Bayes' Theorem (Carlin & Louis, 2000). This states that the probability of the model is proportional to the likelihood multiplied by the 'prior' probability of the model, $\pi(\boldsymbol{\theta})$, or

$$p(\theta \mid y) = p(y \mid \theta) \cdot \pi(\theta) \cdot \frac{1}{D} \quad (1)$$

where D is the marginal probability of the data, across all possible models: $D = \int p(y \mid \theta)\pi(\theta)d\theta$. The probability density function $p(\theta \mid y)$ is the 'posterior' density of the unknowns. It is the weighted average of the 'prior' probability and the weights are the likelihoods. When prior knowledge is unavailable, $\pi(\boldsymbol{\theta})$ is set equal for the entire parameter space **θ** (a 'non-informative' prior).

When D is known the posterior probability density is said to be available in 'closed form' and the Gibbs sampler makes use of standard density functions (e.g. Gamma, Beta etc.) where the same algebraic form exists for the prior, the likelihood and the posterior. An example is the Beta distribution for proportion data y/n, used by Forrester et al. (2007) to estimate MRSA test sensitivity. The Gamma distribution is used for count data, the Inverse Gamma for variances (Carlin & Louis, 2000).

For more complex models D may be impossible to compute, and the Hastings-Metropolis approach can be used instead (Metropolis et al., 1953). A likelihood function is considered for each unknown parameter in turn, conditional on the data and the other unknown parameters. This is equivalent to the full likelihood with all other unknown parameters fixed, e.g. $p(y,\theta_1 \mid \theta_2, \theta_3)$. The algorithm works by iteratively sampling a 'candidate' parameter value, say θ_1^*, from a 'proposal distribution' which may be the prior density function, $\pi(\theta)$, or a multivariate normal density with means $\mu = (\theta_1, \theta_2, \theta_3)$ and some variance-covariance matrix Σ (Carlin & Louis, 2000). The candidate density is then accepted with probability r where

$$r = \min\left[\frac{p(y,\theta_1^* \mid \theta_2,\theta_3).p(\theta^*)}{p(y,\theta_1 \mid \theta_2,\theta_3).p(\theta)},1\right] \qquad (2)$$

The list of accepted parameter values makes up the Markov chain. No matter what starting values for $\boldsymbol{\theta}$, the chain converges to the posterior distribution. When discarding the first 500 iterates or so we obtain an 'ergodic' chain whose distribution can be used to measure confidence intervals for the estimates.

Forrester et al. (2007) applied a mixture of MCMC approaches to MRSA carriage data from a patient cohort admitted to a 12-bed ITU with 2 isolation rooms. Their parameter space, $\boldsymbol{\theta} = (\beta_0, \beta_1, \beta_2, \varphi, \rho)$ is represented by a background infection rate (β_0) and transmission coefficients β_1 (from other patients) and β_2 (from patients in isolation rooms), as well as the probability of colonization on admission to the ITU (φ) the sensitivity of the MRSA screening test (ρ), the time of MRSA colonization, c_i, for patient i. The data were dates of admission (a_i), first positive swab (v_i), isolation (q_i) and discharge (r_i). For a discussion of results see Section 4. Similar approaches have been used for *Stapylococcus aureus* (McBryde et al., 2007), VRE (Cooper et al., 2008) and swine flu (Hohle et al., 2005).

There is a philosophical problem with more realistic (and complex) models. The model may never fit the precise circumstances of the data, and estimated parameters may not be truly representative of the target situation. This is the case of norovirus outbreaks (section 5), with rare epidemics involving small numbers of cases, each on different wards with their own idiosyncratic sets of infection control approaches and patient management. Even when epidemic data are available for such a specific settings it is by no means certain that they are representative of a common 'true' underlying model. A pragmatic approach is to illustrate a point by using a set of parameter values vaguely consistent with observation.

4. Some conclusions from the literature

4.1 Screening and surveillance

The advantage of screening is three-fold: 1) detection protects the positive case when measures are taken to clear carriage; 2) isolation of positives prevents transmission to other inpatients; 3) removal of carriage from the community means less imported cases in future re-admissions. Bootsma et al. (2006) used a stochastic model to compare six infection control components that are part of what is known as the "search and destroy" approach, including the passive treatment and isolation of known MRSA carriers, the screening of all patients and health-care staff in affected wards, and the eradication of colonization at discharge. They find that treatment of known carriers and screening of contact patients can bring down prevalence from 15% and maintain low endemicity (<1%), but additional screening (such as of staff in affected wards) does not offer additional benefit.

The paradox is that when HAI screening is successful it becomes less cost effective (Raboud et al., 2005; Hubben et al., 2011). Raboud et al. modelled a Canadian hospital ward with 1.3% MRSA prevalence and showed that culture-based MRSA screening is cost-effective so long as there is at least 1 case for every 2 to 3 years, but MRSA infection is too infrequent to justify a more expensive molecular test. Hubben et al. compared two settings: high prevalence (15%) vs. medium prevalence (5%) of MRSA carriage. The molecular test was more cost effective at high prevalence, whereas the culture based chromatogenic test was more cost effective at medium prevalence, in spite of the advantages of molecular tests (high sensitivity, result in hours).

Robotham et al. (2007) use a stochastic model and find random screening (at rate φ per patient per day) more effective at detecting MRSA carriers than screening a proportion ω of all admissions. While this is a more realistic model as it assumes limited isolation capacity (20 rooms), the bizarre result is more likely the result of the unrealistic assumption of a homogeneous inpatient population and randomly distributed MRSA carriers within it. Their baseline 40% prevalence is an extreme exaggeration (5 to 10% would be more likely) and the assumption of no infection control other than isolation is unrealistic. Ultimately admission screening is reputed successful, partly because it targets prevalence in the fraction of the catchment population re-admission risk and partly because it targets patients in ITU, an important reservoir "for generating and then seeding the rest of the hospital with MRSA-colonized patients" (Edgeworth, 2011).

4.2 Isolation

The practice of isolation originates at least from the 1600s, when those affected by the plague were isolated in secluded buildings (Cipolla, 1973). The evidence in favour of isolation on the hospital ward may depend on the type of ward. Cooper et al. (2003, 2004b) carried out a Cochrane review and identified 46 studies that addressed the issue. Not one study was fully clear of methodological shortcomings. The authors subsequently designed and carried out a new study to address such study design problems (Cepeda *et al.,* 2005). They chose ITU inpatients, a study population with special issues around the act of switching off life support machinery in order to move patients to isolation facilities and measured acquisition of MRSA carriage and infection over a period of 12 months as outcome. They applied a quasi-experimental cross-over design comparing isolation with no isolation, and controlled for numerous potential confounders such as nursing hours per patient, severity of underlying disease and antibiotic usage. No beneficial effect of isolation was detected (multivariate relative risk of infection for non-isolation: 0.73, 95% confidence intervals: 0.49-1.10). Unfortunately their design lacked adequate temporal controls leaving conclusions open to uncertainty. Hand-hygiene compliance in staff was also low (21%) and isolation was not expected to work anyway (Huskins & Goldmann, 2005).

By contrast, Cooper et al. (2004a) used a stochastic model of MRSA in a homogeneous 1000 bed-hospital and showed that 20-bed isolation units are successful in controlling and eradicating MRSA from hospital inpatients, so long as $R_0 < 1.3$, although this can take as much as 15 years to achieve. This is consistent with "search and destroy" being effective only in low-prevalence situations such as in Denmark and the Netherlands (Wertheim et al., 2004). In high endemic countries (e.g. USA and UK), isolation alone is not sufficient, especially if isolation is not 100% efficient. Forrester et al. (2007), estimate non-zero transmission rates from isolated inpatients (β_2=0.0045), although smaller than for non-isolated patients (β_1 = 0.0131).

4.3 Antimicrobial resistance

Early models of antibiotic resistance were deterministic and concerned large host populations (Levin, 2002). Austin *et al.* (1999b) modelled bacterial carriage, where individuals may be colonized with one of two possible variants (one susceptible and one resistant to antibiotics) and may or not be treated with antibiotics. The absence of a co-carrier state means the two variants compete for colonization space. In the absence of antibiotics the sensitive variant has a selective advantage (greater transmission coefficient). They fitted the model to β-lactam resistance in *Moraxella catarrhalis* from Finland (where cephalosporin usage increased), and to penicillin-resistance in pneumococci from Iceland (where antibiotic usage declined) and found that significant reductions in resistance require equally significant reductions in drug consumption.

Lipsitch et al. (2000) used a similar deterministic model for antibiotic resistance in the hospital, with the addition of categories of 'history of past usage'. They found that when reductions in antibiotic usage are implemented, the response is rapid—weeks to months—the dynamics being driven by replacement of resistant variants by sensitive admissions. Unfortunately this prediction is not always consistent with observation (Enne et al., 2001; Sundqvist et al., 2010; Cook et al., 2004), possibly due to compensatory mutations that counter genetic costs of resistance (Wijngaarden et al., 2004; Besier et al., 2005) or because resistance to one antibiotic is genetically linked to resistance to other antibiotics that are still in use (Enne et al., 2004; Fraser et al., 2005). The expectation of a 'rapid' response may also be explained by the implicit assumption of 100% competition for 'susceptible space' between variants. The inclusion of a co-carrier state in the model would allow for milder forms of competition, and slower responses to changes in antibiotic usage.

Similar work focused on optimal empirical treatment strategy, when sensitivity knowledge is absent or delayed. Haber et al. (2010) used a stochastic, model and concluded that antimicrobial resistance should drop within months (rather than years) when a switch to second-line drugs is made. Kouyos et al. (2011) modelled MRSA carriers and infections on a 20-bed ward assuming clinicians can choose between two broad spectrum antibiotics (A and B) while they wait for antibiotic sensitivity results from the laboratory (so that a narrow-spectrum drug can be given). They compared the performance of a number of empirical treatment strategies: mixing (simultaneous use of different drugs in different patients), cycling (sequential use of different drugs), and informed switching strategies (ISS) which can take many forms. Sensitivity analyses showed the optimal strategy to be ISS with deployment of drugs at frequencies inversely proportional to their respective resistance frequencies, especially if historical data are used (their ISS_7).

4.4 Barrier precautions and cohorting

Sebillé et al. (1997) used a deterministic model of *S aureus*, and showed that it takes >60% hand hygiene compliance to reduce prevalence from 30% to below 20%. Austin et al. (1999a) used a deterministic model of VRE where patients and staff infect each other by direct contact. They find the role of barrier precautions (gowns, gloves and hand-hygiene) and cohorting of major importance in controlling VRE infection. This is probably because they ignore the effect of environmental contamination on transmission, a choice based on pulse field gel electrophoresis of bacteria isolated from patients, HCWs and the environment

(Bonten et al., 1996). Raboud et al. (2005) used a similar model and made compliance dependent on the type of contact: with non-isolated patients (low-risk visits, 34% vs. high-risk visits, 74%), and isolated patients (low-risk visits, 75% vs. high-risk visits, 85%). They show that increasing hand-hygiene compliance by just 10% can result in a 50% reduction in the number of MRSA cases. Grundmann et al. (2002) applied the same model of Austin et al. to MRSA, and conclude that a 10% increase in hand-hygiene compliance might compensate the ill effects of staff shortage, though very difficult to achieve because above a certain level of compliance hand-hygiene gets in the way of life-saving action.

Beggs et al. (2008) use a modified version of an earlier model used by Cooper et al. (1999) where the patient-staff contact structure is explicitly modelled (as in Austin et al. 1999a), except that they distinguish between hand-hygiene *compliance* from hand-hygiene *efficacy*. They argue that a low hand-hygiene rate (20-40%) is enough to control *S aureus* infections, and additional improvements in compliance yield diminishing returns. Their deterministic model is however not ideal for a population of 20 inpatients and 3 staff members. The assumption of equal patient-staff and staff-patient contact rates is unrealistic (Ong et al., 2008). Beggs et al. (2009) reach similar conclusions with a stochastic approach. In each simulation the HCW makes 100 journeys from patient A (the source of MRSA) to patient B. MRSA is transmitted from A to HCW (with probability p′) and from HCW to patient B (with probability p). The integer of a normally distributed random number gives the number of hand hygiene events out of 100 journeys. Each batch of journeys is repeated 1000 times. Should transmission occur between A and B, the risk of infection is 1 if no hand hygiene event takes place, and $1-\lambda$ otherwise (λ is hand-hygiene efficacy). They use $p' = 0.4$ and $p = 0.1$ as estimated for VRE in the intensive care unit (Austin et al., 1999a), an odd choice given that it is meant for MRSA (supposedly 0.15 and 0.01 respectively; Grundmann et al., 2002). The hand-hygiene efficacy was either $\lambda = 0.58$ (antibacterial soap) or $\lambda = 0.83$ (alcohol-based solution). No indication is given as to how the standard deviations were chosen. They suggest that when hand hygiene compliance is low the alcohol-based solution confers little advantage. Their model seems unrealistic as infection is only allowed in one direction, there are only 4 patients at most, and the HCW is not allowed to infect multiple patients.

5. Norovirus on a UCLH elderly care ward

In January 2009 a 63-bed ward in a UCLH hospital had an outbreak of norovirus affecting 39 cases (only 19 of which were laboratory confirmed). The time-line of the outbreak is shown in Figure 2.

5.1 The model

In collaboration with the HPA work began to gather data to inform a MCMC model of norovirus spread among inpatients and staff on a ward stratified into bays. The idea was to build an outbreak simulator flexible enough to help members of the infection control office make decisions during an outbreak. On a day-to-day basis, they would alter the settings so as to match the ward 'state', as well as specifying the infection control strategy of interest. Figure 3 illustrates in more detail the spatial structure of the ward affected by the outbreak: 13 bays (3-4 beds each), and 7 isolation rooms. Users could then run batches of simulations and learn from the outcome.

Date	Day of outbreak	Bay: North Side							South Side									
		(1-4)	(5-8)	(9-12)IR	(14-18)	(19-22)	(23-26)	(27-31)	(32-36)	(37-40)	41IR	(42-45)	(46-49)	(50-51)IR	(52-55)	(56-59)	(60-63)	STAFF
30/12/2008	0							**1**										
31/12/2009	1						1											1
01/01/2009	2						2	**2**		1					1	**3**		
02/01/2009	3		1	**2**														
03/01/2009	4		**1**										1					
04/01/2009	5												**1**					
05/01/2009	6				**1**					2		3						1
06/01/2009	7					**1**												
07/01/2009	8												**1**	1				
08/01/2009	9					1	1									**2**		
09/01/2009	10																	
10/01/2009	11																	
11/01/2009	12																	
12/01/2009	13																**1**	
13/01/2009	14									**2**		1				1		
14/01/2009	15	1					1		1									
15/01/2009	16																	
16/01/2009	17																	
17/01/2009	18																	
18/01/2009	19		**1**															
19/01/2009	20									1								2
20/01/2009	21																	
21/01/2009	22																	
22/01/2009	23																	
23/01/2009	24																	
24/01/2009	25																	
25/01/2009	26																	
26/01/2009	27																	

Fig. 2. Time-line of UCLH outbreak. IR = isolation room, each column represents one bay (beds numbered in brackets); numbers are cases (laboratory confirmed if in a bold square). Bays were closed to admission (grey squares), turned into isolation wards (blue squares) and deep cleaned (black squares).

The model concerns the infectious status of individuals (inpatients and staff) and inpatients are mapped on beds nested within bays. Patient and HCW movements are implicitly modelled via transmission coefficients stratified so as to distinguish between contacts within a bay (β_0), across bays (β_1) and with HCWs (β_2). Transmission from isolation rooms is assumed nil. The β_s were chosen so as to match the known distribution of outbreak sizes, and attack rates in inpatients and staff from UK hospitals (Lopman et al., 2004; Harris et al., 2010), matching interquartile ranges for outbreak sizes (6 to 92 days) and attack rates (6% to 65% for inpatients and 18% to 43% for staff). Each Member of staff is assigned a selection of bays. Bed occupancy may be under 100% and discharged patients are immediately replaced with a new admission (not necessarily to the same bed as the dischargee). Cases may not be discharged until they have recovered. Staff members 'rotate' shifts of 5 working days each and 2 days leave in between. Diarrhoea caused by agents other than norovirus (e.g. antibiotics, other viruses) affects 5% of inpatients.

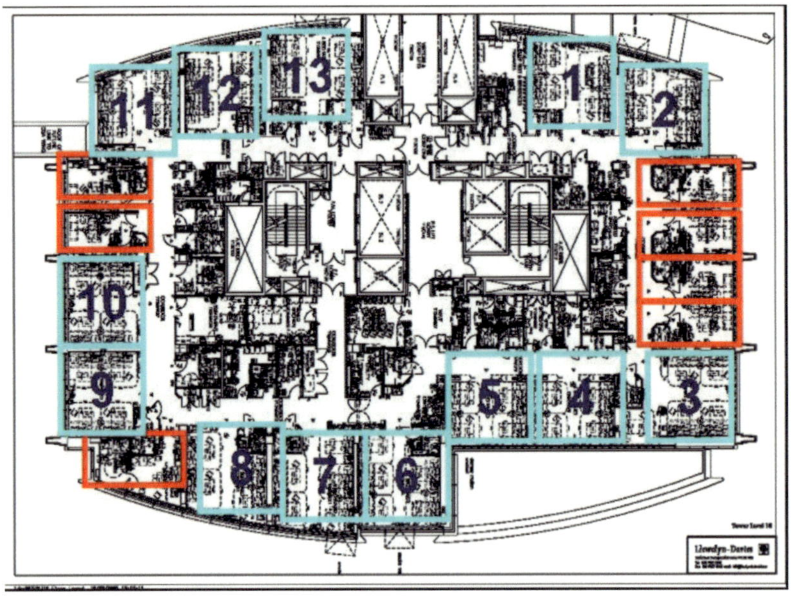

Fig. 3. Layout of the UCLH geriatric ward affected by the norovirus outbreak (blue squares indicate bays, and red rectangles are isolation rooms).

A 60 day simulation period is split into 'time steps' of width Δt (starting with Δt = 3 hours). For some events (acquisition of norovirus, detection of norovirus in the laboratory, acquisition and recovery of norovirus-unrelated diarrhoea) we used exponentially distributed waiting-time probability methods, equivalent to Poisson distributed numbers of events per time step (Ross, 2006). When the probability of two or more events per time step exceeded 0.01, we halved Δt. For other events, we sampled from exact distributions. Times to discharge are sampled from the observed distribution of length of stay on this ward for January 2008 (mean 7.2 days), in the absence of an outbreak. Times to onset of symptoms come from experimental studies on US convicts (mean 36 hours, Wyatt et al., 1974) and times to recovery come from observational work from the Avon region, UK (Lopman et al., 2004). Immunity to norovirus was initially set to 30% in patients and 60% in staff members.

Each simulation begins with the introduction of an infectious individual admitted to a random bed. Not all seeding events result in an outbreak. Most outcome measures (attack rates, outbreak durations, bed days lost to closing bays or wards to new admissions) are obtained from the subset of 200 simulations where an outbreak did take place. On acquisition individuals incubate norovirus, then become infectious and finally recover into the immune category. Two definitions of a norovirus 'case' were investigated: a) laboratory confirmed positives with 50% sensitivity (Vinjé et al., 2003; de Bruin et al., 2006) and a 1 day average delay to laboratory result, or b) acquisition symptoms (diarrhoea and/or vomiting).

Infection control measures take place 3 days after an outbreak is declared (two cases within seven days of each other) and include i) isolation of 'cases' into one of the isolation rooms, depending on availability (initially assumed fully occupied); ii) closure of affected bays to admissions until the last bay patient has recovered; iii) closure of the whole ward to readmission until the last case of the outbreak has recovered; iv) affected staff are sent home and may not return to work until 48 hours after recovery; v) restriction of patient-staff assortment (baseline: 6 staff members look after beds 1-31, the other 6 look after beds 32-63, as observed on the UCLH ward).

5.2 Results and discussion

The outcomes of three control strategies are shown in Fig. 4. In comparing strategies, medians are not as meaningful as ranges. Waiting for laboratory confirmation is equivalent to no control, because of the delay to the laboratory results, and low test sensitivity (half the cases missed). Acting on symptoms works best, except that in wards with non-specific symptoms it leads to unnecessary bay closures (Fig. 4b). Closing the ward leads to short term losses in patient-days, but control is swift and the outbreak is soon over, with little variability in outbreak sizes. These strategies are extremes and serve only for illustration. In real life managers are more likely to adopt mixed strategies: closing the ward for a few days using laboratory confirmation, and as cases become rare switching to closing only affected bays (Fig. 2). The model could be made more realistic, allowing for mixed strategies. Transmission could be made dependent on actual distance between bays. This may not be necessary when patients do not move (e.g. ITU) and when they move 'too much' (physical distance being no distance). Environmental contamination could be added, allowing

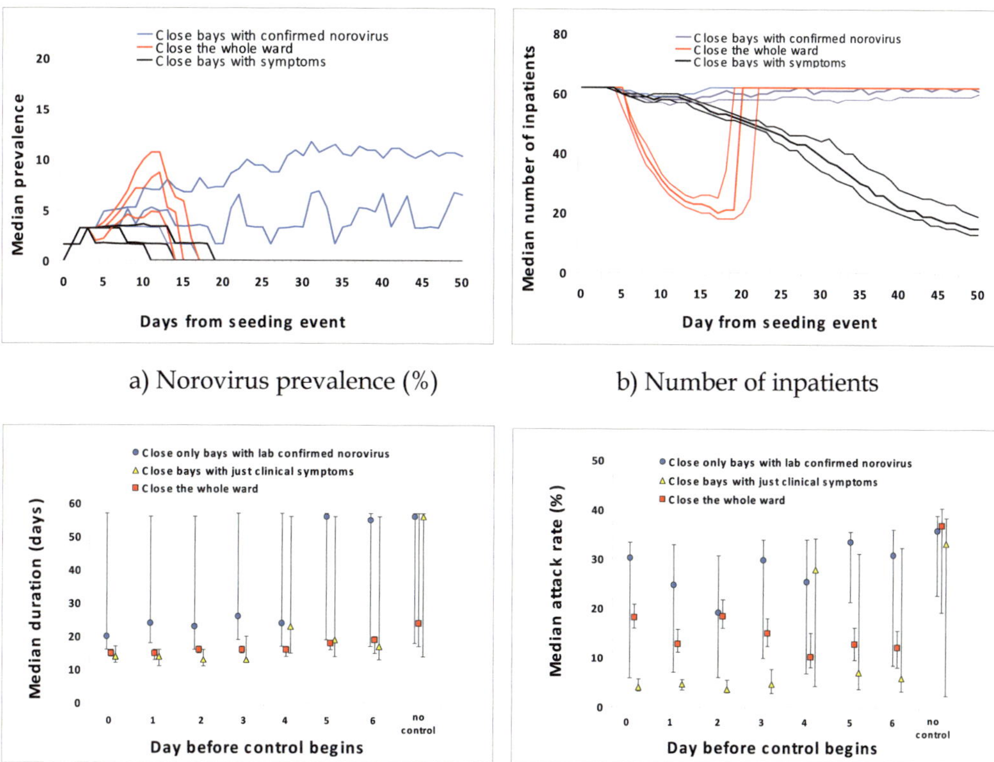

a) Norovirus prevalence (%) b) Number of inpatients

c) Outbreak duration (days) d) Attack rates (% patients)

Fig. 4. Output of the stochastic model. Lines and error bars represent the median, 10th and 90th centiles.

investigation of the impact of deep cleaning. Another aspect is building design. In our case we had an open ward where patients could infect other patients ($\beta_0 > \beta_1 > 0$). Some wards have physical barriers (rooms rather than bays), and HCWs become the main transmission vectors, allowing barrier precautions as well as relative cohorting to be much more effective.

6. Conclusions

The ideal HAI model is stochastic, simulates patient movement between wards of a set of hospitals, stratifies model parameters according to ward location (ITU, AAU, surgical, geriatric, infectious diseases wards etc.), stratifies the extramural population by re-admission rate, stratifies by different categories of HCW, accounts for surveillance and delays in diagnosis, includes antibiotic usage, contaminated environment, and allows for all possible forms of infection control. In reality this level of complexity is not necessary to address questions for a specific setting. Most HAI models deal with MRSA in ITU, a mere fraction of all HAIs. The main lesson is there is no universal answer. Success depends on local conditions (e.g. epidemic/endemic setting, patient mobility, aetiological agent, treatment and intervention costs).

7. Acknowledgments

Thanks to Annette Jeanes and the UCLH Infection Control team for their insights into the management of hospital outbreaks, to Ben Lopman for his support in model development, to David Ramlakhan for introducing me to the Perl programming language, assisting me in the implementation of its functionalities, the provision and management of SQL databases and for storing and accessing infection records.

8. References

Aitkin, M. (1998). Profile likelihood, In: *Encyclopedia of Biostatistics*, Armitage, P. & Colton, T., pp. 3534–3536, John Wiley & Sons, ISBN 0-471-97576-1, Chichester, United Kingdom

Anderson, R.M. & May, R.M. (1991). *Infectious Diseases of Humans, Dynamics and Control*, Oxford Science Publications, ISBN 0-19-854599-1, Oxford

Asoh, N.; Masaki, H.; Watanabe, H.; Watanabe, K.; Mitsusima, H.; Matsumoto, K.; Oishi, K. & Nagatake, T. (2005). Molecular characterization of the transmission between the colonization of methicillin-resistant *Staphylococcus aureus* to human and environmental contamination in geriatric long-term care wards. *Internal Medicine*, Vol. 44, No. 1, (January 2005), 41-5, ISSN 0918-2918

Austin, D.J. & Anderson, R.M. (1999). Transmission dynamics of epidemic methicillin-resistant *Staphylococcus aureus* and vancomycin-resistant enterococci in England and Wales. *Journal of Infectious Diseases*, Vol. 4, No. 4, (April 1999), pp. 883-91, ISSN 0022-1899

Austin, D.J.; Bonten, M.J.; Weinstein, R.A.; Slaughter, S. & Anderson, R.M. (1999a). Vancomycin-resistant enterococci in intensive-care hospital settings: transmission dynamics, persistence, and the impact of infection control programs. *Proceedings of the National Academy of Sciences, U S A*, Vol. 96, No. 12 (June 1999), pp. 6908-13 ISSN 0027-8424

Austin, D.J.; Kristinsson, K.G. & Anderson, R.M. (1999b). The relationship between the volume of antimicrobial consumption in human communities and the frequency of resistance. *Proceedings of the National Academy of Sciences, U S A*, Vol. 96, No. 3, (February 1999), pp. 1152-6, ISSN 0027-8424

Aziz, R.K. & Kotb, M. (2008). Rise and persistence of global M1T1 clone of *Streptococcus pyogenes*. *Emerging Infectious Diseases*, Vol. 14, No. 10, (October 2008), pp. 1511-7, ISSN 1080-6059

Bailey, N.T.J. (1975). *The Mathematical Theory of Infectious Diseases and its Application*, Griffin, ISBN 978-0195205640, London

Beggs, C.B.; Shepherd, S.J. & Kerr, K.G. (2008). Increasing the frequency of hand washing by healthcare workers does not lead to commensurate reductions in staphylococcal infection in a hospital ward. *BMC Infectious Diseases*, Vol. 8, No. 114, (September 2008), pp. 1-11, ISSN 1471-2334

Beggs, C.B.; Shepherd, S.J. & Kerr, K.G. (2009). How does healthcare worker hand hygiene behaviour impact upon the transmission of MRSA between patients? An analysis using a Monte Carlo model. *BMC Infectious Diseases*, Vol. 9, No. 64, (May 2009), pp. 1-9, ISSN 1471-2334

Beggs, C.B.; Shepherd, S.J. & Kerr, K.G. (2010).Potential for airborne transmission of infection in the waiting areas of healthcare premises: stochastic analysis using a Monte Carlo model BMC Infectious Diseases, Vol. 10, (August 2010), pp. 1-8, ISSN 1471-2334

Besier, S.; Ludwig, A.; Brade, V. & Wichelhaus, T.A. (2005). Compensatory adaptation to the loss of biological fitness associated with acquisition of fusidic acid resistance in *Staphylococcus aureus*. *Antimicrobial Agents and Chemotherapy*, Vol. 49, No. 4, (April 2005), pp. 1426-31, ISSN 0066-4804

Bode, L.G.; Wertheim, H.F.; Kluytmans, J.A.; Bogaers-Hofman, D.; Vandenbroucke-Grauls, C.M.; Roosendaal, R.; Troelstra, A.; Box, A.T; Voss, A.; van Belkum, A.; Verbrugh. H.A. & Vos, M.C. (2011). Journal of Hospital Infectinon, Vol. 2011 Jul 13. [Epub ahead of print] Sustained low prevalence of meticillin-resistant Staphylococcus aureus upon admission to hospital in The Netherlands.

Bonten, M.J.; Hayden, M.K.; Nathan, C.; van Voorhis, J.; Matushek, M.; Slaughter, S.; Rice, T. & Weinstein, R.A. Epidemiology of colonisation of patients and environment with vancomycin-resistant enterococci. *Lancet*, Vol. 348, No. 9042, (December 1996), pp. 1615-9, ISSN 0140-6736

Bonten, M.J.; Austin, D.J. & Lipsitch, M. (2001). Understanding the spread of antibiotic resistant pathogens in hospitals: mathematical models as tools for control. *Clinical Infectious Diseases*, Vol. 33, No. 10, (November 2001), pp. 1739-46 ISSN 1058-4838

Bootsma, M.C.; Diekmann, O. & Bonten, M.J. (2006). Controlling methicillin-resistant *Staphylococcus aureus*: quantifying the effects of interventions and rapid diagnostic testing. *Proceedings of the National Academy of Sciences, USA*, Vol.103, No. 14, (April 2006), pp. 5620-5, ISSN 0027-8424

Bootsma, M.C.; Bonten, M.J.; Nijssen, S.; Fluit, A.C. & Diekmann, O. (2007). An algorithm to estimate the importance of bacterial acquisition routes in hospital settings.

American Journal of Epidemiology, Vol. 166, No. 7, (October 2007), pp. 841-51, ISSN 0002-9262

Bryan, C.S. & Reynolds, K.L. (1984). Hospital-acquired bacteremic urinary tract infection: epidemiology and outcome. *Journal of Urology*, Vol. 132, No. 3, (September 1984), pp. 494-8, ISSN 0022-5347

Carlin, B.P. & Louis, T.A. (2000). *Bayes and Empirical Bayes Methods for Data Analysis* (second edition), Chapman & Hall/CRC, ISBN 1-58488-170-4, Florida, USA

Cepeda, J.A.; Whitehouse, T; Cooper, B.; Hails, J.; Jones, K.; Kwaku, F.; Taylor, L.; Hayman, S.; Cookson, B.; Shaw, S.; Kibbler, C.; Singer, M.; Bellingan, G. & Wilson, A.P. (2005). Isolation of patients in single rooms or cohorts to reduce spread of MRSA in intensive-care units: prospective two-centre study. *Lancet*, Vol. 365, No. 9456, (January 2005), pp. 295-304, ISSN 1474-547X

Cipolla, C.M. (1973). *Cristofano and the Plague. The Study of the History of Public Health in the Age of Galileo*, Collins, ISBN 0002111918, London

Coello, R.; Glynn, J.R.; Gaspar, C.; Picazo, J.J. & Fereres, J. (1997). Risk factors for developing clinical infection with methicillin-resistant Staphylococcus aureus (MRSA) amongst hospital patients initially only colonized with MRSA. *Journal of Hospital Infection*, Vol. 37, No. 1, (September 1997), pp. 39-46, ISSN 0195-6701

Coen, P.G. (2007). How mathematical models have helped to improve understanding the epidemiology of infection. *Early Human Development*, Vol. 83, No. 3, (February 2007), pp. 141-8, ISSN 0378-3782

Cook, P.P.; Catrou, P.G.; Christie, J.D.; Young, P.D. & Polk, R.E. (2004). Reduction in broad-spectrum antimicrobial use associated with no improvement in hospital antibiogram. *Journal of Antimicrobial Chemotherapy*, Vol. 53, No. 5, (May 2004), pp. 853-9, ISSN 0305-7453

Cooper, B.S.; Medley, G.F. & Scott, G.M. (1999). Preliminary analysis of the transmission dynamics of nosocomial infections: stochastic and management effects. *Journal of Hospital Infection*, Vol. 43, No. 2, (October 1999), pp. 131-47, ISSN 0195-6701

Cooper, B. & Lipsitch, M. (2004). The analysis of hospital infection data using hidden Markov models. *Biostatistics*, Vol. 5, No. 2, (April 2004), pp. 223-37, ISSN 1465-4644

Cooper, B.S.; Stone, S.P.; Kibbler, C.C.; Cookson, B.D.; Roberts, J.A.; Medley, G.F. *et al.* (2003). Systematic review of isolation policies in the hospital management of methicillin-resistant *Staphylococcus aureus*: a review of the literature with epidemiological and economic modelling. *Health Technology Assessment*, Vol. 7, No. 39, (December 2003), ISSN 1366-5278

Cooper, B.S.; Medley, G.F.; Stone, S.P.; Kibbler, C.C.; Cookson, B.D.; Roberts, J.A.; Duckworth, G.; Lai, R. & Ebrahim, S. (2004a). Methicillin-resistant *Staphylococcus aureus* in hospitals and the community: stealth dynamics and control catastrophes. *Proceedings of the National Academy of Sciences, USA*, Vol. 101, No. 27, (July 2004), pp. 10223-8, ISSN 0027-8424

Cooper, B.S.; Stone, S.P.; Kibbler, C.C.; Cookson, B.D.; Roberts, J.A.; Medley, G.F.; Duckworth, G.; Lai, R. & Ebrahim, S. (2004b) Isolation measures in the hospital management of methicillin resistant *Staphylococcus aureus* (MRSA): systematic review of the literature. *British Medical Journal*, Vol. 329, No. 7465, (September 2004), pp. 1-8, ISSN 1468-5833

Cooper, B.S.; Medley, G.F.; Bradley, S.J. & Scott, G.M. (2008). An augmented data method for the analysis of nosocomial infection data. *American Journal of Epidemiology*, Vol. 168, No. 5, (September 2008), pp. 548-57, ISSN 1476-6256

Cooper, B. & Lipsitch, M. (2004). The analysis of hospital infection data using hidden Markov models. *Biostatistics*, Vol. 5, No. 2, (April 2004), pp. 223-37, ISSN 1465-4644

Cullik, A.; Pfeifer, Y.; Prager, R.; von Baum, H. & Witte, W. A novel IS26 structure surrounds blaCTX-M genes in different plasmids from German clinical *Escherichia coli* isolates. *Journal of Medical Microbiology*, Vol. 59, No. 5, (May 2010), pp. 580-7, ISSN 1473-5644

David, M.Z. & Daum, R.S. (2010). Community-associated methicillin-resistant *Staphylococcus aureus*: epidemiology and clinical consequences of an emerging epidemic. *Clinical Microbiology Reviews*, Vol. 23, No. 3, (July 2010), pp. 616-87, ISSN 1098-6618

Dall'Antonia, M.; Coen, P.G.; Wilks, M.; Whiley, A. & Millar, M. (2005). Competition between methicillin-sensitive and -resistant Staphylococcus aureus in the anterior nares. *Journal of Hospital Infection*, Vol. 61, No. 1, (September 2005), pp. 62-7, ISSN 0195-6701

de Bruin, E.; Duizer, E.; Vennema, H. & Koopmans, M.P. (2006). Diagnosis of Norovirus outbreaks by commercial ELISA or RT-PCR. *Journal of Virological Methods*, Vol. 137, No. 2, (November 2006), pp. 259-64, ISSN 0166-0934

Edgeworth, J.D. (2010). Has decolonization played a central role in the decline in UK methicillin-resistant *Staphylococcus aureus* transmission? A focus on evidence from intensive care. *Journal of Antimicrobial Chemotherapy*, Vol. 66, Suppl. 2, (April 2010), pp. ii41-ii47, ISSN 1460-2091

Edwards, A.W.F. (1972). *Likelihood*. Cambridge University Press, Cambridge, ISBN 0-521-31871-8, Cambridge

Enne, V.I.; Livermore, D.M.; Stephens, P. & Hall, L.M. (2001). Persistence of sulphonamide resistance in *Escherichia coli* in the UK despite national prescribing restriction. *Lancet*, Vol. 357, No. 9265, (April 2001), pp. 1325-8, ISSN 0140-6736

Enne, V.I.; Bennett, P.M.; Livermore, D.M. & Hall, L.M. (2004). Enhancement of host fitness by the sul2-coding plasmid p9123 in the absence of selective pressure. *Journal of Antimicrobial Chemotherapy*, Vol. 53, No. 6, (April 2004), pp. 958-63, ISSN 0305-7453

Feil, E.J.; Cooper, J.E.; Grundmann, H.; Robinson, D.A.; Enright, M.C.; Berendt, T.; Peacock, S.J.; Smith, J.M.; Murphy, M.; Spratt, B.G.; Moore, C.E & Day, N.P. (2003). How clonal is *Staphylococcus aureus*? *Journal of Bacteriology*, Vol. 185, No. 11, (June 2003), pp. 3307-16, ISSN 0021-9193

Fraser, C.; Hanage, W.P. & Spratt, B.G. (2005). Neutral microepidemic evolution of bacterial pathogens. *Proceedings of the National Academy of Sciences, USA*, Vol. 102, No. 6, (February 2005), pp. 1968-73, ISSN 0027-8424

Fukutome, A.; Watashi, K.; Kawakami, N. & Ishikawa, H. (2007). Mathematical modeling of severe acute respiratory syndrome nosocomial transmission in Japan: the dynamics of incident cases and prevalent cases. *Microbiology and Immunology*, Vol. 51, No. 9, (June 2007), pp. 823-32, ISSN 0385-5600

Forrester, M.L.; Pettitt, A.N. & Gibson, G.J. (2007). Bayesian inference of hospital-acquired infectious diseases and control measures given imperfect surveillance data. *Biostatistics*, Vol. 8, No. 2, (April 2007), pp. 383-401, ISSN 1465-4644

Griffiths, D.; Fawley, W.; Kachrimanidou, M.; Bowden, R.; Crook, D.W.; Fung, R.; Golubchik. T.; Harding, R.M.; Jeffery, K.J.; Jolley, K.A.; Kirton, R.; Peto, T.E.; Rees, G.; Stoesser, N.; Vaughan, A.; Walker, A.S.; Young, B.C.; Wilcox, M. & Dingle, K.E. Multilocus sequence typing of *Clostridium difficile*. *Journal of Clinical Microbiology*, Vol. 48, No. 3, (March 2010), pp. 770-8, ISSN 0095-1137

Grigg, O.A.; Farewell, V.T. & Spiegelhalter, D.J. (2003). Use of risk-adjusted CUSUM and RSPRT charts for monitoring in medical contexts. *Statistical Methods in Medical Research*, Vol. 12, No. 2, (March 2003), pp. 147-70, ISSN 0962-2802

Grundmann, H.; Hori, S.; Winter, B.; Tami, A. & Austin, D.J. (2002). Risk factors for the transmission of methicillin-resistant *Staphylococcus aureus* in an adult intensive care unit: fitting a model to the data. *Journal of Infectious Diseases*, Vol. 185, No. 4, (February 2001), pp. 481-8, ISSN 0022-1899

Grundmann, H.; Livermore, D.M.; Giske, C.G.; Canton, R.; Rossolini, G.M.; Campos, J.; Vatopoulos, A.; Gniadkowski, M.; Toth, A.; Pfeifer, Y.; Jarlier, V.; Carmeli, Y. & CNSE Working Group (2010). Carbapenem-non-susceptible Enterobacteriaceae in Europe: conclusions from a meeting of national experts. *Eurosurveillance*, Vol. 15, No. 46, (November 2010), pp. 1-13, ISSN 1560-7917

Haber, M.; Levin, B.R. & Kramarz, P. (2010). Antibiotic control of antibiotic resistance in hospitals: a simulation study. *BMC Infectious Diseases*, Vol. 10, (August 2010), pp. 1-10, ISSN 1471-2334

Hamilton, D.; Foster, A.; Ballantyne, L.; Kingsmore, P.; Bedwell, D.; Hall, T.J.; Hickok, S.S.; Jeanes, A.; Coen, P.G. & Gant, V.A. (2010). Performance of ultramicrofibre cleaning technology with or without addition of a novel copper-based biocide. *Journal of Hospital Infection*, Vol. 74, No. 1, (January 2010), pp. 62-71, ISSN 1532-2939

Harris, J.P.; Lopman, B.A. & O'Brien, S.J. (2010). Infection control measures for norovirus: a systematic review of outbreaks in semi-enclosed settings. *Journal of Hospital Infection*, Vol. 74, No. 1, (January 2010), pp. 1-9, ISSN 1532-2939

Health Protection Agency (2011a). *Protocol for the Surveillance of Surgical Site Infection*, Version 5, April 2011, Retrieved from <http://www.hpa.org.uk>

Health Protection Agency (2011b). *Clostridium difficile* Ribotyping Network (CDRN) for England and Northern Ireland, 2009/10 Report, Retrieved from <http://www.hpa.org.uk>

Health Protection Agency (2011c). PVL-Staphylococcal infections an update. *Health Protection Report*, Vol. 5, No. 7, Retrieved from <http://www.hpa.org.uk>

Höhle, M.; Jørgensen, E. & O'Neill, P.D. (2005). Inference in disease transmission experiments by using stochastic epidemic models. *Journal of the Royal Statistical Society: Series C (Applied Statistics)*, Vol. 54, No. 2, (January 2005), pp. 349-366, ISSN 1467-9876

Hospital Infection Society & Infection Control Nurses Association (2007). *The third prevalence survey of healthcare associated infection in acute hospitals, 2006. Preliminary results from England*, Retrieved from: <http://www.his.org.uk>

Hubben, G.; Bootsma, M.; Luteijn, M.; Glynn, D., Bishai, D.; Bonten, M. & Postma, M. (2011). Modelling the costs and effects of selective and universal hospital admission screening for methicillin-resistant *Staphylococcus aureus*. *PLoS One*, Vol. 6, No. 3, (March 2011), pp. 1-11, ISSN 1932-6203

Huskins, W.C. & Goldmann, D.A. (2005). Controlling meticillin-resistant *Staphylococcus aureus*, aka "Superbug". *Lancet*, Vol. 365, No. 9456, (January 2005), pp. 273-5, ISSN 1474-547X

Jeanes, A.; Macrae, B. & Ashby, J. (2011). Isolation prioritization tool: revision, adaptation and application. *British Journal of Nursing*, Vol. 20, No. 9, pp. 540-544, ISSN 0966-0461

Jernigan, J.A.; Titus, M.G.; Gröschel, D.H.; Getchell-White, S. & Farr, B.M. (1996). Effectiveness of contact isolation during a hospital outbreak of methicillin-resistant *Staphylococcus aureus*. *American Journal of Epidemiology*, Vol. 143, No. 5, (March 1996), pp. 496-504, ISSN 0002-9262

Johnson, S.; Clabots, C.R.; Linn, F.V.; Olson, M.M.; Peterson, L.R. & Gerding, D.N. (1990). Nosocomial *Clostridium difficile* colonisation and disease. *Lancet*, Vol. 336, No. 8707, (July 1990), pp. 97-100, ISSN 0140-6736

Kouyos, R.D.; Abel Zur Wiesch, P. & Bonhoeffer, S. (2011). Informed switching strongly decreases the prevalence of antibiotic resistance in hospital wards. *PLoS Computational Biology*, Vol. 7, No. 3, (March 2011), pp. 1-10, ISSN 1553-7358

Kypraios, T.; O'Neill, P.D.; Huang, S.S.; Rifas-Shiman, S.L. & Cooper, B.S. (2010). Assessing the role of undetected colonization and isolation precautions in reducing methicillin-resistant *Staphylococcus aureus* transmission in intensive care units. BMC Infectious Diseases, Vol. 10, No. 29, (February 2010), pp. 1-10, ISSN 1471-2334

La Force, F.M. (1987). The Control of Infections in Hospitals: 1750 to 1950, In: *Prevention and Control of Nosocomial Infections*, R.P. Wenzel (Ed.), pp.1-12, Williams & Wilkins, Baltimore, USA, ISBN 0-683-08923-4

Levin, B.R. (2002). Models for the spread of resistant pathogens. *Netherlands Journal of Medicine*, Vol. 60, No. 7, (August 2002), pp. 58-64, ISSN 0300-2977

Lipsitch, M.; Bergstrom, C.T. & Levin, B.R. (2000). The epidemiology of antibiotic resistance in hospitals: paradoxes and prescriptions. *Proceedings of the National Academy of Sciences, USA*, Vol. 97, No. 4, (February 2000), pp. 1938-43, ISSN 0027-8424

Livermore, D.M.; Winstanley, T.G. & Shannon, K.P. (2001). Interpretative reading: recognizing the unusual and inferring resistance mechanisms from resistance phenotypes. *Journal of Antimicrobial Chemotherapy*, Vol. 48, Suppl. 1, (July 2001), pp. 87-102, ISSN 0305-7453

Lopman, B.A.; Reacher, M.H.; Vipond, I.B.; Sarangi, J. & Brown, D.W. (2004). Clinical manifestation of norovirus gastroenteritis in health care settings. *Clinical Infectious Diseases*, Vol. 39, No. 3, (July 2004), pp. 318-324, ISSN 1537-6591

Lu, P.L.; Chin, L.C.; Peng, C.F.; Chiang, Y.H.; Chen, T.P.; Ma, L. & Siu, L.K. (2005). Risk factors and molecular analysis of community methicillin-resistant *Staphylococcus aureus* carriage. Journal of Clinical Microbiology, Vol. 43, No. 1, (January 2005), pp. 132-9, ISSN 0095-1137

McBryde, E.S.; Pettitt, A.N. & McElwain, D.L. (2007). A stochastic mathematical model of methicillin resistant *Staphylococcus aureus* transmission in an intensive care unit: predicting the impact of interventions. *Journal of Theoretical Biology*, Vol. 245, No. 3, (April 2007), pp. 470-81, ISSN 0022-5193

Metropolis, N.; Rosenbluth, A.W.; Rosenbluth, M.N.; Teller, A.H. & Teller, E. (1953). Equations of State Calculations by Fast Computing Machines. *Journal of Chemical Physics*, Vol. 21, No. 6, pp. 1087–1092, ISSN 0021 9606

Milkman, R. & Bridges, M.M. (1990). Molecular evolution of the *Escherichia coli* chromosome. III. Clonal frames. *Genetics*, Vol. 126, No. 3, (November 1990), pp. 505-17, ISSN 0016-6731

Oie, S.; Yanagi, C.; Matsui, H.; Nishida, T.; Tomita, M. & Kamiya, A. (2005). Contamination of environmental surfaces by Staphylococcus aureus in a dermatological ward and its preventive measures *Biological & pharmaceutical bulletin*, Vol. 28, No. 1, (January 2005), pp. 120-3, ISSN 0918-6158

Ong, B.S.; Chen, M.; Lee, V. & Tay, J.C. (2008). An individual-based model of influenza in nosocomial environments, In: *Proceedings of the 8th international conference on Computational Science, Part I*, pp. 590-599, Springer-Verlag, ISBN 978-3-540-69383-3, Berlin

Pelupessy, I.; Bonten, M.J. & Diekmann, O. (2002). How to assess the relative importance of different colonization routes of pathogens within hospital settings. *Proceedings of the National Academy of Sciences, USA*, Vol. 99, No. 8, (April 2002), pp. 5601-5, ISSN 0027-8424

Pelupessy I, Bonten MJ, Diekmann O. Phillips, G.; Tam, C.C.; Rodrigues, L.C. & Lopman, B. (2010). Prevalence and characteristics of asymptomatic norovirus infection in the community in England. *Epidemiology and Infection*, Vol. 138, No. 10, (October 2010), pp. 1454-8, ISSN 1469-4409

Pittet, D.; Mourouga, P. & Perneger, T.V. (1999). Compliance with handwashing in a teaching hospital. Infection Control Program. *Annals of Internal Medicine*, Vol. 130, No. 2, (January 1999), pp. 126-30, ISSN 0003-4819

Plowman, R.; Graves, N.; Griffin, M.; Roberts, J.A.; Swan, A.; Cookson, B. *et al.* (1999). The socio-economic burden of hospital acquired infection, In: Department of Health (date of access: 15th September 2011), Available from: http://www.doh.gov.uk.

Press, W.H.; Teukolsky, S.A.; Vetterling, W.T. & Flannery, B.P. (1994). *Numerical Recipes in Fortran, the Art of Scientific Computing* (second edition), Cambridge University Press, ISBN 0-521-43064-X

Raboud, J.; Saskin, R.; Simor, A.; Loeb, M.; Green, K.; Low, D.E. & McGeer, A. (2005). Modeling transmission of methicillin-resistant Staphylococcus aureus among patients admitted to a hospital. Infection Control Hospital Epidemiology, Vol. 26, No. 7, (July 2005), pp. 607-15, ISSN 0899-823X

Renshaw, E. (1991). *Modelling Biological Populations in Space and Time*, Cambridge University Press, ISBN 0-521-44855-7, Cambridge

Robotham, J.V., Jenkins, D.R. & Medley, G.F. (2007). Screening strategies in surveillance and control of methicillin-resistant *Staphylococcus aureus* (MRSA). *Epidemiology and Infection*, Vol. 135, No. 2, pp. 328-42, ISSN 0950-2688

Ross, S.M. (2006). *Simulation*, (4th edition), Academic Press, ISBN 0-12-598063-9

Scott, M.E & Smith, G. (1994). *Parasitic and Infectious Diseases, Epidemiology and Ecology*, Academic Press, ISBN 0-12-633325-4

Sébillé, V.; Chevret, S. & Valleron, A.J. (1997). Modeling the spread of resistant nosocomial pathogens in an intensive-care unit. *Infection Control and Hospital Epidemiology*, Vol. 18, No. 2, (February 1997), pp. 84-92, ISSN 0899-823X

Smith, J.M.; Smith, N.H.; O'Rourke, M. & Spratt, B.G. (1993). How clonal are bacteria? *Proceedings of the National Academy of Sciences, USA*, Vol. 90, No. 10, (May 1993), pp. 4384-8, ISSN 0027-8424

Smith, D.L.; Dushoff, J.; Perencevich, E.N.; Harris, A.D. & Levin, S.A. (2004). Persistent colonization and the spread of antibiotic resistance in nosocomial pathogens: resistance is a regional problem. *Proceedings of the National Academy of Sciences, USA*, Vol. 101, No. 10, (March 2004), pp. 3709-14, ISSN 0027-8424

Sneader, W. (2005). *Drug Discovery, a History*, Wiley, ISBN 0-471-89979-8

Stewart, G.P. & Holt, R.J. (1963). Evolution of natural resistance to the new penicillins. *British Medical Journal*, Vol. 1, No. 5326, pp. 308-11, ISSN 0007-1447

Sundqvist, M.; Geli, P.; Andersson, D.I.; Sjölund-Karlsson, M.; Runehagen, A.; Cars, H.; Abelson-Storby, K.; Cars, O. & Kahlmeter, G. *Journal of Antimicrobial Chemotherapy*, Vol. 65, No. 2, (February 2010), pp. 350-60, ISSN 1460-2091

van Schaik, W. & Willems, R.J. (2010). Genome-based insights into the evolution of enterococci. *Clinical Microbiology of Infection*, Vol. 16, No. =6, (June 2010), pp. 527-32, ISSN 1469-0691

Vinjé, J.; Vennema, H.; Maunula, L.; von Bonsdorff, C.H.; Hoehne, M.; Schreier, E.; Richards, A.; Green, J.; Brown, D.; Beard, S.S.; Monroe, S.S.; de Bruin, E.; Svensson, L. & Koopmans, M.P. (2003). International collaborative study to compare reverse transcriptase PCR assays for detection and genotyping of noroviruses. *Journal of Clinical Microbiology*, Vol. 41, No. 4, (April 2003), pp. 1423-33, ISSN 0095-1137

Warny, M.; Pepin, J.; Fang, A.; Killgore, G.; Thompson, A.; Brazier, J.; Frost, E. & McDonald, L.C. (2005). Toxin production by an emerging strain of *Clostridium difficile* associated with outbreaks of severe disease in North America and Europe. *Lancet*, Vol. 366, No. 9491, (September 2005), pp. 1079-84, ISSN 0140-6736

Wertheim, H.F.; Vos, M.C.; Boelens, H.A.; Voss, A.; Vandenbroucke-Grauls, C.M.; Meester, M.H.; Kluytmans, J.A.; van Keulen, P.H. & Verbrugh, H.A. (2004). Low prevalence of methicillin-resistant *Staphylococcus aureus* (MRSA) at hospital admission in the Netherlands: the value of search and destroy and restrictive antibiotic use. *Journal of Hospital Infection*, Vol. 56, No. 4, (April 2004), pp. 321-5, ISSN 0195-6701

Wijngaarden, P.J.; van den Bosch, F.; Jeger, M.J. & Hoekstra, R.F. (2005). Adaptation to the cost of resistance: a model of compensation, recombination, and selection in a haploid organism *Proceedings of the Royal Society, London (Biological Sciences)*, Vol. 272, No. 1558, (January 2005), pp. 85-9, ISSN 0962-8452

Wyatt, R.G.; Dolin, R.; Blacklow, N.R.; DuPont, H.L.; Buscho, R.F.; Thornhill, T.S.; Kapikian, A.Z. & Chanock, R.M. (1974). Comparison of three agents of acute infectious nonbacterial gastroenteritis by cross-challenge in volunteers. *Journal of Infectious Diseases*, Vol. 129, No. 6, (June 1974), pp. 709-14, ISSN 0022-1899

Zagheni, E.; Billari, F.C.; Manfredi, P.; Melegaro, A.; Mossong, J. & Edmunds, W.J. (2008). Using time-use data to parameterize models for the spread of close-contact infectious diseases. *American Journal of Epidemiology*, Vol. 168, No. 9, (November 2008), pp. 1082-90, ISSN 1476-6256

Zhao, F.; Bai, J.; Wu, J.; Liu, J.; Zhou, M.; Xia, S.; Wang, S.; Yao, X.; Yi, H.; Lin, M.; Gao, S.; Zhou, T.; Xu, Z.; Niu, Y. & Bao, Q. (2010). Sequencing and genetic variation of multidrug resistance plasmids in *Klebsiella pneumoniae*. *PLoS One*, Vol. 5, No. 4, (April 2010), pp. 1-9, ISSN 1932-6203

4

Infection Control in Developing World

Lul Raka and Gjyle Mulliqi-Osmani
Faculty of Medicine, University of Prishtina & National Institute of Public Health of Kosova, Prishtina
Kosova

1. Introduction

Infectious diseases are a global concern and the second commonest cause of death in the world. Of the annual 15 million deaths, 95% occur in the developing world, with predominance of acute respiratory infections, diarrhoeal diseases, measles, AIDS, malaria and tuberculosis (World Health Organization, 2008). More than 1 billion inhabitants in this part of the world do not have access to safe water and basic sanitation (Moe & Rheingans, 2006).

Health care-associated infections (HCAIs) constitute an important health challenge worldwide and pose a major threat to patient safety. Risks for acquiring infections during health care delivery have increased dramatically with advances in diagnostic and treatment procedures. In developing world this challenge is more highlighted because infection prevention and control policies are either nonexistent, poorly adapted or insufficiently funded by governments (Ponce-de-Leon & Macias, 2003). Therefore, infections are between 2-6 times higher than those in developed world.

Hospitals are main facilities for the risk of acquiring an infection during the delivery of care. Therefore infection control and prevention activities are focused mainly at the hospital level. The rates of HCAIs within a hospital represent the best indicator for the quality of services offered, where a high frequency of HCAIs is evidence of a poor quality of health service delivery. But, nowadays their occurrence is increasing in outpatient clinics and in nursing homes as well.

HCAIs impact on the population in many ways. They affect patients directly, causing increased morbidity and mortality; they may lead to disability and may reduce quality of life (Pittet et al., 2008). They also impact on the healthcare system by extending hospitalization of affected patients and driving up the costs of diagnosis and treatment. HCAIs may be transmitted from healthcare settings into the community. They also may be a subject of indictment by the treated patients in hospitals, decreasing the reputation of healthcare institutions in the eyes of the public.

The endemic burden of HCAIs is significantly higher in developing countries, in particular in patients admitted to intensive care units and in neonates (Raka, 2008). Most developing countries lack surveillance systems for HCAI. They usually have limited and low quality data (Allegranzi et al., 2011). In developing world there are many determinants, which are specific to settings with limited resources described below.

2. Challenges of infection control in developing countries

2.1 Health care and hospitals in developing world - Constraints and outcomes

2.1.1 Resources and incomes

Resources and incomes are unequally distributed throughout the world. Country economies are divided among income groups according to 2008 gross national income (GNI) per capita, calculated using the World Bank Atlas method. Countries with low income ($975 or less) and lower middle income ($976–3,855) are referred to as developing countries and they represent more than 75% of the world population. Prevention and control in low and middle income countries differs substantially from that in the developed world with high income. Limited resources represent the main challenge for governments in developing countries (Lynch et al., 2007). There may be a lack of commitment to healthcare by policy-makers in the developing world and allocation of funds is often disproportionate to the priorities set by providers. Priority in the allocation of funds is often directed to visible targets within society such as schools, infrastructure and security. Healthcare frequently is far behind. Even in countries where the healthcare budget is given high priority, the proportion devoted to prevention of HCAIs is usually insufficient.

2.1.2 Health care system and society

Health systems in developing countries are hospital-dominated, with 50-80% of resources allocated to hospitals in urban centres, which often have tertiary academic affiliations. On the other hand a large number of people present to the other regional hospitals, which have inadequate resources, staff training, and motivation with an impact on the health of millions of people (Duke et al., 2006).

Corruption and nonformal payments are frequent in developing countries. Inadequate salaries lower the healthcare workers' motivation for quality care. Information systems are not fully developed. There are limited grants available for research and no legislation mandating accreditation of hospitals and infection control programmes. In-service training for employees is highly variable and often minimal. Patients and their families may be required to provide care materials such as syringes, surgical gowns, and drugs. Frequent movement of patients and staff between hospitals wards results in an increased risk of transmission of multidrug-resistant microorganisms (Clements et al., 2008). Such transmission is often exacerbated by overcrowding, with patients sometimes sharing beds and supplies.

During the last few decades, infection control activities in developing countries have increased, particularly in South America, South East Europe and countries of the former Soviet Union (Morris, 2008). Public pressure to improve the quality of hospital care, the increased cost of HCAIs in healthcare systems, the emergence of multiresistant microorganisms, the approach of occupational hazards have played an important role in this development.

In many hospitals of developing countries adequate supplies to control and prevent infections are not available. Compliance with hand hygiene is often very low. Many other problems abound; for example, sterilisation departments are not centralised and there is lack of quality control in disinfection and sterilisation. Although many hospitals in the developing countries may have infection control programmes and committees on paper, in practice they barely exist. Inadequate numbers of trained personnel work in infection control, and face continual resistance from clinical staff. This litany of problems means that the response to common outbreaks of disease in high risk units by management and staff is mainly reactive rather than proactive. Lack of ongoing surveillance results in delays in detecting outbreaks, with increasing costs and mortality.

Baseline endemic infection rates are not established by the hospital authorities in vast majority of developing countries and usually there is no anticipation of the possible risks of acquiring a HCAI. Infection control does not exist as a medical or nursing speciality, and formal training programmes on infection control are not available in medical schools of developing world. In addition to mentioned constraints, frequent malnutrition and other types of infection and diseases contribute to increase the risk of HCAIs in developing countries. Poverty, war, economic and political disturbances all significantly increases HCAIs (Lynch et al., 2007). As a result of the weakness and problems outlined above, developing countries face the challenge of high rates of HCAIs and frequent outbreaks.

2.2 Blood and injection safety

Transfusion and injections may pose a risk for transmission of HIV and hepatitis in developing world. Between 5% and 10% of human immunodeficiency virus (HIV) infections worldwide are transmitted through transfusion of contaminated blood and blood products. Over 16 billion injections are administered each year in developing countries and the proportion of injections given by syringes and needles that are reused without sterilization ranges from 1.5 to 69.4% (Simonsen et al., 1999). Improper waste disposal is present in 18-64% of health care facilities of developing countries (World Health Organization, 2005). The 2000 Global Burden of Disease study, death and disability from injection-associated infections by hepatitis B virus (HBV), hepatitis C virus (HCV) and HIV revealed that patients received an average of 3.4 injections per year, 39.3% of which were given with reused equipment. Contaminated injections caused an estimated 21 million HBV infections, 2 million HCV infections and 260 000 HIV infections, accounting for 32%, 40% and 5%, respectively, of new infections (Hauri et al., 2004).

2.3 The burden and impact of health care-associated infections

HCAIs represent one of the commonest adverse event during delivery of health care, complicating 5-10% of admissions to acute care hospitals in industrialised countries. Pooled prevalence of HCAI in Europe is 7.1% with range 3.5- 11.3% (ECDC, 2008). More than 4 million patients are affected by HCAI every year in Europe and 1.7 million in USA. In developed countries, approximately 25-30% of patients admitted to Intensive Care Unit (ICU) are affected by HCAI. Urinary tract infections constitute a predominant portion of HCAIs with 30-40% of the overall infections.

In developing countries the global picture of the burden of HCAI is unknown due to lack of reliable data and the use of different definitions and methodologies. Many developing countries have not conducted any surveillance studies regarding HCAIs and few studies provide information on etiology and risk factors for HCAIs (Allegranzi et al., 2011). Only 23 developing countries of 147 (15.6%) reported a functioning HCAI national surveillance system in 2010. Hospital-wide prevalence of HCAI in developing countries varied from 5.7% to 19.1%. A review of several studies in developing world showed that increased length of stay associated with HCAI varied between 5 and 29.5 days.

Surgical site infection (SSI) is the most surveyed and most frequent type of infection in developing countries with incidence rates ranging from 1.2 to 23.6 per 100 surgical procedures and a pooled incidence of 11.8%. By contrast, SSI rates vary between 1.2% and 5.2% in developed countries (Allegranzi et al., 2011). Incidence of ICU-acquired infection is at least 2–3 fold higher than in high-income countries; device-associated infection densities up to 13 times higher than in the USA were reported in some studies.

Ventilator-associated pneumonia (VAP) is a leading cause of death in hospitalised patients. A meta-analysis of articles concerning VAP in developing countries in MEDLINE (January 1966 to April 2007) showed rates from 10 to 41.7 per 1000 ventilator-days; crude mortality ranged from 16% to 94% and with increased length of stay in intensive care (Arabi et al., 2008). VAP attributable costs was US$ 10 000–25 000 per case.

Many studies have shown the importance of HCAI among neonates in developing countries, where an average of 4384 children die every day of these infections (WHO, 2007). In a major review, reported rates of neonatal infections were 3-20 fold higher than those reported in industrialised countries (Zaidi et al., 2005). Neonatal infections are estimated to cause 1.6 million deaths annually, 40% of all neonatal deaths in developing countries (Lawn, 2004). From microbiological prospective of HCAI in developing world the most frequent microbial pathogens were *S. aureus* in mixed patient populations, and *Acinetobacter spp.* in high-risk patients.

The costs of HCAIs are substantial everywhere, although they varies between countries due to different health care systems. In countries with prospective payment systems based on diagnosis- related groups, hospitals lose from $583 to $4,886 for each HCAI. Annual economic impact of HCAIs in Europe is about 7 billion euro per year and 16 million extra-days of hospital stay(ECDC, 2008). In the USA, associated costs are approximately US$ 6.5 billion (Klevens et al., 2007). The cost to the government of Trinidad and Tobago for HCAIs was estimated at $697,000 annually. In Mexico, the annual cost approaches $1.5 billion; in Mexican ICUs, overall average cost of a HCAI episode was calculated at US$ 12 155 (Higuera et al., 2007). In Thailand 10% of the annual hospital budget is spent on HCAIs (WHO, 2005). Some investigators have attempted to measure costs related to hospital outbreaks of HCAIs caused by multiresistant organisms. In a study of infections caused by MRSA it was estimated that average cost was $4000 per infection, whereas costs of C. difficile-associated diarrhea was approximately $4500 per patient (Stone, 2009). In an university hospital in Malaysia the cost of antibiotics prescribed to treat HCAI was estimated at US$ 521 000 per year (Hughes et al., 2005).

2.4 Antimicrobial resistance

Resistance to antimicrobial agents is a global challenge in all healthcare facilities. In developing countries inappropriate and uncontrolled use of antibiotics is very common and antimicrobials are frequently available over the counter in pharmacies. In many developing countries resistance among common pathogens to cheap antimicrobials has already increased drastically, resulting in limited effectiveness. The quality and potency of antibiotics are often suspected, with unregulated import, registration and distribution. Another factor contributing to resistance is lack of antibiotic policies or basic recommendations at governmental level or within hospitals. Between 20% and 50% of a hospital budget is spent on antimicrobials, which are used to treat more than half of all patients. Even in developed countries >50% of antimicrobials are prescribed incorrectly, either administered in suboptimal doses or for incorrect duration (Wenzel, 2000). Misuse has been identified as an important factor in the emergence of antimicrobial resistance (Kollef, 2001). In turn, this resistance makes the clinical management of the patients more difficult.

The use of antimicrobials in the veterinary area had an important impact on increase of antimicrobial resistance. Other factors contributing to increase of antimicrobial resistance are: limited number of new classes of antibiotics in pipeline by pharmaceutical companies and globalization, which enabled the rapid spread of multiresistant microorganisms worldwide (Okeke, 2005).

	Pooled mean (range) (interquantile range, 25-75%)	**Pooled mean(range) (interquantile range, 25-75%)**
Antibiotic resistant pathogen	**INICC 2002-2007**	**US NNIS 1992-2004**
Methicillin-resistant Staphylococcus aureus (MRSA)	80.8 (50.0-100.0)	52.9 (32.7-603)
Methicillin-resistant coagulase-negative staphylococci	75.2 (64.0-100.0)	76.6 (69.4-83.8)
Vancomycin-resistant enterococcus species	9.4 (0.0-6.3)	13.9 (5-24.3)
Ciprofloxacin/ofloxacin-resistant Pseudomonas aeruginosa	52.4 (40.0-75.0)	34.8 (17.4-41.3)
Imipenem-resistant P aeruginosa	36.6 (0.0-52.4)	19.1 (8.3-25.5)
Ceftazidime-resistant P aeruginosa	51.7 (33.3-72.7)	13.9 (5-16.9)
Piperacillin-resistant P aeruginosa	50.8 (36.4-75.0)	17.50 (7.5-19.5)
Ceph3-resistant Enterobacter species	56.8 (30.8-80.0)	27.70 (17.4-36.4)
Carbapenem-resistant Enterobacter species	8.5 (0.0-0.0)	0.70 (0.0-0.0)
Ceph3-resistant Klebsiella pneumoniae	68.2 (33.3-85.7)	6.20 (0.0-8.0)
Ceph3-resistant Escherichia coli	53.9 (11.1-80.0)	1.3 (0.0-2.6)
Ciprofloxacin/ofloxacin-resistant E coli	42.6 (12.7-78.9)	7.30 (0.0-8.2)

Table 1. Comparison of antimicrobial resistance rates (%) in the ICUs of the International Nosocomial Infection Control Consortium (INICCC) and the U.S. National Nosocomial Surveillance System (NNIS) (Rosenthal et al., 2010).

Table 1 presents overview of antimicrobial reisistance rates in ICU between INICC and NNIS system. The frequencies of resistance of *Staphylococcus aureus* isolates to methicillin (MRSA) (80.8% vs 52.9%), Enterobacter species to ceftriaxone (50.8% vs 17.8%), and *Pseudomonas aeruginosa* to fluoroquinolones (52.4% vs 34.8%) were also far higher in the Consortium's ICUs.

2.5 Consequences

As a result of the weakness and problems outlined above, developing countries face the challenge of high rates of HCAI and frequent hospital outbreaks. Another consequence of insufficient infection control infrastructure is the spread of multidrug-resistant organisms, such are meticillin-resistant *Staphylococcus aureus* (MRSA), vancomycin-resistant *Enterococcus spp.* (VRE), extended-spectrum b-lactamase-producing Gram-negative bacilli, multidrug-resistant *Mycobacterium tuberculosis* and fluconazole-resistant *Candida spp.*

3. Solutions and perspectives for prevention and control

In order to improve the effectiveness of infection control in developing countries, a multifactorial initiatives needs to be implemented (Borg, 2010). Some of these initiatives are cheap and cost-effective, whereas others have a budget implications for governments.

3.1 Prevention comes first

Most countries address the problem of HCAI differently. As healthcare systems vary widely, so preventive strategies must be designed accordingly. The key component of solution is infection prevention. The prevention and control of HCAIs requires a triangle partnership between health care workers (HCW), government and community. Most HCAIs can be prevented with readily available and relatively inexpensive strategies. The Study on the Efficacy of Nosocomial Infection Control in 1974 showed that effective infection control programmes could reduce infection rates by as much as 32% and be cost-effective (Haley, 1980). In an overview of published reports on the effect of infection control programmes from 1990 to 2002, Harbarth et al. found that between 10% and 70% of HCAIs were preventable (Harbarth, 2003). In the Hospital Sao Paulo in Brazil, there was a 71% decline in all HCAIs in the ICU when an infection control programme was implemented, saving about US $2 million (Cavalcante, 2001). Many other successful strategies have been documented.

3.2 Political commitment and support

In developing countries, the risk of patients and HCWs acquiring HCAIs could be significantly reduced if governments make infection control a high priority. Administrative controls are amongst the most important steps in prevention and control of HCAIs. Therefore a political support and commitment is essential in effectiveness of all other measures. National authorities must understand that without the proper resources, hospitals can be high risk areas. Therefore health care authorities must establish and support a comprehensive, effective national programme. Such a programme should set national objectives, and develop strategies, guidelines and policies for specific infection control issues, which are regularly updated. Many countries already have such programmes. If these programmes are not available, those from the developed world should be adopted. Since developing countries have their own characteristic problems, these must be taken into account when formulating recommendations and policies (Raza et al.,2004). Due to their contact with patients or infected material from patients, many health care workers are at risk for exposure and possible transmission of infectious agents. Therefore occupational health and immunisation of HCWs is an essential part of prevention and infection control programmes (Randle, 2006). Moreover, education of HCWs and behavioural models complete the mosaic for prevention and control of HCAIs.

3.3 Hand hygiene

Hand hygiene remains the simplest and the primary measure to prevent HCAI and reduce spread of multidrug resistant organisms. Although hand hygiene is a simple measure, the lack of compliance among healthcare workers is problematic worldwide, averaging <40% (Boyce & Pittet 2002). In 2002, the CDC recommended the use of alcoholic hand rubs which have the advantage that they can be placed at the bedside (Hugonet et al., 2003). Also, where hand-washing facilities are primitive or scarce, it is often easier to provide a hand rub than sinks with running water and a functioning sewage system. Introduction of alcohol- based hand rub has led to increased hand hygiene compliance among healthcare workers and fewer HCAIs (Rosenthal et al., 2005). Today, many developing countries use WHO based formulation for alcoholic hand rub. In some developing countries, implementation of education, process surveillance, and performance feedback has considerably enhanced hand hygiene compliance (Damani, 2008).

3.4 Surveillance

Surveillance is an essential component in HCAIs prevention, with the aims of outbreak identification, establishment of endemic baseline rates of infection and the evaluation of control measures. Surveillance data can be used to identify preventable infections in high risk areas, so that resources are targeted to high priority areas. Surveillance of most important HCAIs should be accompanied by surveillance of antimicrobial use and resistance pattern. There is good evidence that antibiotic stewardship programmes have been successful in modifying antimicrobial prescribing practices, resulting in most instances in reduction of use (Gould, 1999). Unfortunately, such programmes are often lacking in developing countries, and antimicrobial resistance problems emphasise the importance of clinical microbiology laboratory services (Pfaller & Herwalt, 1997).

3.5 The bundle approach

In order to meet the required level of prevention, multiple strategies must be implemented simultaneously. Care bundles are part of a set of multiple intervention strategies to improve patient outcomes. They have been introduced in the USA by Institute for Healthcare Improvement and through the Saving Lives initiative produced by the UK Department of Health as hight impact interventions. Bundles are directed generally at aseptic procedures that carry a high risk of HCAI if not done properly (Westwell, 2008). These usually represent a set of three to five practices that, when performed collectively, reliably, and continuously have been proven to improve patient outcomes. Bundles also incorporate a simple audit tool to check that they are being implemented. The bundles are focused on the most important HCAIs: catheter-associated bloodstream infection, catheter-associated UTI, ventilator-associated pneumonia and SSI.

Bundled interventions using systems quality improvement approaches for improved infection control in developing countries face many obstacles. Limited resources, poor infrastructure, insufficient equipment, lack of national guidelines, policies and evidence are key difficulties in successful implementation of bundle approach.

3.6 Global initiatives: World alliance for patient safety

Improving the safety of patient care is now a global issue. A growing awareness of HCAIs and patient safety prompted the World Health Organization (WHO) to promote the creation of the World Alliance for Patient Safety to coordinate, spread and accelerate improvements in patient safety (Allegranzi et al., 2007). Prevention of HCAI is the target of the Alliance's First Global Patient Safety Challenge, 'Clean Care is Safer Care', launched in October 2005. Implementation strategies include the integration of multiple interventions in the areas of blood safety, injection safety, clinical procedure safety, and water, sanitation and waste management, with the promotion of hand hygiene in healthcare as the cornerstone. The main target of the campaign is 'Five Moments for Hand Hygiene' approach. It defines the key moments for hand hygiene with united vision. Various tools and resources have been developed to complement the Five Moments approach including localized country specific tool (Allegranzi & Pittet, 2009).

3.7 Research

One measure to improve the knowledge base of infection control is through research and development. Research resources for addressing infection control problems of developing countries remain disproportionately low compared with the disease burdens borne by these countries. National economies in developing countries remains too weak to support research and development. Research activities are sporadic and marginal, based mainly on individual initiatives in the university sector and with almost no support from governments. There is a need to focus these limited resources on research that will optimize health benefits with cost-effective interventions. Research priorities of developing countries in the field of HCAI are different compared to developed world. Research infrastructure should be focused on evaluating costs of HCAIs, risk factors for developing HCAI, hand hygiene, gather surveillance data on HCAI, study on antibiotic consumption and resistance patterns and monitor impact of infection control programmes. Publications from developing countries are increasing daily. An important window for research in developing countries arose through the International Nosocomial Infection Control Consortium (INICC). The INICC is the first multinational research network established to control HCAIs in hospitals in limited-resource countries. It has developed from South American hospitals in 1998 to a dynamic network of 450 healthcare centers in 108 cities, from 36 countries of 4 continents. It is the only source of aggregate standardized international data on HCAIs epidemiology in intensive care.

INICC published a surveillance study from January 2003 through December 2008 in 173 ICUs in Latin America, Asia, Africa, and Europe. During the 6- year study, using CDC

NNIS/NHSN definitions for device-associated healthcare-associated infection, prospective data were collected from 313,008 patients hospitalized in the consortium's hospital ICUs for an aggregate of 2,194,897 days (Rosenthal et al., 2011). Despite the fact that the use of devices in the developing countries' ICUs was remarkably similar to that reported in US ICUs in the CDC's NHSN, rates of device-associated nosocomial infection were significantly higher in the ICUs of the INICC hospitals; the pooled rate of central line-associated bloodstream infection in the INICC ICUs of 6.8 per 1,000 central line-days was more than 3-fold higher than the 2.0 per 1,000 central line-days reported in comparable US ICUs. The overall rate of ventilator-associated pneumonia also was far higher (15.8 vs 3.3 per 1,000 ventilator-days), as was the rate of catheter-associated urinary tract infection (6.3 vs. 3.3 per 1,000 catheter-days) and the crude unadjusted excess mortalities of device-related infections ranged from 7.3% (for catheter-associated urinary tract infection) to 15.2% (for ventilator-associated pneumonia).

	INICC 2004-2009 Pooled Mean (95% CI)	**U.S. NHSN 2006-2008 Pooled Mean (95% CI)**
Medical Cardiac ICU		
CLAB	6.2 (5.6 - 6.9)	2.0 (1.8 - 2.1)
CAUTI	3.7 (3.2 - 4.3)	4.8 (4.6 - 5.1)
VAP	10.8 (9.5 - 12.3)	2.1 (1.9 - 2.3)
Medical-surgical ICU		
CLAB	6.8 (6.6 - 7.1)	1.5 (1.4 - 1.6)
CAUTI	7.1 (6.9 - 7.4)	3.1 (3.0 - 3.3)
VAP	18.4 (17.9 - 18.8)	1.9 (1.8 - 2.1)
Pediatric ICU		
CLAB	4.6 (3.7 - 5.6)	3.0 (2.7 - 3.1)
CAUTI	4.7 (4.1 - 5.5)	4.2 (3.8 - 4.7)
VAP	6.5 (5.9 - 7.1)	1.8 (1.6 - 2.1)
Newborn ICU (1501-2500 g)		
CLAB	11.9 (10.2 - 13.9)	1.5 (1.2 - 1.9)
VAP	10.1 (7.9 - 12.8)	0.8 (0.04 - 1.5)

CI, confidence interval; ICU, intensive care unit; DA-HAI, device associated health care associated infection; INICC, International Nosocomial Infection Control Consortium; NHSN, National Healthcare Safety Network; CAUTI, catheter-associated urinary tract infections; CLAB, central line-associated blood stream infection; VAP, ventilator-associated pneumonia.

Table 2. Device associated infections (DAI) rates (per 1000 device-days) in the ICUs of the low income countries participating in International Nosocomial Infection Control Consortium (INICC) and the U.S. National Healthcare Safety Network(NHSN)(Rosenthal et al., 2011).

3.8 Environment

Isolation precautions with disinfection and sterilization comprise another important brick in the wall of infection control. Isolation precautions are important step in preventing transmission of infectious agents within the hospital wards. Isolation systems enable health care workers to identify patients who need to be isolated and undertake appropriate precautions. In developing world there is a lack of isolation rooms and usually patients with infections caused by same microorganisms are cohorted in same rooms. Personal protective equipment support achievement of this objective. Education of healthcare workers regarding standard precautions and safe and appropriate use of injections are important for prevention and control of HCAI. Important steps in prevention of HCAI are introduction of validated processes for decontamination, cleaning and sterilisation or high level disinfection of soiled instruments and other items; and improving safety in operating rooms and other high risk areas (Rutala & Webber, 2004).

3.9 Infection control societies

Many countries have not yet established infection control societies or associations, and general professional societies of physicians, nurses, and laboratory staff are not effectively engaged in infection control and prevention activities. The International Federation of Infection Control (IFIC) is an umbrella organisation of societies and associations of healthcare professionals in infection control and related fields worldwide including majority of them coming from developing countries. Currently IFIC has 66 members from 51 countries, and provides guidelines and educational material. Many regional and international networks throughout the world also participate in IFIC.

3.10 Microbiology laboratory support for infection control

Clinical microbiology laboratory plays a pivotal role in patient care providing information on a variety of microorganisms with clinical significance and is an essential component of an effective infection control program (Kalenic & Budimir, 2009). Laboratory plays important duties in prevention of HCAIs, which include: surveillance of HCAIs and antimicrobial resistance, rapid communication of laboratory data relevant to infection control, epidemiology typing of isolated pathogens, storing laboratory data and isolates, outbreak investigation and management. A variety of methods can be used to identify microorganisms in clinical specimens, although in developing countries diagnostic capabilities are insufficient. Partnership between the infection preventionist and the clinical microbiology laboratory staff is crucial in combating against HCAIs.

3.11 Combating antibiotic resistance

There is good evidence that antibiotic stewardship programmes have been successful in modifying antimicrobial prescribing practices, resulting in most instances in reduction of use. Unfortunately, such programmes are often lacking in developing countries, and antimicrobial resistance problems emphasise the importance of clinical microbiology laboratory services(Sosa et al.,2010) . Key actions in prevention and control of antimicrobial resistance are: empower the surveillance systems of antibiotic use and antibiotic resistance, prudent use in clinical practice (governmental measures, increase awareness of the public and health care workers, upgrading diagnostic capabilities), prudent use in veterinary, infection control in hospitals and community, implementation of Information technology, applied research and international cooperation.

4. Conclusion

HCAIs represent a major threat to patient safety and quality healthcare in developing countries. In many hospitals of developing world infection control activities are limited by many constraints in all levels of health care. As a consequence, these countries are facing the challenges of higher rates of hospital infections, frequent outbreaks, unsafe care and spread of infections in acute care facilities and community. The best solution for this challenge entail a multifactorial initiatives, which have to be sustainable in order to have a great impact on outcomes. Through focusing on infection control, countries with limited resources can improve the quality of healthcare in the future.

5. References

Allegranzi B, Pittet D. Role of hand hygiene in health care-associated infection prevention. J Hosp Infect 2009; 73(4): 305-15.

Allegranzi B, Storr J, Dziekan G, et al. The First Global Patient Safety Challenge "Clean Care is Safer Care": from launch to current progress and achievements. J Hosp Infect 2007; 65(Suppl 2): 115-23.

Allegranzi B et al. Burden of endemic health care-associated infection in developing countries: systematic review and meta-analysis. Lancet, 2011, 377:228–241.

Annual epidemiological report on communicable diseases in Europe 2008. Report on the state of communicable diseases in the EU and EEA/EFTA countries. Stockholm, European Centre for Disease Prevention and Control, 2008.

Arabi Y, Al-Shirawi N, Memish Z, Anzueto A. Ventilatorassociated pneumonia in adults in developing countries: a systematic review. Int J Infect Dis 2008; 12: 505-12.

Boyce JM, Pittet D. Guideline for hand hygiene in healthcare settings. Am J Infect Control 2002; 30: 1-46.

Burke J. Infection control e a problem for patient safety. N Engl J Med 2003; 348: 651-6.

Cavalcante MD, Braga OB, Teofilo CH, Oliveira EN, Alves A. Cost improvements through the establishment of prudent infection control practices in a Brazilian general hospital, 1986-1989. Infect Control Hosp Epidemiol 1991; 12: 649-53.

Centers for Disease Control. Public health focus: surveillance, prevention and control of nosocomial infections. Morb Mortal Wkly Rep 1992; 41: 783-7.

Clements C, Halton K, Graves N, et al. Overcrowding and understaffing in modern health-care systems: key determinants in meticillin-resistant Staphylococcus aureus transmission. Lancet Infect Dis 2008; 8: 427-34.

Corona A, Raimondi F. Prevention of nosocomial infection in the ICU setting. Minerva Anestesiol 2004; 70(5): 329-37.

Damani N. Surveillance in countries with limited resources. Int J Infect Control 2008; 4: 1.

Ducel G, Fabry J, Nicolle L, et al. Prevention of hospital-acquired infections. A practical guide. World Health Organ 2002; 9.

Duke T, Kelly J, Weber M, English M, Campbell H. Hospital Care for Children in Developing Countries: Clinical Guidelines and the Need for Evidence. J Trop Pediatr 2006; 52(1): 1-2

Editorial. Blood supply and demand. Lancet 2005; 365: 2151.

European Center for Disease Control, Commision Disease Report 2008.

Global patient safety challenge. Clean care is Safe care. World Health Organ 2005.

Gould IM. A review of the role of antibiotic policies in the control of antibiotic resistance. J Antimicrob Chemother 1999; 43: 459-65.

Haley RW, Quade D, Freeman HE, Bennet JV. The SENIC project: Study on the Efficacy of Nosocomial Infection Control. Am J Epidemiol 1980; 111: 472-85.

Harbarth S, Sax H, Gastmeier P. The preventable proportion of nosocomial infections: an overview of published reports. J Hosp Infect 2003; 54: 258-66.

Hauri AM, Armstrong GL, Hutin YJ. The global burden of disease attributable to contaminated injections given in health care settings. Int J STD AIDS 2004; 15: 7-16.

Higuera F et al. Attributable cost and length of stay for patients with central venous catheterassociated bloodstream infection in Mexico City intensive care units: a prospective, matched analysis. Infection Control and Hospital Epidemiology, 2007, 28:31–35.

Horan TC, Emori TG. Definitions of key terms used in the NNIS system. Am J Infect Control 1997; 25: 112-6.

Hughes AJ et al. Prevalence of nosocomial infection and antibiotic use at a university medical center in Malaysia. Infection Control and Hospital Epidemiology, 2005, 26:100–104.

Hugonnet S, Perneger TV, Pittet D. Alcohol-based handrub improves compliance with hand hygiene in intensive care units.Arch Intern Med 2002; 62: 1037-43.

Kalenic S, Budimir A. The role of microbiology laboratory in healthcare-associated infection prevention. Int J Infect Control 2009; v5: i2.

Klevens RM et al. Estimating health careassociated infections and deaths in U.S. hospitals, 2002. Public Health Reports, 2007, 122:160–166.

Kollef M. Optimizing antibiotic therapy in intensive care unit setting. Crit Care 2001; 5: 189-95.

Lawn JE, Cousens S, Bhutta ZA, et al. Why are 4 million newborn babies dying each year? Lancet 2004; 364: 399-401.

Lynch P, Pittet D, Borg MA, Mehtar S. Infection control in countries with limited resources. J Hosp Infect 2007; 65: 148-50.

Lynch P, Rosenthal V, Borg M, Eremin S. Infection control in developing countries. In: Jarvis WR, Ed. Bennett and Brachman's Hospital Infections. Philadelphia: Lippincott Williams & Wilkins 2007; pp. 240-55.

Miller MA, Pisani E. The cost of unsafe injections. Bull World Health Organ 1999; 77(10).

Moe CL, Rheingans RD. Global challenges in water, sanitation and health. J Water Health 2006; 4 Suppl 1: 41-57.

Morris K. Global control of health-care associated infections. Lancet 2008; 372: 1941-2.

Okeke IN, Laxminarayan R, Bhutta ZA, et al. Antimicrobial resistance in developing countries. Lancet Infect Dis 2005; 8: 481- 493.
Pfaller M, Herwalt L. The clinical microbiology laboratory and infection control: emerging pathogens, antimicrobial resistance and new technology. Clin Infect Dis 1997; 25: 858-70.
Pittet D, Allegranzi B, Storr J, et al. Infection control as a major World Health Organization priority for developing countries. J Hosp Infect 2008; 68(4): 285-92
Ponce-de-Leon-Rosales S, Macias A. Global perspectives of infection control. In: Wenzel RP, Ed. Prevention and control of nosocomial infections. 4th ed. Philadelphia-Lippincott Williams & Wilkins 2003; 14-33.
Raka L. Lowbury lecture- Infection control and limited resources : Searching for the best solutions. Journal of Hospital Infections May 2009;72:292-298
Ramirez JA. Controlling multiple-drug-resistant organisms at the hospital level. Expert Opin Pharmacother 2006; 7(11): 1449-55.
Randle J, Clarke M, Storr J. Hand hygiene compliance in healthcare workers. J Hosp Infect 2006; 64: 205-9.
Raza MW, Kazi BM, Mustafa M, Gould FK. Developing countries have their own characteristic problems with infection control. J Hosp Infect 2004; 57: 294-9.
Rosenthal VD, Guzman S, Safdar N. Reduction in nosocomial infection with improved hand hygiene in intensive care units of a tertiary care hospital in Argentina. Am J Infect Control 2005; 33:392-7.
Rosenthal VD, Maki DG, Jamulitrat S, et al. International Nosocomial Infection Control Consortium (INICC) report, data summary for 2003-2008, issued June 2009. Am J Infect Control 2010; 38(2): 95-104.
Rutala WA, Weber DJ. Disinfection and sterilization in health care facilities: what clinicians need to know. Clin Infect Dis 2004; 39:702-9.
Simonsen L, Kane A, Lloyd J, Zaffran M, Kane M. Unsafe injections in the developing world and transmission of bloodborne pathogens: a review. Bull World Health Organ 1999; 77: 789-800.
Sosa, A. de J.; Byarugaba, D.K.; Amábile-Cuevas, C.F.; Hsueh, P.-R.; Kariuki, S.; Okeke, I.N. (Eds.) Antimicrobial Resistance in Developing Countries, 2010
Stone PW. Economic burden of healthcare-associated infections: an American perspective. Expert Rev Pharmacoecon Outcomes Res 2009; 9(5): 417-22.
Vagholkar S, Ng J, Chan RC, Bunker JM, Zwar NA. Healthcare workers and immunity to infectious diseases. Aust NZ J Public Health 2008; 32: 367-71.
Wenzel RP, Edmond MB. Managing antibiotic resistance. N Engl J Med 2000; 343: 1961-63.
Westwell S. Implementing a ventilator care bundle in an adult intensive care unit. Nurs Crit Care 2008; 13: 203-7.
World Alliance for Patient Safety. Global patient safety e clean care is safer care. Geneva: World Health Organ 2005; 3-16.
World Bank. World Bank Classification of Economies. vol 2008.
World Health Organization. (2008) WHO global burden of disease: 2004 update. Available from:

www.who.int/healthinfo/global_burden_disease/2004_report_update/en/index.html

Zaidi AK, Huskins WC, Thaver D, et al. Hospital-acquired neonatal infections in developing countries. Lancet 2005; 365: 1175-88.

Part 2

Preventive Strategies

5

Prevention of Catheter-Related Bloodstream Infections in Patients on Hemodialysis

Dulce Barbosa, Mônica Taminato, Dayana Fram, Cibele Grothe and Angélica Belasco
Federal University of São Paulo/UNIFESP
Brazil

1. Introduction

Fourteen percent of deaths among patients with endstage kidney disease (ESKD) are due to infections, preceded only by cardiovascular diseases (USRDS,2006). According to The United States Renal Data System (USRDS), the number of patients receiving hemodialysis in the United States of America (USA) was 328,000 in 2006(USRDS,2008). Secondary to multiple defects in the ability to kill bacteria, infectious complications are more frequent in the Chronic Kidney Disease (CKD) and dialysis populations. (USRDS,2010).

Data from Brazilian Society of Nephrology reported that the number of patients on dialysis treatment in Brazil was 77.589 in 2009 and 90.8% of those patients were receiving hemodialysis (SBN,2010). The estimated prevalence and incidence rates of chronic renal failure on maintenance dialysis were 405 and 144 patients per million population, respectively. The estimated number of new patients starting dialysis program in 2010 was 49,077. The annual gross mortality rate was 17.1%. For prevalent patients, 39.9% were aged 60 years or older, 89.6% were on hemodialysis and 10.4% on peritoneal dialysis, 30,419 (39.2%) were on a waiting list of renal transplant, 27% were diabetics, 37.9% had serum phosphorus > 5.5 mg/dL and 42.8% hemoglobin < 11 g/dL. A venous catheter was the vascular access for 12.4% of the hemodialysis patients.

CVC (CVC) as vascular access are considered inferior to other means of vascular access with 2006 K/DOQI guidelines recommending less than 10% prevalence rate. However, despite these recommendations the Dialysis Outcomes and Practice Patterns Study (DOPPS II), reports that 46% to 70% of European and Canadian ESKD patients commencing maintenance haemodialysis do so via a CVC. This dependence on CVC is also reflected in the prevalence rates which range from 18% (Europe) to 34% (Canada) (Mendelssohn DC 2006). This over reliance on catheters may be attributed to late referrals to nephrologists, delay in access formation, lack of sufficient time for an AVF to mature or an ever increasing older ESKD population who experience higher rates of vascular disease and diabetes resulting in an inadequate vasculature for AVF formation (Butterly DW 2001 ; Letourneau I 2003 ; Mendelssohn DC 2006).

Data from the USA National Healthcare Safety Network demonstrated that bloodstream infection rates in 2006 varied according to the site of vascular access: 0.5% arteriovenous fistula (AVF), 0.9% AV grafts, 4.2% long-term central venous catheter and 27.1% short-term central venous catheter per month, respectively.

Chronic kidney disease (CKD) is a syndrome caused by many diseases that have in common the progressive reduction of glomerular filtration. Regardless of the initial insult caused by the underlying disease, the lesion progresses to glomerulosclerosis and interstitial fibrosis, resulting in established chronic kidney disease (ECKD). The ECKD treatment depends on the evolution of the disease and may be conservative with medication use, diet and fluid restriction, when such treatment becomes insufficient, you need to start dialysis to replace, in part, the kidney's function, or even apply to a kidney transplant (Mason J et al, 2008).

Conservative treatment aims to help reduce the rate of progression of the renal disease, using the dietary guidelines that aim to promote adequate nutritional status, metabolic control and uremic symptoms (20), with the improvement in organ dysfunction and comorbid conditions such as infection, contributing to better outcomes related to dialysis and transplantation (Klevens RM et al, 2008).

Despite advances in dialysis mortality remains high in ECKD. The infection continues to be a major cause of morbidity and the second most frequent cause of mortality (14%), preceded only by cardiovascular events as the first cause of death (Klevens RM et al, 2008).

Most microorganisms detected in the blood culture were considered to be a skin contaminant *coagulase-negative Staphylococcus*. Forty two percent (42%) of *Staphylococcus aureus* were resistant to methicillin and 39% of *Enterococcus* spp were resistant to vancomycin (Klevens et al,2008). Patients receiving hemodialysis have high risk for infection due to immunosuppression caused by ESKD, comorbidities, inadequate diet and the need for maintaining the venous access for long periods. In dialysis clinics many patients are submitted to this procedure at the same time, leading to the dissemination of microorganisms through direct or indirect contact with the devices, equipment, contaminated surfaces or the hands of health professionals.

In a study conducted at the Federal University of São Paulo (UNIFESP) it was found an incidence of infection of the bloodstream of 61% among patients with ESKD in use of central venous catheter associated with a mortality rate of 29% (Grothe C et al, 2009).

American data show that the main agents of bloodstream infections in hemodialysis patients were methicillin-resistant *Staphylococcus aureus* (MRSA), *Staphylococcus coagulase negative* (SCN) and vancomycin-resistant *Enterococcus spp* (VRE) (Klevens RM, 2008).

S. aureus is an important etiologic agent of both community-acquired infections and healthcare associated infections (HAI). In community-acquired infections are responsible for infections of skin and soft tissues, but is also responsible for invasive infections such as pyomyositis, osteomyelitis, necrotizing fasciitis, pneumonia and severe sepsis (King MD et al, 2006; Bocchini CE et al 2006; PV Adem et al , 2005). This agent is an important colonizer of the skin and mucous membranes. Although many sites of the human body can be colonized, nasal colonization is the most common. Studies show that approximately 20% of health professionals have persistent colonization and 80% intermittent colonization by this microorganism, nasal colonization is the biggest risk factor for the development of most endogenous infections (Van Belkum A et al, 2009 ; Wertheim HF et al, 2004; Von Eiff C et al, 2001).

Following the acquisition of MRSA colonization during hospitalization, patients with chronic renal failure on conservative treatment may persist as carriers for prolonged periods even after discharge from hospital and readmittance, may reintroduce the bacteria in the hospital (Roberts S et al, 2004)

The risk of transmission occurs most often because the patient is not identified as a carrier. A retrospective analysis that used information from hospital patients for eight years evaluated the risk of acquiring MRSA in patients who shared the same room with other hospital patients colonized with MRSA, unidentified. The study found a 13% incidence of infection by the same strain of MRSA among colonized patients (Moore C et al, 2008). Another study that evaluated the prevalence of MRSA on admission identified that 49% of patients would not have been identified without screening on admission (VCC Cheng et al, 2008).

Faced with complications that occurred due to infection in patients on dialysis treatment, Barbosa et al (D Barbosa et al, 2004; MCS Freitas et al, 2006) assessed the prevalence of colonization by vancomycin-resistant *Enterococcus* (VRE) in 300 patients in program dialysis and 280 transplant recipients treated in this service. It was found a prevalence rate of 14.5% in dialysis patients and 14% in renal transplanted patients, which proves to be quite high in relation to the rate documented in American services, which is around 7% (Tokars JI et al, 2000). The molecular typing of these samples was recently performed and it made possible the important detection of cross-transmission of VRE among patients treated at the Department of Dialysis and Transplantation of UNIFESP, and Fram et al observed the occurrence of vancomycin-resistant *Enterococcus* (VRE) cross-transmission between two patient groups (long-term dialysis and kidney transplant patients) Fram D et al, 2010.

In Europe and the United States the increase in infections caused by VRE in patients with ESKD have contributed to an increased morbidity and mortality in this patients population, which has generated a great concern in the nephrology services (Perencevich EM et al, 2004). Data from the National Healthcare Safety Network show that VRE was isolated in 26% of dialisys patients' blood cultures (Rom Klevens, 2008).

In the 90s, there was a significant increase in the prevalence of VRE infection in hospitals, particularly among immunosuppressed patients, such as those with chronic diseases, infectious diseases and renal transplants (Brady JP et al, 1998). Currently, VRE is between the second and third most frequent cause in the IRAS, due to its rapid spread, high associated mortality and limited treatment options, besides the possibility of transfer of the *vanA* resistance gene to other virulent organisms and more prevalent as the *S . aureus* (Chang S et al, 2003; & Salgado CD Farr BM, 2003).

The glycopeptide resistance may be mediated by several genes, *vanA, vanB, vanC, vanD, vanE, vanG* and *vanL*. Resistance mediated by mobile elements, called plasmids, may be transferred from one strain of VRE to another (Werner G et al, 2008; Arthur M, 1993)

The increased risk of VRE colonization and infection has been associated with the indiscriminate use of antibiotics, prolonged hospital stay, underlying diseases, transplantation, invasive treatments such as intra-abdominal surgery, presence of central venous catheterization and proximity to colonized patients. Studies done in the UNIFESP's nephrology service demonstrated the presence of VRE in dialysis patients and kidney transplantation. Among dialysis patients, the colonization prevalence was 14.5% and the identified risk factors were: dialysis type (hemodialysis), number of hospitalizations and length of hospital stay. Similar rate was found among patients undergoing renal transplantation, where the prevalence was 14%, although no risk factor was identified (Barbosa D et al, 2004; MCS Freitas et al, 2006).

Considering the emergence of new microorganisms, *Klebsiella pneumoniae* producing carbapenemases (KPC) has been highlighted as an important pathogen in healthcare related infections. Due to the great ability to spread and limited therapeutic options, the introduction of surveillance of this pathogen in the study group is necessary. According to a recent study by Ji-Young Rhee (2010), the isolation of bacteria *K. pneumoniae* producing carbapenemases (KPC) in hemodialysis patients with chronic renal failure demonstrated that the infection caused by multidrug-resistant pathogen that affected the patient's prognosis. Another study in Chicago showed that the implementation of a bundle that includes: surveillance cultures, team education, contact precautions, chlorhexidine bathing and environment cleaning greatly reduced the horizontal transmission of this pathogen (Mimoz O, 2007).

Microbial resistance should be considered because patients on dialysis treatment are often hospitalized and exposed to multi-resistant microorganisms and to broadspectrum antimicrobial therapy. (Klevens et al, 2008; Fram et al, 2010; Horl Wh 1999;Descamps-Latscha B & Herbelin A, 1993; MMWR,2001). On the one hand, the quality of dialysis and thus patients. well being and survival depend on the venous access; on the other hand, this is considered the major risk factor for infection and especially bacteremia in this group of patients(Mangini et al, 2005). In a study performed at Universidade Federal de São Paulo, 61% of patients with ESKD using central venous catheter presented bacteremia. Risk factors for bacteremia were: catheter insertion in the subclavian vein, duration of catheter use and the hospitalization period. The mortality rate in these patients was 29% and for patients who developed endocarditis it was 55.5%(Groethe C et al, 2010). As this population is exposed to a high infection risk which can be prevented in most cases by health professionals, a systematic review of literature was performed to establish standard measures to prevent catheter associated infections in hemodialysis patients.

1.2 Epidemiology

Twenty months of epidemiological surveillance data in the USA demonstrated that the risk for bacteremia was 32 times higher when short-term venous catheter was used, and 19 times higher when long-term venous catheter was used compared to the use of arteriovenous fistula (AVF). Similar data were observed in a study conducted in 11 dialysis centers in Canada (George A et al, 2006). A prospective survey with 35,000 randomized patients between the years of 1996 and 2007 treated in about 300 dialysis units in 12 countries demonstrated a great variation on AVF utilization. AVF use declined in elderly, obese, diabetic and patients with cardiovascular diseases or recurrent cellulitis. Considering the high mortality caused by the use of catheters, the best option for these patients is AV graft. However, in some countries there was an increase in catheter use and a proportional decrease in the use of AV grafts in patients with the characteristics mentioned (LoboRD et al, 2005). Measures to prevent catheter associated infections in hemodialysis patients must be considered taking into account the reduction in the use of central venous catheter (CVC), giving priority to the use of AVF whenever possible. However, in patients with impaired vessels, obesity and diabetes, where access through AVF or graft can be difficult, long-term CVC use is recommended(MMWR, 2001).

2. Methods

The present study was carried out through a review of the literature encompassing the issue of preventing catheter-associated bloodstream infections in hemodialysis patients. Studies published from 1990 to 2011 have been selected through electronic search in the following databases: *Cochrane Library,CINAHL, WEB OF SCIENCE, Medline, SciELO, Embase, Lilacs,* works presented in congresses, reviews and guidelines. The search strategy used for Medline presented the following steps: .Catheterization, Central Venous. [Mesh] AND .Infection. [Mesh]) AND .Renal Dialysis. [Mesh]) AND .Renal Dialysis/education. [Mesh] AND .Infection Control. [Mesh]. To select articles, two independent reviewers assessed the titles and abstracts of the publications found. All studies in the issue meeting the criteria for review have been included regardless of the language or design. Photocopies of the articles have been obtained and a standard form has been used to extract data.

3. Results

Two hundred and ninety three articles were found according to the used descriptors, 50 of them were literature reviews. After a previous selection, we included some studies that met the inclusion criteria were selected according to the assessment of the two independent reviewers. Among the studies analyzed we included (chart 1) systematic reviews, prospective cohorts, experimental study, meta-analysis review, controlled randomized clinical essays, cross-sectional randomized clinical trial and guidelines.

It was clear that surveillance is the essential issue for an infection control program and also for improving quality of care. A prospective study carried out in London between 2002 and 2004 with 112 patients (3418 patients per month) demonstrated reduction in bacteremia rate from 6.2% to 2.0% per month, reduction in hospitalizations due to bacteremia from 4.0% to 1.4% per month and also a significant downward trend was seen in bacteremia rates and antibiotic usage after the introduction of a surveillance scheme with patients. risk stratification, definition of denominators, type of access performed by physicians and nurses from the service, team training, preventive measures of infections, dissemination of data and use of results to optimize the actions introduced (George A et al, 2006). The training and education of health professionals, patients and care givers is recommended by the Center for Disease Control and Prevention (CDC) to prevent dialysis infections and must be compatible with the available knowledge from the personnel involved(9). A study conducted in a university hospital from São Paulo demonstrated 40% reduction in catheter-associated bloodstream infections (CABSI) after the implementation of an educational intervention with staff members (Lobo RD et al, 2005)

There are some standard precautions based on strategies to prevent transmission of infections that health professionals must use in patients. care: hand washing before and after

Author, year of publication and country	Design	Participants	Type of intervention	outcomes
George A, 2006- England	Prospective cohort	112 patients	Surveillance system	
Lobo RD, 2005- Brazil	Experimental	75 professionals	Health professional educational program	
Guideline CDC, 2001- USA	Systematic review	206 references	Recommendations for dialysis infection Prevention	
Guideline CDC, 2007- USA	Systematic review	1102 references	Care Recommendations	
Guideline CDC, 2002- USA	Systematic review	293 references	Recommendations to prevent catheterrelated infections	
Mimoz O, 2007- France	Controlled randomized clinical trial	538 catheters	Use of chlorhexidine versus polyvinylpyrrolidone-iodine solution (PVP-I)	P=0,002 Statistically significant reduction in bloodstream infection chlorehexidine group (1.4 versus 3.4 PVPI)
Gillies D, 2011 Australia	Systematic review and Meta-Analysis	6 studies	To compare gauze and tape and transparent polyurethane central venous catheter dressings	
Sesso R, 1998- Brazil	Controlled randomized clinical trial	136 patients	Use of mupirocin on catheter insertion	Odds:0,18
Johnson DW, 2002- Australia	Controlled randomized clinical trial	50 patients	Use of mupirocin on catheter insertion	Odds:0,08
Taminato M, 2011 Brazil	Systematic Review and Meta-Analysis	3 studies	Use of Mupirocin in Central Venous Catheter for Hemodialysis	
Roth PE, 2006 Spain	Cross-sectional	375 strains	Mupirocin resistance	
Bleyer AJ, 2007- USA	Systematic review	34 studies	Use of antimicrobial lock solutions	
Safdar N, 2006- USA	Systematic review with meta-analysis	7 studies	Use of a vancomycin-lock solution to reduce bacteremia	
Ethier J, 2008 multicenter	Prospective cohort	35000 patients	Venous access effectiveness	
McCann M & Moore ZEH	Systematic Review and Meta-Analysis	10 studies	INTERVENTIONS FOR PREVENTING INFECTIOUS COMPLICATIONS IN HAEMODIALYSIS PATIENTS WITH CENTRAL VENOUS CATHETERS	
Safdar N & Maki DG, 2006	Systematic Review and Meta-Analysis	4 studies	LOCK OF ANTIMICROBIAL IN HAEMODIALYSIS WITH CENTRAL VENOUS CATHETER	

Chart 1. Summary of the studies included

the contact, use of gloves, masks, protection glasses and laboratory coats when there is risk of contact with biological material, be careful with sharp-edged and hollow-pointed devices, environmental cleaning, adequate use of materials and equipments and health professionals immunization. When patients present suspicion or confirmation of a more severe infection, additional measures must be taken in addition to those mentioned above (Ethier J et al 2008). According to national and international recommendations, catheter insertion has to be conducted under sterile conditions and maximum barrier: masks, laboratory coats, gloves and sterile drapes (Descamps-Latscha B & Herbelin A, 1993; MMWR 2001; O.Grady NP et al, 2002). Alcoholic chlorhexidine 2% (drug of choice) or polyvinylpyrrolidone-iodine solution (PVP-I) 10% has to be used for skin antisepsis before catheter insertion and before dressing changes (MMWR, 2001; Mimoz O et al, 2007).

A CVC can be non-tunnelled or tunnelled. A non-tunnelled catheter - sometimes referred to in the literature as non-cuffed, temporary, short-term or acute - is intended for short-term haemodialysis use. On the other hand tunnelled catheters - also known as cuffed, chronic, long-term or permanent catheters - are generally used when patients require more than two to three weeks haemodialysis (Frankel, 2006). However, the reported use of these different catheters suggest that tunnelled catheters have been used for periods of short duration and, although not recommended, non-tunnelled catheters have been used for periods of long duration (months or years) (Ash SR, 2001; KDOQI 2006; Oliver MJ 2001; Ponikvar R, 2005).

A Cochrane systematic review with meta-analysis, published in 2003 compared the use of gauze and micropore film *versus* sterile transparent semipermeable polyurethane (Opsite ® (Smith & Nephew Healthcare Ltd), Tegaderm ® (3M) and Opsite IV3000 ®) to cover the catheter central venous . The transparent film covers so classified as highly permeable and permeable polyurethane polyurethane. The outcomes analyzed in this review were: catheter-related sepsis, infection at the catheter insertion site and colonization of catheter between the different types of coverage, but there was no statistical difference in any outcome analysis. One of the observations made by the plaintiff was an insufficient number of randomized clinical trials that could be included in the study (Gillies D et al, 2003)

A randomized study(Sesso R et al, 1998) highlighted that use of chlorhexidine before catheter insertion and during dressing changes is associated with less colonization and occurrence of CABSI when compared to the use of alcoholic PVP-I. Gauze or sterile transparent film are recommended to dress the site of catheter insertion. After bathing or showering it is important to inspect the insertion site, protecting it and replacing the catheter-site dressing when it becomes damp, loosened, or soiled (Descmaps-Latscha B & Herbelin A,1993; MMWR 2001; Ethier et al, 2008). A study (Sesso R et al 1998) demonstrated that mupirocin use in the catheter insertion site reduces significantly the risk of *S aureus* colonization and bacteremia. The same result was obtained in a study carried out in Australia (Johnson DW et al 2.002).

The meta-analysis of a profhylatic use of Mupirocin in central venous catheter for hemodialysis indicates that the use of topical mupirocin has been effective to reduce episodes of infections among patients increasing the usage time of the catheter in addition to significantly reducing the infections by *S aureus*, the most prevalent in this population (Taminato M et al, 2011).

Other systematic review (McCann M & Moore ZEH, 2008) shws that topical antimicrobial ointments compared to no ointment or placebo had a significant favourable effect on catheter removal due to infection caused by all types of organisms (RR 0.35, 95% CI 0.25 to 0.50). Catheter removal due to S. aureus was significantly reduced by topical antimicrobial.

However, the emergence of resistant strains must be considered as demonstrated in a Spanish study where pandemia of methicillin-resistant *Staphylococcus aureus* was associated to high-level mupirocin resistance (Johnson et al, 2002; Perez-Roth E et al, 2006).

Another prevention strategy is the use of gentamicin, cephalosporin or vancomycin lock solution, taking into account the possibility of the emergence of resistant microorganisms when vancomycin is used (Bleyer AJ, 2007; Safdar N & Maki DG, 2006).

The study Al-Kwiesh & Abdulla Khalaf, showed that the administration of vancomycin catheter lock via intralumenal was superior compared to the peripheral intravenous administration, where the results showed that the experimental group of 28 patients that used the vancomycin catheter lock had only one (3%) catheter removal, in contrast, the control group of 39 patients that had peripheral intravenous antibiotics had 22 (56%) catheter removals.

In a meta-analysis, authors demonstrated that in highrisk patients treated with long-term catheters the use of vancomycin lock solution reduces the risk of bacteremia(Safdar N & Maki DG, 2006). CDC does not recommend the regular use of antimicrobial lock solution to prevent bloodstream infection. The use is recommended only in special circumstances (e.g. patient with a long-term catheter or patients with clinical data of recurrent infections despite optimal maximal adherence to aseptic technique (O´Grady et al, 2002).

4. Conclusion

The authors conducted extensive review to suggest that catheter-associated bloodstream infection can be reduced when prevention measures are adequately taken they are: proper choice of insertion site, local antisepsis, personnel appropriate attire, infection surveillance, care and maintenance of the catheter or remove as well as the use of new technologies. Topical mupirocin ointment significantly reduced the risk of *S. aureus* exit site infection and catheter-related bacteraemia. The risk of catheter removal and episodes of hospitalisation due to *S. aureus* were also significantly reduced in those patients who used topical mupirocin ointment. Taking into account that this is a population at high risk for infection, the emergence of multi-resistant microorganisms must be considered, and if a severe case occurs, additional prevention measures must be taken to avoid an outbreak in this population. All personnel involved in the process of catheter insertion, maintenance and removal must be aware of the importance of excellent care for infection prevention therefore this chapter may contribute to infection control book.

5. Acknowledgment

We thank the research groups of Nephrology Nursing UNIFESP-Group and the systematic review and meta-analysis of the, UNIFESP.

We thank of Cochrane Brazil Colaboration.

6. References

[1] Adem PV, Montgomery CP, Husain AN, Koogler TK, Arangelovich V, Humilier M, et al. *Staphylococcus aureus* sepsis and the Waterhouse-Friderichsen syndrome in children. N Engl J Med. 2005; 353: 1245–1251.

[2] Al-Hwiesh AK, Abdul-Rahman IS. Successful Prevention of Tunneled, Central Catheter Infection by Antibiotic Lock Therapy Using Vancomycin and Gentamycin. Saudi J Kidney Dis Transpl [serial online] 2007 [cited 2011 Aug 16];18:239-47.

[3] Arthur M, P Courvalin. Genetics and mechanism of glycopeptide resistance in enterococci. Antimicrob Agents Chemother 1993; 37(8): 1563- 1571.

[4] Ash SR. The evolution and function of central venous catheters for dialysis. Seminars in Dialysis 2001;14:416-24.

[5] Barbosa D, Lima L, Silbert S, Sader H, Cendoroglo M, Draibe S et al. Evaluation of the prevalence and risk factors for colonization by vancomycin-resistant *Enterococcus* among patients on Dialysis. Am J Kidney Dis 2004; 44: 337-343.

[6] Brady JP, Snyder JW, Hasbargen JA. Vancomycin-resistant *Enterococcus* inend-stage renal disease. Am J Kidney Dis. 1998; 32(3):415-8.

[7] Brasilian Society of Nefrology (SBN). National sense 2007 [Internet]. São Paulo: SBN; 2010. [link: 2011 September 19]. Acess: http://www.sbn.org.br/Censo/2010/censo_SBN_2010.ppt

[8] Bleyer AJ. Use of Antimicrobial Catheter Lock Solutions to Prevent Catheter-Related Bacteremia. Clin J Am Soc Nephrol. 2007; 2: 1073-1078.

[9] Bocchini CE, Hulten KG, Mason EO, Jr., Gonzalez BE, Hammerman WA. (2006) Panton-Valentine leukocidin genes are associated with enhanced inflammatory response and local disease in acute hematogenous Staphylococcus aureus osteomyelitis in children. Pediatrics 117: 433–440.

[10] Butterly DW, Schwab SJ. Catheter access for hemodialysis: an overview. Seminars in Dialysis 2001;14:411-5.

[11] Chang S, Sievert DM, Hageman JC, Boulton ML, Tenover FC, Downes FP, et al. Brief report. Infection with vancomycin-resistant *Staphylococcus aureus* containing the *van*A resistance gene. N Engl J Med 2003; 348(14):1324-1347.

[12] Cheng V C C, Li I W S, Wu A K L, Tang B S F, Ng K H L, To K K W, Tse H, Que T L, Ho P L, Yuen K Y. Effects of antibiotics on de bacterial load of meticillin-resistant *Staphylococcus aureus* colonisation in anterior nares. Journal of Hospital Infection. 2008; 70: 27-34.

[13] Clinical practice guidelines and clinical practice for vascular access, update 2006.

[14] Descamps-Latscha B, Herbelin A. Long-term dialysis and cellular immunity: a critical survey. Kidney Int Suppl. 1993;41:S135-42.

[15] Ethier J, Mendelssohn DC, Elder SJ, Hasegawa T, Akizawa T, Akiba T, et al. Vascular access use and outcomes: an international perspective from the Dialysis Outcomes and Practice Patterns Study. Nephrol Dial Transplant. 2008;23(10):3219-26. Erratum in: Nephrol Dial Transplant. 2008;23(12):4088.

[16] Fram D, Castrucci FM, Taminato M, Godoy-Martinez P, Freitas MC, Belasco A, Sesso R, Pacheco-Silva A, Pignatari AC, Barbosa D. Cross-transmission of vancomycin-resistant *Enterococcus* in patients undergoing dialysis and kidney transplant. Braz J Med Biol Res. 2010; 43(1):115-9.

[17] Frankel A. Temporary access and central venous catheters. European Journal of Vascular & Endovascular Surgery 2006;31:417-22.
[18] Freitas MCS, Silva AP, Barbosa D, Silbert S, Sader H, Sesso R et al. Prevalence of vancomycin- resistant *Enterococcus* fecal colonization among kidney transplant patients. BCM Infectious Diseases 2006; 6:133.
[19] George A, Tokars JI, Clutterbuck EJ, Bamford KB, PuseyC, Holmes AH. Reducing dialysis associated bacteraemia, and recommendations for surveillance in the United Kingdom: prospective study. BMJ. 2006;332(7555):1435.
[20] Gilles D, Carr D, Frost J, O'Riordan R, O'Brien I. Gauze and tape and transparent polyurethane dressings for central venous catheters. Cochrane Database of Systematic Reviews 2003.
[21] Grothe C, Belasco A, Bettencourt A, Diccini S, Vianna L, Sesso R, Barbosa D. High incidence of bacteremia among patients undergoing hemodialydis. Rev Latinoam Enferm. 2009; 18 (1): (8 telas).
[22] Hörl WH. Neutrophil function and infections in uremia. Am J Kidney Dis. 1999;33(2):xlv.xlviii.
[23] Johnson DW, MacGinley R, Kay TD, Hawley CM, Campbell SB, Isbel NM, Hollett P. A randomized controlled trial of topical exit site mupirocin application in patients with tunnelled, cuffed haemodialysis catheters. Nephrol Dial Transplant. 2002;17(10):1802-7.
[24] Klevens RM, Edwards JR, Andrus ML, Peterson KD, Dudeck MA, Horan TC; NHSN Participants in Outpatient Dialysis Surveillance. Dialysis Surveillance Report: National Healthcare Safety Network (NHSN) - data summary for 2006. Semin Dial. 2008;21(1):24-8.
[25] King MD, Humphrey BJ, Wang YF, Kourbatova EV, Ray SM, et al. Emergence of community-acquired methicillin-resistant Staphylococcus aureus USA 300 clone as the predominant cause of skin and soft-tissue infections. Ann Intern Med. 2006; 144: 309–317.
[26] Letourneau I, Ouimet D, Dumont M, Pichette V, Leblanc M. Renal replacement in end-stage renal disease patients over 75 years old. American Journal of Nephrology 2003;23:71-7.
[27] Lobo RD, Levin AS, Gomes LMB, Cursino R, Park M, Figueiredo VB, et al. Impact of an educational program and policy changes on decreasing catheter-associated bloodstream infections in a medical intensive care unit in Brazil. Am J Infect Control. 2005;33(2):83-7.
[28] Mangini C, Camargo LFA, coordenadores. Prevenção de infecção relacionada à diálise. São Paulo: APECIH - Associação Paulista de Estudos e Controle de Infecção Hospitalar; 2005.
[29] Mason J, Khunti K, Stone M, Farooqi A, Carr S. Educational Interventions in Kidney Disease Care: A systematic review of randomized trials. Am J of Kidney Dis. 2008;51(6):933-51.
[30] Mendelssohn DC, Ethier J, Elder SJ, Saran R, Port FK, Pisoni RL. Haemodialysis vascular access problems in Canada: results from the dialysis outcomes and practice patterns study (DOPPS II). Nephrology Dialysis Transplantation 2006;21:721-8.
[31] McCann M & Moore ZEH. Interventions for preventing infectious complications in haemodialysis patients with central venous catheters. Cochrane Database of

Systematic Reviews. In: *The Cochrane Library,* Issue 08, Art. No. CD006894. DOI: 10.1002/14651858.CD006894.pub1

[32] Mimoz O, Villeminey S, Ragot S, Dahyot-Fizelier C, Laksiri L, Petitpas F, Debaene B. Clorhexidine-based antiseptic solution vs alcohol-based povidone-iodine for central venous catheter care. Arch Intern Med. 2007;167(19):2066-72.

[33] Moore C, Dhaliwal J, Tong A, Eden S, Wigston C, Willey B, McGeer A. Risk factors for methicillin-resistant Staphylococcus aureus (MRSA) acquisition in roommate contacts of patients colonized or infected with MRSA in an acute-care hospital. *Infect Control Hosp Epidemiol.* 2008;29:600–606.

[34] O.Grady NP, Alexander M, Dellinger EP, Gerberding JL, Heard SO, Maki DG, et al. Guidelines for the prevention of intravascular catheter-related infections. Centers for Disease Control and Prevention. MMWR Recomm Rep. 2002;51(RR-10):1-29.

[35] Oliver MJ. Acute dialysis catheters. Seminars in Dialysis 2001;14:432-5.

[36] Pérez-Roth E, López-Aguilar C, Alcoba-Florez J, Méndez-Alvarez S. High-level mupirocin resistance within methicillin-resistant staphylococcus aureus pandemic lineages. Antimicrob Agents Chemother. 2006;50(9):3207-11.

[37] Perencevich EN, Fisman DN, Lipsitch M, Harris AD, Morris JG Jr, Smith DL. Projected benefits of active surveillance for vancomycin-resistant enterococci inintensive care units. Clin Infect Dis. 2004; 15 38(8):1108-15.

[38] Ponikvar R. Hemodialysis catheters. Therapeutic Apheresis & Dialysis: Official Peer-Reviewed Journal of the International Society for Apheresis, the Japanese Society for Apheresis, the Japanese Society for Dialysis Therapy 2005;9:218-22.

[39] Recommendations for preventing transmission of infections among chronic hemodialysis patients. MMWR Recomm Rep. 2001;50(RR-5):1-43.

[40] Rhee JY, Park KY, Shin JY, Choi JY, Lee MY,Peck KR et al. KPC-producing extreme drug-resistant Klebsiella pneumoniae isolate from a patient with diabetes mellitus and chronic renal failure on hemodialysis in South Korea. Agents Chemother. 54;(5):2278-9, 2010.

[41] Roberts S, West T, Morris A. Duration of methicillin-resistant *Staphylococcus aureus* colonization in hospitalised in patients. New Zeland Medical Journal. 2004; 117: 1195.

[42] Salgado CD, Farr BM. Outcomes associated with vancomycin-resistant enterococci: a meta-analysis. Infect Control Hosp Epidemiol. 2003; 24(9):690-8.

[43] Safdar N, Maki DG. Use of vancomycin-containing lock or flush solutions for prevention of bloodstream infection associated with central venous access devices: a meta-analysis of prospective, randomized trials. Clin Infec Dis. 2006;43(4):474-84.

[44] Sesso R, Barbosa D, Leme IL, Sader H, Canziani ME, Manfredi S, et al. Staphylococcus aureus prophylaxis in hemodialysis patients using central venous catheter: effect of mupirocin ointment. J Am Soc Nephrol. 1998;9(6):1085-92.

[45] Siegel JD, Rhinehart E, Jackson M, Chiarello L, Healthcare Infection Control Practices Advisory Committee. 2007 Guideline for Isolation Precautions: Preventing Transmission of Infectious Agents in Healthcare Settings [Internet]. CDC; 2007.[cited 2011 september 12]. Available from: http://www.cdc.gov/ncidod/dhqp/pdf/isolation2007.pdf

[46] Taminato M, Fram DS, Groethe C, Belasco A, Barbosa DA. Prophilatic Use of Mupirocin in Central Venous Catheter for Hemodialysis: Systematic Review and Meta-Analysis. Acta Paulista de Enfermagem. 2012 : 25 (1):(in press).

[47] Tokars JI, Frank M, Alter MJ, Arduino MJ. National surveillance of dialysis-associated diseases in the United States, 2000. Semin Dial. 2002; 15(3):162-71.

[48] U.S. Renal Data System, USRDS 2006 Annual Data Report: Atlas of End-Stage Renal Disease in the United States, National Institutes of Health, National Institute of Diabetes and Digestive and Kidney Diseases, Bethesda, MD, 2006.

[49] U.S. Renal Data System, USRDS 2008 Annual Data Report: Atlas of Chronic Kidney Disease and End-Stage Renal Disease in the United States, National Institutes of Health, National Institute of Diabetes and Digestive and Kidney Diseases, Bethesda, MD, 2008.

[50] U.S. Renal Data System, USRDS 2010 Annual Data Report: Atlas of Chronic Kidney Disease and End-Stage Renal Disease in the United States, National Institutes of Health, National Institute of Diabetes and Digestive and Kidney Diseases, Bethesda, MD, 2010.

[51] Wertheim HF, Vos MC, Ott A, van Belkum A, Voss A, Kluytmans J, et al. Risk and outcome of nosocomial *Staphylococcus aureus* bacteraemia in nasal carriers versus non-carriers. Lancet 2004 364: 703–705.

[52] Werner G, Coque TM, Hammerum AM, Hope R, Hryniewicz W, Johnson A, et al. Emergence and spread of vancomycin resistance among enterococci in Europe. Euro Surveill. 2008; 13: 1-11.

[53] Van Belkum A, Verkaik NJ, de Vogel CP, Boelens HA, Verveer J. Reclassification of *Staphylococcus aureus* nasal carriage types. J Infect Dis. 2009; 199:1820–1826.

[54] Von Eiff C, Becker K, Machka K, Stammer H, Peters G. Nasal carriage as a source of *Staphylococcus aureus* bacteremia. Study Group. N Engl J Med. 2001; 344: 11–16.

6

Implementation of MRSA Infection Prevention and Control Measures – What Works in Practice?

Jobke Wentzel, Nienke de Jong,
Joyce Karreman and Lisette van Gemert-Pijnen
Center for eHealth Research and Disease Management
University of Twente
The Netherlands

1. Introduction

There have been increasing numbers of media reports about careless behaviour by healthcare workers, mainly involving insufficient cleaning practices and the absence of hand hygiene measures (Boyce, 2009). Although adherence to infection prevention and control measures has received a lot of attention in the media and in scientific literature, surprisingly little attention has been given to the implementation of the infection prevention and control strategies in healthcare practices. In the medical literature the focus is on the availability of national or regional MRSA surveillance data and guidelines for prevention and control. To date hardly any data has been made available about the kinds of interventions that have been successful in implementing infection prevention and control.

Research has shown that an intensive infection prevention programme could prevent about one-quarter to one-third of all hospital infections (Sengers et al., 2000). An example of such a successful policy is the 'search-and-destroy' strategy that has been introduced in the Netherlands, to prevent the spread and outbreak of infections caused by multi-resistant bacteria such as Methicillin Resistant Staphylococcus Aureus (MRSA). However, adherence to this policy still remains a problem. It is known from prior research (van Gemert et al., 2005; Verhoeven et al., 2009) that healthcare workers are insufficiently aware of infection control measures; they do not understand the rationale behind these measures and think that infection control is not their problem, that it is mainly an issue for hygiene experts.

Research in the social sciences has shown that improving safety in hospitals requires a tailored strategy to persuade people to change their attitudes and behaviours (Fogg, 2003). Furthermore, changing routines and habits in healthcare is not easy: it requires an integral approach, with activities addressing human behaviour, culture, incentives and other managerial reinforcement activities, and of course adequate information about safety regulations (Foy et al., 2001; Van Gemert et al., 2005; Verhoeven et al., 2009). A multifaceted implementation strategy might be a solution (Foy et al., 2001, Pittet et al.,

2000). Such a strategy should include interventions aimed at different levels: the management of healthcare institutions, the behaviour of healthcare workers and the quality of the infection control guidelines. However, what empirical evidence exists for a multi-faceted implementation strategy? And how successful are these strategies? To investigate this, we conducted a systematic literature review. This review will be used to develop an implementation strategy that fits the habits and culture of hospital-based healthcare workers (HCWs) in hospital care settings. In this review, we searched for empirical studies to investigate and identify effective implementation strategies for improving adherence to MRSA prevention and control measures. The following questions guided our review of the literature:

- What implementation strategies are used?
  - What is the foundation of these strategies (theories, experience, etc.)?
- What research designs were used to measure the effects of the implementation strategies?
- What effects are reported?
  - On adherence to the measures?
  - On the reduction of costs?
  - On the reduction of MRSA?

2. Method of the systematic review

The York protocol for systematic reviews (Centre for Reviews and Dissemination, 2001) was used to guide the review process. Literature searches were carried out in the online databases Scopus, ISI Web of Knowledge and the Cochrane Library. In addition, we hand-searched the indexes of the *Journal of Hospital Infection* (JHI), the *American Journal of Infection Control* (AJIC) and *Clinical Microbiology and Infection* (CMI) for relevant publications. We searched for studies describing the implementation of MRSA prevention or control measures. The publications were included in the review if they met the inclusion criteria listed in Table 1. Most important was that the publications described an implementation strategy and implementation outcomes. Two independent reviewers (NdJ, JW) applied the inclusion criteria to the publications in a title screening round, followed by an abstract and a full-text screening round. After each round, the reviewers compared their judgments and resolved discrepancies through discussion. The included studies are summarized in a data table, and the study features and results are summarized and compared. Due to the heterogeneity of the data and the limited number of included studies, no meta-analysis was performed.

3. Results of the systematic review

3.1 Article screening

The search strategy resulted in 661 potentially relevant publications (after duplicates were removed). The screening process and outcomes are shown in Figure 1; 29 publications were included in the review. The characteristics of these publications are summarized in Table 2. The characteristics and outcomes of the included studies are discussed in the following sections. The numbers we cite correspond to the publications summarized in Table 2.

Inclusion Criteria
Publication Type
(Scientific) Journal article, published between 2005-2010
Scope of Studies
Implementation of an evidence-based MRSA prevention or control measure. The implementation strategy must be described.
Study Settings
Primary-/secondary-care facilities, long-term care facilities, nursing homes
Outcome measure
Implementation outcomes (mostly behavioural) must be given. • Behavioural (e.g. adherence to implemented measure, knowledge) • Clinical (e.g. prevalence rates, infection rates, deaths) • Organizational (e.g. changes in Length of Stay (LoS), expenditures, costs)

Table 1. Inclusion Criteria

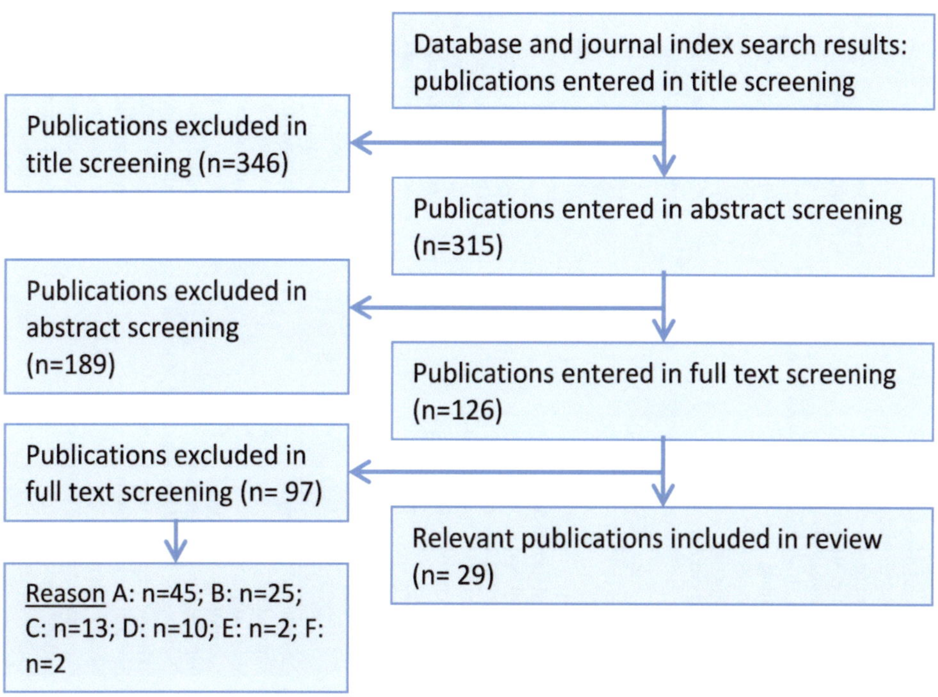

A: Insufficient implementation strategy information. B: No Compliance rates; no implementation results described. C: Article is a Viewpoint/Review. D: Article was not written in English. E: Article is a report of Conference Proceedings. F: Other.

Fig. 1. Results of the screening process

Author, Year, Country	Implementation strategy	Reported Findings (behavioural, clinical, financial)
1: Baldwin, et al., 2010, Ireland	Educational meetings Local opinion leaders Audit and feedback Technology supported *Implementation foundation* Theoretical: absence of IC research in nursing home setting *Infection control measure* Hand hygiene Environmental hygiene Personal protective equipment *Design* RCT	**Behavioural** *In-person observations* Mean audit score was higher in the intervention than in the control homes at 3 months, 6 months and 12 months. **Clinical** MRSA positive screenings were similar in intervention and control homes at 3 months, 6 months and 12 months. MRSA prevalence rates among staff were similar in intervention and control group at 3 months, 6 months and 12 months.
2: Bassetti, et al., 2009, Italy	Audit and feedback AB permission Formulary restrictions Clinical multidisciplinary teams *Infection control measure* Medication *Design* Time series design	**Behavioural** Significant reduction in cephalosporins use. Significant increase in ciprofoxacin use. **Clinical** Significant reduction in MRSA due to intervention. An increase in susceptibility to piperacillin/ tazobactam observed during the pre-intervention period in P. aeruginosa isolates ceased after the change in antibiotic policy. Increase in susceptibility to ciprofloxacin in K. pneumoniae isolates after the intervention began, although an abrupt change in the percentage of susceptible isolates followed termination of the intervention. Decrease in susceptibility to piperacillin/tazobactam and imipenem in K. pneumoniae isolates and an increase in susceptibility to ciprofloxacin in P. aerugionosa isolates was observed during the entire surveillance period, with no significant changes due to intervention.
3: Burkitt, et al., 2010, United States	Educational meetings Reminders Mass media Technology-supported *Implementation foundation* Theoretical: lack of measurement of actual changes in knowledge due to education *Infection control measure* Hand hygiene Personal protective equipment Patient screening Patient isolation *Design* Before and after design	**Behavioural** *Questionnaires* Significant increase in proportion of respondents who reported using alcohol-based hand rubs rather than soap and water to clean their hands. Significant increase in mean number of knowledge questions answered correctly. Significant increase in proportion of respondents who agreed or strongly agreed that MRSA was a problem in their unit. Significant increase in proportion of respondents who reported being comfortable reminding other staff about proper hand hygiene and contact precautions. Significant decrease in job satisfaction. Significant increase in proportion of respondents who reported using prevention practices. Significant increase in proportion of respondents reporting at least one barrier to proper hand hygiene, primarily because they feared that hand rubs or soap damages the skin or because they forgot to perform hand hygiene.

Author, Year, Country	Implementation strategy	Reported Findings (behavioural, clinical, financial)
4: Camins & Fraser, 2005, United States	Distribution of educational materials Educational meetings Local opinion leaders Audit and feedback Reminders Rewards *Implementation foundation* Theoretical: CDC Hand Hygiene Task Force recommendations *Infection control measure* Hand hygiene *Design* Before and after design	**Behavioural** *Observations in person* Hand hygiene compliance increased from 1st to 4th quarter of 2004. (Details on material use or observed compliance not given).
5: Carboneau, et al., 2010, United States	Distribution of educational materials Educational meetings Local opinion leaders Audit and feedback Reminders Mass media Changes in physical structure, facilities and equipment Technology-supported *Implementation foundation* Theoretical: prior research solutions, including scientific articles and at other hospital *Infection control measure* Hand hygiene *Design* Before and after design	**Behavioural** *Observations in person* Hand hygiene compliance increased from 17-months pre-intervention to 7 months post-intervention. **Clinical** Decrease in MRSA-positive cases from 17 months pre-intervention to 7 months post-intervention and decrease in invasive MRSA cases. **Financial** Net dollar savings due to MRSA infection prevention of US $276,500 over study period (August 1, 2006 to September 30, 2007) 41 MRSA infections were prevented during study period, thereby decreasing length of stay, resulting in a savings of $354,276, a net hard-dollar savings of $276,500. Increased hand sanitizer costs of $40,000 per year.
6: Cheng et al., 2009, China	Educational meetings Educational outreach Audit and feedback (trained auditors) Reminders Mass media Clinical multidisciplinary teams Changes in physical structure, facilities and equipment *Infection control measure* Hand hygiene Patient isolation *Design* Before and after design Time series design	**Behavioural** *Observations in person* Increased hand hygiene adherence. Increased use of alcohol-based hand rub. **Clinical** Decreased MRSA infection rates Change in ICU onset MRSA infections between phase 1 and 2 (ICU renovation) and between phase 2 and 3 (hand hygiene campaign).

Author, Year, Country	Implementation strategy	Reported Findings (behavioural, clinical, financial)
7: Davis, 2010, United Kingdom	Reminders Mass media *Duration* 6 months *Infection control measure* Hand hygiene *Design* Before and after design	**Behavioural** *Video observations* Significant increase in hand hygiene compliance of HCWs but no significant increase for patients. **Clinical** Decrease in MRSA incidence (from 2 to 0 cases during 6-month periods), reference unit: increase in MRSA incidence (from 0 to 2 cases during 6-month periods).
8: Eveillard, et al., 2006, France	Educational meetings Educational outreach Audit and feedback Reminders Mass media Changes in physical structure, facilities and equipment *Implementation foundation* Empirical: existing programme to limit the spread of MRSA was not effective *Infection control measure* Hand hygiene Patient screening *Design* Before and after design Time series design	**Behavioural** Increase in use of waterless alcohol-based hand disinfectants. In 2004, the use of alcohol-based hand disinfectants was twice as high in high-risk wards than in low-risk wards. *Questionnaire* 46% of 450 employees declared they had attended at least one educational session. Number of patients screened on admission or after intra-hospital transfer increased **Clinical** Decrease in the incidence of newly acquired MRSA infections in high-risk wards. Decrease in the incidence of risk of acquisition. Decrease in proportion of acquired MRSA. Number of MRSA carriage on admission did not increase. Proportion of MRSA/total S. aureus within the first 48 hours decreased.
9: Fowler, et al., 2010, England	Audit and feedback Reminders *Implementation foundation* Theoretical: systematic reviews on improving AB prescribing and feedback *Infection control measure* Medication *Design* Time series design	**Behavioural** Significant decrease in targeted ABs: Cephalosporins and Amoxicillin/clavulanate Significant increase in the long-term trend of benzyl penicillin. Significant increase in level of amoxicillin. Non-significant change in trend (not reversed long-term). Non-significant change in level and trend of trimethoprim. **Clinical** Significant decrease in CDI (clostridium difficile infection) and Incident Rate Ratio. Non-significant change in MRSA infections. Non-significant change in crude mortality. **Financial** No change in length of stay throughout study.

Author, Year, Country	Implementation strategy	Reported Findings (behavioural, clinical, financial)
10: Gagné, et al., 2010, Canada	Distribution of educational materials Educational outreach Patient-mediated interventions Mass media *Implementation foundation* Empirical: own observation that MRSA kept spreading despite staff decontamination *Infection control measure* Hand hygiene *Design* Before and after design	**Behavioural** *Observations in person* Increase in overall staff hand hygiene compliance. **Clinical** Decrease in MRSA infections vs. positive screenings. Decrease in MRSA infections. **Financial** Based on comparative year, 51 cases of infection were prevented in study year, resulting in net savings of CAN$688,843.
11: Gillespie, et al., 2007 Australia	Audit and feedback Reminders Mass media Changes in physical structure, facilities and equipment *Infection control measure* Hand hygiene Patient screening *Design* Before and after design	**Behavioural** Exact compliance rate unclear, but all staff/family entering was send back by 'door monitor' in case of non-compliance; compliance is assumed to be close to 100% **Clinical** MRSA acquisition rate decreased. Resistance increased, due to a clonal outbreak of rifampicin-resistant MRSA.
12: Goodman, et al., 2008, United States	Educational meetings Audit and feedback Changes in physical structure, facilities and equipment *Implementation foundation* Other: development of a novel and nontoxic tracking marker that is visible only under UV lamp *Infection control measure* Environmental hygiene *Design* Before and after design	**Behavioural** *Observations in person* Mark removal was more frequent during the intervention period than during baseline period. Additional predictors of mark removal included type of ICU and type of surface. No difference in the effect of the intervention between surgical and medical ICUs. **Clinical** Type of ICU was predictive of positive surface-culture results, as was type of surface. Multivariate models showed significant intervention effect, with reduced environmental MRSA and VRE contamination when cultures were used as the unit of analysis and data were clustered by room. No direct association between the removal of the mark from a specific surface and the likelihood that the surface culture would yield MRSA or vancomycin-resistant enterococci (VRE). Multivariate models assessing the proportion of marks removed showed that there were 30% fewer positive cultures for every 10% increase in the proportion of removed marks.

Author, Year, Country	Implementation strategy	Reported Findings (behavioural, clinical, financial)
13: Grayson, et al., 2008, Australia	Distribution of educational materials Educational meetings Audit and feedback Mass media Technology-supported *Implementation foundation* Empirical: prior success of a single-site HHCCP *Infection control measure* Hand hygiene *Design* Before and after design Time series design	**Behavioural** *Observations in person* Pilot programme: significant increase in hand hygiene compliance. After an initial increase, some sites showed some transient declines in compliance (related to changes of project officers). Pilot programme: alcohol-based hand rubs (ABHRS) increased, but correlated poorly with hand hygiene compliance. *Observations in person* State-wide: significant increase in hand hygiene compliance after 4 months and after 11-12 months. *Material use* State-wide: ABHRS increased, but correlated only roughly with HH compliance rates. **Clinical** Pilot group: significant decrease of patients with MRSA bacteremia. Significant reduction of the total number of clinical MRSA cases. State-wide: decrease in patients with MRSA bacteremia. Significant decrease in the number of clinical MRSA isolates, but this trend had already started before HHCCP.
14: Harrington, et al., 2007, Australia	Educational meetings Audit and feedback *Duration* 24 months *Infection control measure* Hand hygiene Other (sign put up in case of MRSA) *Design* Time series design	**Behavioural** *Observations in person* Overall rate of usage of the standard of all products increased. **Clinical** New patients with MRSA in the ICU decreased. Hospital-wide rate of new patients with MRSA decreased. MRSA central line-associated bloodstream infection (CLABSI) rates in ICU decreased. Decrease in hospital-wide rate of episodes of MRSA bacteremia.
15: Holder & Zellinger, 2009, United States	Educational meetings Educational outreach Local opinion leaders Audit and feedback *Duration* 2 months *Infection control measure* Medication (chlorhexidine baths) *Design* Time series design	**Behavioural** *Patient documentation* Compliance with bathing procedure increased. **Clinical** Bloodstream infection (BSI) rates decreased after implementation of the chlorhexidine bath procedure. Rate of MRSA/VRE colonization decreased after implementation of the chlorhexidine bath procedure. **Financial** 75% reduction in BSIs over 6 months and increased costs per bath led to a projected cost savings of $1.56 million per year if chlorhexidine baths were used in all hospital ICUs.

Author, Year, Country	Implementation strategy	Reported Findings (behavioural, clinical, financial)
16: Huang, et al., 2006, United States	Educational meetings Audit and feedback Reminders Rewards Changes in physical structure, facilities and equipment *Duration* Sterile CVC placement: 10 months. Alcohol-based hand rubs: 1 month. Hand hygiene campaign: 14 months. Routine surveillance: 12 months *Infection control measure* Hand hygiene Personal protective equipment Patient screening Patient isolation *Design* Before and after design Time series design	**Behavioural** *Observations in person* ABHR institution and hand hygiene campaign increased compliance in the first campaign year, but decreased thereafter. *Lab statistics (PD)* Routine MRSA surveillance caused increase in compliance after institution of daily physician orders for admission and weekly nares cultures. **Clinical** Campaign to promote sterile CVC precautions caused substantial decrease in all-cause catheter-associated bacteremia in ICUs. Among the interventions, only routine ICU MRSA surveillance was associated with a significant decrease in the incidence density of MRSA bacteremia. After 16 months, routine screening was associated with a decrease in hospital-associated incidence density in ICUs, in non-ICUs, and hospital-wide. Routine screening was associated with a decrease in hospital-associated incidence density in ICUs, in non-ICUs, and hospital-wide. All findings were statistically significant. Routine surveillance caused significant reduction in MRSA acquisition in ICUs when comparing the first and last halves of the intervention period, exclusive of the phase-in period. This was despite a stable MRSA importation rate into ICUs. No significant secular trend and no impact of any infection control interventions on rates of methicillin-susceptible S. aureus (MSSA) bacteremia.
17: Johnson, et al., 2005, Australia	Distribution of educational materials Audit and feedback Reminders Mass media Technology-supported *Implementation foundation* Theoretical: scientific articles *Duration* 36 months *Infection control measure* Hand hygiene Environmental hygiene Patient screening HCW screening Environmental screening *Design* Time series design	**Behavioural** *Observations in person* Overall hand hygiene compliance improved at 4 months, and was maintained at the same level at 12 months. In individual sentinel areas, compliance rates improved significantly between pre-intervention and 4 months post-intervention in all areas. Use of ABHRS products increased in all sentinel areas. **Clinical** MRSA colonization rates did not change in any of the sentinel areas during OCS. Rate of healthcare worker MRSA colonization did not decrease in sentinel areas except in the ICU. Environmental contamination did not change significantly during Operation Clean Start (OCS). Significant decline in total clinical MRSA infections per 100 patient-discharges over 36 months. For patient episodes of MRSA bacteremia, the monthly rate during the 28-month pre-intervention period was static, but fell significantly in the post-intervention period. By the 36th month, the monthly rate of MRSA bacteremia had decreased. Total clinical isolates per month of ESBLs increased during the 28 months before intervention, but had fallen by more than 90% by the 36th month of OCS.

Author, Year, Country	Implementation strategy	Reported Findings (behavioural, clinical, financial)
18: Kho, et al., 2008, United States	Reminders Technology-supported *Implementation foundation* Theoretical: low compliance (delay) associated with manual/paper-based information systems; computerized reminders appear promising *Duration* 12 months *Infection control measure* Patient isolation *Design* Before and after design	**Behavioural** *Computer logs* Significant increase in proportion of correct contact isolation order. Mean time between ward arrival and isolation order decreased Acceptance of the reminder increased. *Questionnaire* 19/20 survey respondents reported that the reminder either had no negative effect on workflow or saved them time. 25/27 agreed with automatic contact isolation, and half of these would simultaneously request surveillance swabs. **Clinical** *Lab statistics* During the intervention period, the number of patients with known MRSA or VRE increased which reflected an increased ability of the IC service to both identify patients and update the list. National trend of MRSA/VRE increased during the study (no significant difference between baseline and post-intervention **Financial** Annual isolation gown expenditures increased 23% from the same time period a year earlier (from US$167,000 to US$205,000). No calculations of cost savings in prevented nosocomial infections made.
19: Kurup, et al., 2010, Singapore	Educational meetings Audit and feedback Reminders Mass media *Duration* 12 months *Infection control measure* Hand hygiene Patient screening: Active Surveillance Testing (AST) Patient isolation *Design* Before and after design	**Behavioural** Between groups: compliance in performing all study-related swab activities appeared better in the Surgical ICU (SICU), but the difference between the ICUs was not statistically significant **Clinical** AST detected MRSA in at least 137 of the 653 patients (21.0%). In contrast, clinical cultures for MSRA were positive in only 12 patients (1.8%). No significant overall improvement in detection rate when including axilla and groin sites in the AST. No improvement in detection rate in patients admitted to Medical ICU (MICU), slight improvement in SICU. Inclusion of axilla and groin sites did not affect the MRSA detection rate during the ICU stay and at discharge, both overall and when the ICUs were analysed individually. Between groups: the rate of MRSA colonization detected by AST during the ICU stay or at ICU discharge was higher in SICU than MICU. No significant difference in MRSA infection rate pre- and post-intervention in both ICUs combined or when analysed individually. Less variability in MRSA rates post-intervention; the 95% CI at post-intervention was narrower than that at pre-intervention. Septic shock at ICU admission was more common in MRSA-colonized patients than in non-colonized patients. **Financial** Detection of MRSA at any point was associated with longer pre-ICU length of stay, longer duration of antibiotic therapy, and longer ICU length of stay.

Author, Year, Country	Implementation strategy	Reported Findings (behavioural, clinical, financial)
20: Lederer, et al., 2009, United States	Distribution of educational materials Audit and feedback Reminders Mass media Clinical multidisciplinary teams *Implementation foundation* Theoretical and empirical: CDC recommendations and observed low compliance *Duration* 10 months *Infection control measure* Hand hygiene *Design* Before and after design Time series design	**Behavioural** Increased hand hygiene compliance with sustained rates greater than 90%. **Clinical** MRSA healthcare-associated rate decreased, representing a 54% reduction associated with improved compliance.
21: Lee, et al., 2009, Canada	Educational meetings Technology-supported *Implementation foundation* Empirical: SARS outbreak in Toronto in 2003, the Ontario Ministry of Labour mandated an IC education programme for all Mount Sinai Hospital staff *Duration* 1 month *Infection control measure* Hand hygiene Personal protective equipment *Design* Before and after design	**Behavioural** Non-significant increase in hand hygiene compliance on inpatient medical units. Annual volume of ABHRS purchased by the hospital. **Clinical** Significant decrease in nosocomial MRSA acquisition rate per 100 admission MRSA exposure days. Significant decrease in nosocomial MRSA acquisition rate per 100 unprotected MRSA exposure days.
22: Liebowitz & Blunt, 2008, United Kingdom	Educational meetings Audit and feedback Clinical multidisciplinary teams *Implementation foundation* Theoretical: prior research, no studies have been published in which the use of both classes of antibiotics has been discouraged. No foundation for content educational activity. *Duration* 2 months *Infection control measure* Medication *Design* Time series design	**Behavioural** Hospital-wide decrease in level of dispensing of intervention drugs. ICU-specific decrease in level of dispensing of intervention drugs. **Clinical** Decrease in level of MRSA-positive screenings (no statistical test). MRSA colonization in screening specimens from high-risk patients decreased. Decrease in level of MRSA-positive screenings (no statistical test).

Author, Year, Country	Implementation strategy	Reported Findings (behavioural, clinical, financial)
23: Madaras-Kelly, et al., 2006, United States	Reminders Technology-supported *Implementation foundation* Theoretical: The Society for Healthcare Epidemiology of America (SHEA) recommendations *Duration* 12 months *Infection control measure* Medication *Design* Time series design	**Behavioural** Non-significant decrease of overall AB use. Significant decreases in the use of several antibiotics. Significant differences between non-antibiotic variables: purchase of chlorhexidine skin preparation increased; the number of ventilator days, purchase of alcohol foam, and the nursing staff ratio decreased. Total fluoroquinolone and levofloxacin use decreased significantly. **Clinical** Decrease in nosocomial MRSA infections (not statistically tested).
24: Miyachi, et al., 2007, Japan	Local opinion leaders Audit and feedback Mass media *Implementation foundation* Theoretical: prior research on link nurses in large hospitals *Duration* 76 months *Infection control measure* Hand hygiene Other, non-specified *Design* Before and after design	**Behavioural** Significant increase in arithmetic mean of monthly consumption of the liquid soap. **Clinical** Percentage of MRSA in Staphylococcus Aureus increased. Monthly counts of new MRSA cases dropped in 15 of 25 wards. Significant decrease in the monthly number of inpatient admissions.
25: Nicastri, et al., 2008, Italy	Educational outreach Clinical multidisciplinary teams *Infection control measure* Medication *Design* Time series design	**Behavioural** Significant reduction of defined daily doses (DDD) of cephalosporins. A clinical audit 12 months after introduction of Antibiotic Stewardship Program (ASP) protocol showed >90% adherence by the physicians (no statistical tests). **Clinical** Significant decrease of MRSA isolations. Significant correlation between MRSA monthly prevalence rates and reduction of crude DDD use of third-generation cephalosporins. Significant reduction of isolation of MRSA from surgical site infection (SSI) and Blood Stream Infection (BSI). Significant decrease in MRSA prevalence among Staphylococcus Aureus associated with SSI. Significant reduction of MRSA prevalence both in Staphylococcus Aureus associated BSI and in the respiratory specimens of patients affected by ventilator-associated pneumonia (VAP) in ICUs.
26: O'Brien, et al., 2008, United States	Educational meetings Reminders Technology-supported *Implementation foundation* Theoretical: SHEA recommendations *Duration* 12 months *Infection control measure* Patient screening *Design* Before and after design	**Behavioural** Post-IT admission culture rate in the telemetry unit was >91% in the ICU and >97% in the Intermediate Care unit. Employee satisfaction with the MRSA surveillance protocol was measured by self-assessment survey; 88% of the respondents were "fully satisfied", the remaining 12% were "satisfied". (No statistical test use). Increased efficiency of staff time use. **Clinical** Overall decrease in the rate of MRSA acquisition in the pre-IT period compared with the post-IT period was statistically significant. Significant decrease in 2 of 3 unit specific comparisons before and after IT implementation.

Author, Year, Country	Implementation strategy	Reported Findings (behavioural, clinical, financial)
27: Peterson, et al., 2010, United States	Distribution of educational materials Educational meetings Educational outreach Local opinion leaders Audit and feedback Reminders Changes in physical structure, facilities and equipment Technology-supported *Implementation foundation* Theoretical: Institute for Healthcare Improvement's (IHI) five components to MRSA control *Duration* 24 months *Infection control measure* Patient screening *Design* Before and after design	**Behavioural** Screening compliance increased to >90%, and sustained >90% after programme. **Clinical** Decrease in MRSA transmission (from colonization to infection). Decrease in overall MRSA BSIs by the end of the first year. **Financial** Programme cost represented a net expense of $15-$16 per admission. Eliminating 50 infections led to a reduction of nearly $1,200,000 in medical expenditures, which was at least cost-neutral.
28: Robert, et al., 2006, France	Distribution of educational materials Reminders Mass media *Implementation foundation* Theoretical: observational studies indicated that isolation precautions were poorly implemented outside ICUs *Duration* 3 months *Infection control measure* Patient isolation (Flagging records) *Design* Before and after design	**Behavioural** Within groups: medical and nursing staff reported that they knew the MRSA status of patients in 87% of cases in the control period, and in 96% of cases in the intervention period. Medical and nursing records were flagged significantly more often in the intervention period than in the control period. The set of four organizational measures was implemented more frequently in the intervention period than in the control period. The same observation was made when each measure was evaluated separately. When considering only ICUs and rehabilitation units, i.e. wards with MRSA rounds, there was also a significant increase in the implementation of isolation precautions; signs posted on the door more often, use of gowns increased, use of dedicated materials increased, availability of alcohol hand rub increased, and proportion of MRSA patients in private rooms increased. There was no significant increase in the proportion of healthcare workers informed of the MRSA status of patients or in the proportion of flagged records.
29: Thomas, et al., 2005, United States	Reminders Mass media *Implementation foundation* Theoretical: research on hand hygiene posters *Duration* 12 months *Infection control measure* Hand hygiene *Design* Before and after design	**Behavioural** Increase in hand hygiene compliance over all units. Participants agreed that, overall, posters had a positive influence on hand hygiene behaviour within the units. More so when poster displayed 'human qualities' or promoted action (instead of just awareness).

Table 2. Characteristics of the studies included in the systematic review

3.2 Study design

Among the included studies, there was one randomized controlled trial (RCT) (1). In eight studies, a time series design was used (2, 9, 14, 15, 17, 22, 23, 25), and in fourteen studies a before and after design was used (3, 4, 5, 7, 10-12, 18, 19, 21, 26-29). Five studies applied a combination of time series and before and after design (6, 8, 13, 16, 20).

3.3 MRSA prevention and control measures

Different measures were implemented to prevent or control MRSA. In some studies a single MRSA prevention or control measure was implemented, in others a bundle of measures was implemented. *Hand hygiene* was implemented as a stand-alone measure in seven studies (4, 5, 7, 10, 13, 20, 29) and as part of a bundle of measures in eleven studies (1, 3, 6, 8, 11, 14, 16, 17, 19, 21, 24). *Environmental hygiene* was implemented as a stand-alone measure in one study (12) and as part of a bundle of measures in two studies (1, 17). The use of *personal protective equipment* such as gloves or gowns was implemented as part of a bundle of measures in four studies (1, 3, 16, 21); it was implemented as a stand-alone measure in none of the studies. *Medication*, or the correct use of antibiotics, was implemented as a stand-alone measure in six studies (2, 9, 15, 22, 23, 25); in none of the included studies was it part of a bundle of measures. In two studies (26, 27), *patient screening* was implemented as a stand-alone measure, and in six studies (3, 8, 11, 16, 17, 19) it formed part of a bundle of measures that was implemented. *HCW screening* was implemented only as part of a bundle of measures, in one study (17). *Patient isolation* was implemented as stand-alone measure in one study (28), and was part of a bundle of measures in five studies (3, 6, 16, 18, 19).

3.4 Implementation strategies and their foundation

Various strategies were used to implement the MRSA prevention and control measures. Most implementation strategies are set up because of the empirical observation of non-adherence to clinical guidelines, thus creating an impediment to successful MRSA control. The theoretical foundation of the chosen strategies is often unclear, or not specified.

Most studies, 24 out of 29, combined different elements (1-17, 19, 20, 22, 24, 25, 26, 27). In five studies the implementation strategy consisted of one component (18, 21, 23, 28, 29). The strategies used are summarized below:

- *Audit and feedback* was performed and given by trained nurses or auditors, infection control specialists, or multidisciplinary teams (nineteen studies: 1, 2, 4-6, 8, 9, 11-17, 19, 20, 22, 24, 27).
- *Reminders* were used in eighteen studies (3-9, 11, 16-20, 23, 26, 27, 28, 29), for example pop-ups, fluorescent tape drawing attention to hand-cleaning facilities, posters or messages clipped to patient charts.
- *Educational meetings* were held, for example to inform HCWs about the measure or to demonstrate new working methods or hygienic practices (seventeen studies: 1, 3-6, 8, 12-16, 19, 21, 22, 26, 27).
- *Mass media* were used in fourteen studies (3, 5-8, 10, 11, 13, 17, 19, 20, 24, 28, 29); posters, and to a lesser extent brochures or flyers, were used to remind or instruct HCWs about the implemented measures. Role models (hospital management or

leaders) were sometimes depicted, or HCWs were involved in the creation of the poster (11, 17, 29).

- *Technology* was used in ten studies (1, 3, 5, 13, 17, 18, 21, 23, 26, 27), in the context of education (PowerPoint presentations, training via DVD), electronic order forms, pop-ups assisting medication choice or screening of patients.
- *Changes in physical structure, facilities and equipment* were applied in eight studies (4, 5, 6, 8, 11, 12, 16, 27). These changes included strategically placed hand disinfectant dispensers, equipping HCWs with pocket bottles of hand disinfectant, or new cleaning materials (cloths), the bundling of protective gear and the availability of a test kit for screening.
- *Educational materials* were distributed in eight studies (4, 5, 8, 10, 13, 17, 20, 27). Brochures, newsletters or instructional pocket cards were given to HCWs, often focused on applying correct (hand) hygiene.
- *Local opinion leaders* guided the implementation process in six studies (1, 4, 5, 15, 24, 27), sometimes by reinforcing good infection control, or acting as a link worker between the professions and management.
- *Clinical multidisciplinary teams* were used in five studies (2, 6, 20, 22, 25) to guide the implementation of a MRSA control measure. Via cooperation or consultation these teams supported the measures taken, for example by approving antibiotic prescriptions.
- *Educational outreach* was carried out in five studies (6, 10, 15, 25, 27) to teach HCWs on-site and sometimes on demand how to apply the implemented measure.
- *Rewards* for correctly performing the implemented measures were given in two studies (4, 16), either to individuals directly after observing correct behaviour, or to groups based on periodic adherence results.
- A *patient-mediated intervention* was implemented in one study (10); patients and visitors were actively addressed to perform the desired hand hygiene behaviour and motivate adherence among staff.
- *AB permission/formulary* was applied in one study (2) where permission to use a certain antibiotic was required.

3.5 Outcomes

We classified the reported effects into three categories: adherence to the measures, reduction of costs and reduction of MRSA.

In twelve studies (1-3, 7, 9, 12, 13, 17, 18, 24, 28) significant improvements (e.g. fewer prescriptions for antibiotics, more correctly executed hand hygiene, reduced expenditure on materials) in adherence to the MRSA control measures were observed. Similar positive results were observed in fourteen studies (4-6, 8, 10, 14-16, 20, 22, 23, 25, 27, 29), although these results were not statistically tested. In one of the studies (16), negative effects were observed: adherence to the measures increased in the first year but decreased thereafter.

Acquiring a hospital-associated infection (HAI) results in a longer length of stay for the patient and poses many additional *costs*. Therefore, reductions in length of stay are an important outcome associated with decreased MRSA infection rates. Cost savings, or at least cost-neutral intervention effects, were observed in four studies (5, 10, 15, 27). On the other hand, increased isolation and increased expenditure also posed costs, as described in one study (18). However, in this study, these increased costs were not compared to possible savings due to prevented infections. In another study (19), improved screening led to increased lengths of stay (pre-ICU and ICU), because MRSA detection increased.

In nine studies (8, 12-14, 16, 17, 21, 25, 26), significant clinical improvements were reported, including MRSA prevalence, MRSA infection rates and susceptibility rates. Positive effects were also observed in eleven other studies (2, 5, 7, 10, 11, 15, 20, 22-24, 27), although these results were not statistically tested.

4. Conclusion and discussion

The results of our review show that in most cases hygiene experts or an infection control team (nurse, infectologist, microbiologist) are the developers of implementation strategies. These strategies are driven by empirical observations and audits. The theoretical foundation of the chosen strategies is often unclear. No references to theories and models of human behaviour are made. However, some articles indicated that a literature search was carried out.

When looking at the implementation strategies, we can conclude that in most cases a multi-faceted strategy was carried out. This strategy entails a combination of several activities:

- Education or training modules for HCWs, sometimes mandatory, taking various forms (DVDs, PowerPoint presentations, posters, meetings, brochures) to improve hand hygiene and compliance with protocols.
- Inspections of the adherence to the safety programme and of hand washing behaviour via audits, on-site instructions, and observations by hygiene experts or trained auditors. Results were communicated to management and demonstrated via feedback meetings.
- Environmental interventions (red lines at the entrance to high-risk wards, talking walls) to remind HCWs to behave safely in that particular area and to provide antibiotic policy support via guidelines and cards.

The implementation pathway consists of *education-inspection-feedback* rounds; unfortunately it is unclear who is responsible for the management of the intervention strategies and who invests in these activities. No business model seems to underpin the entire implementation strategy.

To answer the research question about the effect of the implementation strategies, we reviewed the research designs that were used to measure their effects. In general, quasi-experimental designs (before and after and time series designs) underpin the research activities. Implementation outcomes are usually measured in a before-and-after design, where they do not concern antibiotic use, and therefore provide little insight into temporal changes in implementation results or adherence. HCWs are the main target group in the research designs. It is unclear who these designs seek to manage (researchers, HCWs, management) in their execution or whether a project manager is responsible for this. Trained nurses or infection control teams are sometimes used. In most cases quantitative instruments are used to measure the effects on knowledge and behaviour (questionnaires, self-reporting of behaviour, material use, and hand hygiene) and on a reduction in MRSA and antibiotic doses (lab statistics). The effects on cost/benefits were sometimes measured, addressing utilizations such as reduced length of stay. In general the outcomes are promising. However, the extent to which the outcomes are related to the implementation strategies is not clear, except for the routine screenings and reduced MRSA rates. The outcomes on cost-savings are especially hard to analyse. It remains unclear what is measured, how it is measured and to what purpose. Long-term effects are almost never addressed.

Due to several shortcomings in research designs, the overall impact of the implementation strategies could not be measured sufficiently. Shortcomings in the research designs include, for example, the one-sided focus on HCWs. We know from prior research (Verhoeven et al., 2009) and from behaviour change models that not only is a multifaceted strategy needed to change safety behaviour, but that a multi-perspective stakeholder view (HCWs, infection experts, patients, the safety policy of the management of the organization) is necessary to obtain insight into the cost/benefits of the implementation strategy and to discuss the long-term implications of the strategy for the organization and workflow (Kukafka et al., 2003). This requires a theory or innovation-driven approach that grounds the implementation strategy, enabling an assessment of which activities are successful for whom (patient, HCWs, management) and what the interaction effects of the different components of the strategy are.

Another shortcoming concerns the chosen study designs. Authors of the included studies refer to the difficulties in matching control and intervention groups, the high rates of drop-outs and the low volume of included respondents, and confounding factors that cannot be excluded. These shortcomings are well-known impediments related to RCTs and the self-reported behaviours. In fact, these shortcomings cannot be avoided due to the study of real-time behaviours and contextual factors that influence these behaviours. Therefore, these factors should not be regarded as nuisances, as the authors do; they are the key issues that are important in implementation studies aimed at changing culture and behaviour. For example, some authors reported problems in implementing the activities due to a lack of resources (a result of the economic downturn) to manage the implementation and problems with measuring the effects of each component of the implementation strategy due to financial constraints. A lack of transparent funding models and lack of management support made the participation of different institutes or wards in the research projects problematic, resulting in only small pilot projects being carried out. These financial barriers should not be reported as shortcomings; rather, these factors should be determined by the key stakeholders and considered as critical factors for changing behaviour and the culture of safety in hospitals or other institutions.

In addition, some authors reported a lack of commitment on the part of nursing personnel to participate in the implementation projects. It appeared that some personnel were uncertain about the implications of several measures. For example, they were concerned that patients would not feel as clean after being washed with wipes instead of soap and water. The level of commitment of HCWs and management is one of the main conditions for success in programmes for innovation or change. The impediments indicate that the implementation strategies are expert-driven rather than stakeholder-centred. Changing safety behaviour in hospitals is first and foremost a cultural problem of management and staff, which requires that implementation strategies should address that level.

How to improve the implementation strategies? Given the fact that the implementation strategies influenced the attitude and knowledge of HCWs in a positive way, that intentions to behave safely increased, and that MRSA rates decreased in several studies, the question is how to boost the impact of the implementation strategies. *Education-inspection-feedback* rounds could be one way to do this.

Based on prior experience in infection management control and on information gathered from other studies of innovation management (Cain & Mittman, 2002; Rogers, 2003), we argue that the participation of staff and management is crucial to the development and implementation of interventions, to increase applicability, accountability and ownership and to create a fit between the proposed activities and the culture of the organization (Van Gemert et al., in press). In addition, both positive and negative incentives are needed to encourage staff to do the right things at the right times. Change agents and demonstration of best practices will improve the incorporation of safety behaviour. To enhance the transparency of the implementation programme and strategies, communication of results or key factors for success should be available to staff. Communication should include insights into results related to infection management (prevalence and incidence rates of MRSA, identification of increasing/decreasing trends), the business model underpinning the programme (resources, investments, additional costs) and benchmarking (how are we doing and what are others doing?). It is also important to demonstrate to the management and staff that the investment costs of the intervention can be less than the costs of not adopting an MRSA-infection control programme.

Another point of attention is the use of media to implement the strategies. Even though evidence of the usefulness and effectiveness of computerized decision support or reminders exists (Grimshaw et al., 2004), it is not often used. We found that in ten studies DVDs, PowerPoint presentations, educational programmes available online or on CD-ROM, and electronic alerts or reminders were used. This is rather remarkable in our Internet-driven world. Web-based communications systems in particular can increase staff knowledge and provide access to accurate, adequate and easy to understand information (Kreps & Neuhauser, 2010). In prior and on-going research projects aimed at cross-border infection control (MRSA-net; EurSafety Health-net) we developed stakeholder-driven, web-based communication systems, based on national infection control standards, to support staff and patient behaviours (see for example Verhoeven et al., 2009). This resulted in fewer errors, time savings and also appropriate behaviour by HCWs.

5. References

Baldwin, N. S., Gilpin, D. F., Tunney, M. M., Kearney, M. P., Crymble, L., Cardwell, C., & Hughes, C. M. (2010). Cluster randomised controlled trial of an infection control education and training intervention programme focusing on meticillin-resistant Staphylococcus aureus in nursing homes for older people. *Journal of Hospital Infection,* 76 (1), pp. 36-41.

Bassetti, M., Righi, E., Ansaldi, F., Molinari, M. P., Rebesco, B., McDermott, J. L., Fasce, R., Mussap, M., Icardi, G., Pallavicini, F. B., & Viscoli, C. (2009). Impact of limited cephalosporin use on prevalence of methicillin-resistant Staphylococcus aureus in the intensive care unit. *Journal of Chemotherapy,* 21 (6), pp. 633-638.

Boyce, J. M., Havill, N. L., Dumigan, D. G., Golebiewske, M., Balogun, O., Rizvani, R. (2009). Monitoring the effectiveness of hospital cleaningpractices by use of an adenoise triphosphate bioluminescence assay. *Infection Control and Hospital Epidemiology,* 30 (7), pp. 678-684.

Burkitt, K. H., Sinkowitz-Cochran, R. L., Obrosky, D. S., Cuerdon, T., Miller, L. J., Jain, R., Jernigan, J. A., & Fine, M. J. (2010). Survey of employee knowledge and attitudes before and after a multicenter Veterans' Administration quality improvement initiative to reduce nosocomial methicillin-resistant Staphylococcus aureus infections. *American Journal of Infection Control,* 38 (4), pp. 274-282.

Cain, M. & Mittman, R. (2002). *Diffusion of innovation in health care.* California HealthCare Foundation, 1-929008-97-X.

Camins, B. C., & Fraser, V. J. (2005). Reducing the risk of health care-associated infections by complying with CDC hand hygiene guidelines. *The Joint Commission Journal on Quality and Patient Safety,* 31 (3), pp. 173-179.

Carboneau, C., Benge, E., Jaco, M. T., & Robinson, M. (2010). A lean Six Sigma team increases hand hygiene compliance and reduces hospital-acquired MRSA infections by 51%. *Journal for healthcare quality : official publication of the National Association for Healthcare Quality,* 32 (4), pp. 61-70.

Cheng, V. C. C., Tai, J. W. M., Chan, W. M., Lau, E. H. Y., Chan, J. F. W., To, K. K. W., Li, I. W. S., Ho, P. L., & Yuen, K. Y. (2009). Sequential introduction of single room isolation and hand hygiene campaign in the control of methicillin-resistant Staphylococcus aureus in intensive care unit. *BMC Infectious Diseases,* 10, 263.

Centre for Reviews and Dissemination (2001). CRD's Guidance for those Carrying Out or Commissioning Reviews. In K. S. Khan, G. t. Riet, J. Glanville, A. J. Sowden & J. Kleijnen (Eds.), *Reviews of Research on Effectiveness.* (2nd ed.): University of York.

Davis, C. R. (2010a). Infection-free surgery: How to improve hand-hygience compliance and eradicate methicillin-resistant Staphylococcus aureus from surgical wards. *Annals of the Royal College of Surgeons of England,* 92 (4), pp. 316-319.

Eveillard, M., Lancien, E., De Lassence, A., Branger, C., Barnaud, G., Benlolo, J. A., & Joly-Guillou, M. L. (2006). Impact of the reinforcement of a Methicillin-Resistant Staphylococcus aureus Control Programme: A 3-year evaluation by several indicators in a French University Hospital. *European Journal of Epidemiology,* 21 (7), pp. 551-558.

Fowler, S., Webber, A., Cooper, B. S., Phimister, A., Price, K., Carter, Y., Kibbler, C. C., Simpson, A. J. H., & Stone, S. P. (2007). Successful use of feedback to improve antibiotic prescribing and reduce Clostridium difficile infection: a controlled interrupted time series. *Journal of Antimicrobial Chemotherapy,* 59 (5), pp. 990-995.

Fogg, B. J. (2003). *Persuasive technology: using computers to change what we think and do.* Morgan Kaufmann, 978-1-55860-643-2, San Francisco.

Foy, R., Eccles, M. &Grimshaw, J. (2001) Why does primary care need more implementation research? *Family Practice,* 18(4), pp. 53-355.

Gagné, D., Bédard, G., & Maziade, P. J. (2010). Systematic patients' hand disinfection: impact on meticillin-resistant Staphylococcus aureus infection rates in a community hospital. *Journal of Hospital Infection,* 75 (4), pp. 269-272.

Gillespie, E. E., ten Berk de Boer, F. J., Stuart, R. L., Buist, M. D., & Wilson, J. M. (2007). A sustained reduction in the transmission of methicillin resistant Staphylococcus aureus in an intensive care unit. *Critical care and resuscitation: journal of the Australasian Academy of Critical Care Medicine,* 9 (2), pp. 161-165.

Goodman, E. R., Platt, R., Bass, R., Onderdonk, A. B., Yokoe, D. S., & Huang, S. S. (2008). Impact of an environmental cleaning intervention on the presence of methicillin-resistant Staphylococcus aureus and vancomycin-resistant enterococci on surfaces in intensive care unit rooms. *Infection Control and Hospital Epidemiology,* 29 (7), pp. 593-599.

Grayson, M. L., Jarvie, L. J., Martin, R., Johnson, P. D. R., Jodoin, M. E., McMullan, C., Gregory, R. H. C., Bellis, K., Cunnington, K., Wilson, F. L., Quin, D., & Kelly, A. M. (2008). Significant reductions in methicillin-resistant Staphylococcus aureus bacteraemia and clinical isolates associated with a multisite, hand hygiene culture-change program and subsequent successful statewide roll-out. *Medical Journal of Australia,* 188 (11), pp. 633-640.

Harrington, G., Watson, K., Bailey, M., Land, G., Borrell, S., Houston, L., Kehoe, R., Bass, P., Cockroft, E., Marshall, C., Mijch, A., & Spelman, D. (2007). Reduction in hospitalwide incidence of infection or colonization with methicillin-resistant Staphylococcus aureus with use of antimicrobial hand-hygiene gel and statistical process control charts. *Infection Control and Hospital Epidemiology,* 28 (7), pp. 837-844.

Holder, C., & Zellinger, M. (2009). Daily bathing with chlorhexidine in the ICU to prevent central line-associated bloodstream infections. *Journal of Clinical Outcomes Management,* 16 (11), pp. 509-513.

Huang, S. S., Yokoe, D. S., Hinrichsen, V. L., Spurchise, L. S., Datta, R., Miroshnik, I., & Platt, R. (2006). Impact of routine intensive care unit surveillance cultures and resultant barrier precautions on hospital-wide methicillin-resistant Staphylococcus aureus bacteremia. *Clinical Infectious Diseases,* 43 (8), pp. 971-978.

Johnson, P. D. R., Martin, R., Burrell, L. J., Grabsch, E. A., Kirsa, S. W., O'Keefe, J., Mayall, B. C., Edmonds, D., Barr, W., Bolger, C., Naidoo, H., & Grayson, M. L. (2005). Efficacy of an alcohol/chlorhexidine hand hygiene program in a hospital with high rates of nosocomial methicillin-resistant Staphylococcus aureus (MRSA) infection. *Medical Journal of Australia,* 183 (10), pp. 509-514.

Kho, A. N., Dexter, P. R., Warvel, J. S., Belsito, A. W., Commiskey, M., Wilson, S. J., Hui, S. L., & McDonald, C. J. (2008). An effective computerized reminder for contact isolation of patients colonized or infected with resistant organisms. *International Journal of Medical Informatics,* 77 (3), pp. 194-198.

Kreps, G. L. & Neuhauser, L. (2010). New directions in ehealth communication: opportunities and challenges. *Patient Education and Counseling, 78,* 329-336.

Kukafka, R., Johnson, S. B., Linfante, A., & Allegrante, J.P. (2003). Grounding a new information technology implementation framework in behavioral science: a systematic analysis of the literature on IT use. *Journal of Biomedical Informatics,* 36, pp. 218-227.

Kurup, A., Chlebicka, N., Tan, K. Y., Chen, E. X., Oon, L., Ling, T. A., Ling, M. L., & Hong, J. L. G. (2010). Active surveillance testing and decontamination strategies in intensive care units to reduce methicillin-resistant Staphylococcus aureus infections. *American Journal of Infection Control,* 38 (5), pp. 361-367.

Lederer Jr, J. W., Best, D., & Hendrix, V. (2009). A comprehensive hand hygiene approach to reducing MRSA health care-associated infections. *Joint Commission journal on quality and patient safety / Joint Commission Resources,* 35 (4), pp. 180-185.

Lee, T. C., Moore, C., Raboud, J. M., Muller, M. P., Green, K., Tong, A., . . . Willey, B. (2009). Impact of a mandatory infection control education program on nosocomial acquisition of methicillin-resistant Staphylococcus aureus. *Infection Control and Hospital Epidemiology,* 30 (3), pp. 249-256.

Liebowitz, L. D., & Blunt, M. C. (2008). Modification in prescribing practices for third-generation cephalosporins and ciprofloxacin is associated with a reduction in meticillin-resistant Staphylococcus aureus bacteraemia rate. *Journal of Hospital Infection,* 69 (4), pp. 328-336.

Madaras-Kelly, K. J., Remington, R. E., Lewis, P. G., & Stevens, D. L. (2006a). Evaluation of an intervention designed to decrease the rate of nosocomial methicillin-resistant Staphylococcus aureus infection by encouraging decreased fluoroquinolone use. *Infection Control and Hospital Epidemiology,* 27, pp. 155-169.

Miyachi, H., Furuya, H., Umezawa, K., Itoh, Y., Ohshima, T., Miyamoto, M., & Asai, S. (2007). Controlling methicillin-resistant Staphylococcus aureus by stepwise implementation of preventive strategies in a university hospital: impact of a link-nurse system on the basis of multidisciplinary approaches. *American Journal of Infection Control,* 35 (2), pp. 115-121.

Nicastri, E., Leone, S., Petrosillo, N., Ballardini, M., Pisanelli, C., Magrini, P., Cerquetani, F., Ippolito, G., Comandini, E., Narciso, P., & Meledandri, M. (2008). Decrease of methicillin resistant Staphylococcus aureus prevalence after introduction of a surgical antibiotic prophylaxis protocol in an Italian hospital. *New Microbiologica,* 31 (4), pp. 519-525.

O'Brien, J. M., Greenhouse, P. K., Schafer, J. J., Wheeler, C. A., Titus, A., Pontzer, R. E., O'Neill, M. M., & Wolf, D. (2008). Implementing and improving the efficiency of a methicillin-resistant Staphylococcus aureus active surveillance program using information technology. *American Journal of Infection Control,* 36 (3 SUPPL.).

Peterson, A., Marquez, P., Terashita, D., Burwell, L., & Mascola, L. (2010). Hospital methicillin-resistant Staphylococcus aureus active surveillance practices in Los Angeles County: Implications of legislation-based infection control, 2008. *American Journal of Infection Control,* 38 (8), pp. 653-656.

Pittet, D., Hugonnet, S., Harbarth, S., Mourouga, P., Sauvan, V., & Perneger, T. V. (2000). Effectiveness of a hospital-wide programme to improve compliance with hand hygiene. *The Lancet,* 356 (9238), pp. 1307-1312.

Robert, J., Renard, L., Grenet, K., Galerne, E., Dal Farra, A., Aussant, M., & Jarlier, V. (2006). Implementation of isolation precautions: Role of a targeted information flyer. *Journal of Hospital Infection,* 62 (2), pp. 163-165.

Rogers, E. M. (2003). *Diffusion of innovations* (5th ed.). New York, NY: Free Press.

Sengers, I. J. M., Ouwerkerk, Y. M. v., & Terpstra, S. (Eds.). (2000). *Hygiëne en infectiepreventie* (4th ed.). Maarssen: Elsevier Gezondheidszorg.

Thomas, M., Gillespie, W., Krauss, J., Harrison, S., Medeiros, R., Hawkins, M., Maclean, R., & Woeltje, K. F. (2005). Focus group data as a tool in assessing effectiveness of a hand hygiene campaign. *American Journal of Infection Control,* 33 (6), pp. 368-373.

Van Gemert-Pijnen, J., Hendrix, R., Van der Palen, J., & Schellens, P. J. (2005). Performance of methicillin-resistant Staphyloccus aureus protocols in Dutch hospitals. *American Journal of Infection Control,* 33 (7), pp. 377-384.

Van Gemert-Pijnen J.E.W.C., Nijland N., Ossebaard H.C., et al. (2011). A Holistic framework to improve the uptake and impact of eHealth technologies. *Journal of Medical Internet Research,* 13(4): e111.

Verhoeven, F., Steehouder, M. F., Hendrix, R. M. G., & van Gemert-Pijnen, J. E. W. C. (2009). Factors affecting health care workers' adoption of a website with infection control guidelines. *International Journal of Medical Informatics,* 78 (10), pp. 663-678.

Part 3

Practice Improvement

7

Implementation of a Need Based Participatory Training Program on Hospital Infection Control: A Clinical Practice Improvement Project

Christopher Sudhaker
MCON, Mangalore, Manipal University
India

1. Introduction

Infection control education has been a core component of infection control programs since they were established (*Scheckler et al., 1998; Department of Health and Ageing, 2004*) and remains a constant feature in the modern healthcare context. Education is a pivotal strategy used to address problems identified through surveillance of infection or to improve infection control practice.(*Dubbert et al, 1990; Scheckler et al, 1998; Turner et al, 1999*). It is clear that simple educational efforts are of minimal benefit and that while a number of interventions may achieve a short-term effect, few have a measurable, prolonged effect (Larson, 1997). Research efforts relating to infection control education as a control measure; have focused on evaluating the effectiveness of a variety of strategies (Kim et al, 2001).

While debate continues regarding the extent and quality of infection control education as a component of professional curricula, it is a requisite element of the orientation process in each healthcare facility. This process ensures that all members of the healthcare team are provided with basic infection control education and training on entry to the healthcare organization. Basic infection control information such as standard and additional precautions, safe use and disposal of sharps, waste segregation and minimization and staff health issues such as vaccination should be imparted through continuing education. Research efforts relating to infection control education as a control measure; have focused on evaluating the effectiveness of a variety of strategies (Kim et al., 2001). Studies often describe the effects of educational initiatives in combination with dissemination of data derived from surveillance initiatives such as practice audits (Goetz et al., 1999 and Chandra and Milind, 2001).

Establishing appropriate Infection control staffing levels for hospitals should be considered as a priority in every health care setting (Hoffman, 1997). Multiple logistic regression analysis found that larger hospitals (*OR, 1.6; 95% CI, 1.2-2.0; P = .003) and teaching hospitals (OR, 3.7 95% CI, 1.2- 11.8; P = .02*) were associated with the presence of VRE. Hospitals were less likely to have VRE when infection control staff frequently contacted physicians and nurses for reports of new infections (*OR, 0.5; 95% CI, 0.3- 0.7; P = .02*) and there were in-service programs for updating nursing and ancillary staff on current infection control practices. Prevention of hospital associated infection remains biggest challenge for health care providers in the developed countries where there are adequate resources and trained staff. We can envisage the hard-fought task of countries like India with minimum resources and non-availability of trained infection control personnel. It is almost impossible to have 1.5 infection control practicing nurses for every 200 beds. Most of the Indian hospitals are not even near to the recommended staffing criteria.

All health care professionals are responsible for ensuring that they consistently deliver high quality clinically effective care and protect their patient from the risk of infection. To do this they need clinical credibility, leadership skills, ability to participate and lead relevant practices and whole range of skills associated with implementation of infection control programs. This ability may be enhanced though continuing education. It was observed that infection control practice and ongoing primary surveillance at unit level is the most challenging task and almost impossible with present staffing model.

The Purpose of the study is to empower selected core group nurses with participatory training on hospital infection control with a view to train other nurses in hospital. Thus providing facilities for ongoing training program for sustained improvement in infection control practice.

This study addresses the following questions regarding improving infection control nursing education and practices in the Indian setting;

1. Why educational programs on hospital infection control are a Herculean task to implement?
2. How to develop an effective and sustainable hospital infection control educational program to empower the nurses working in a selected hospital?
3. Will nurses on ward develop ownership and awareness of infection control activities?
4. How does the culture of the clinical environment influence infection control practice?

Present study is conducted in several hospitals like private multi-specialty ,rural suburban and government settings of Udupi and Dhakshina Kannada district of Karnataka, India.

2. Methodology

The main strategy of the participatory training was needs-driven, internally and determined exercises to facilitate this, the approaches included were;

1. Developing human resources by empowering them with the knowledge required to perform infection control practices and transfer this knowledge to other nurses working with them without any extra effort and cost so that individual participants, the organization and the research project would benefit.
2. Inspiring participants, so that they are motivated to use creativity in developing participatory approaches and techniques.

According to Rao et al.,(1997), participation is closely linked to power and Knowledge. Sources of power and the distinction between dominant knowledge and popular knowledge are important to understand to contextualize participation. *Power in the society is exercised through knowledge. The culture of silence associated with powerlessness is essentially related to lack of articulation and domination of dominant knowledge over people's knowledge.* This is possible by building each individual participant's communication, leadership, small group teaching and facilitating skills and finally developing professional approach towards prevention of Hospital associated infections.

The paradigm shift associated with participation, essentially means, providing space and articulation for popular knowledge, practices and analysis. This helps the powerless to exercise their control over knowledge generation, distribution and will be able to control knowledge and power, there by demystifying dominant knowledge. According to Kiessling, (2003) participation is also seen as an integral part of empowerment process. Thus participation is part of empowerment strategy. Continuous professional development also includes learning from others. The word participation stands for the action or state of taking part with others in an activity'. The fundamental basis of all participatory learning methods is that learners are active participants instead of passive listeners or readers.

The present study of participatory education will empower the nurses by building their capacity and to transmit their current knowledge and skill to prevent infection in low resource settings. During participation the nurses will be exposed to in interactive education, participatory seminars, workshops and other nursing education activities. In their true sense, participatory approaches are important tools to promote practice change, develop the capacity for collective action and reflection, and ensure that people involved are in the decision making process especially in Low resource setting and to enhance power to alter professional practice (*Sudhaker, 2005; Kiessling, 2003; Upendranadh,1997; Brigham and Foster; Hodson, 1991*) When adults participate in learning activities, they bring many years of experiences with them. They view new material through the lens of these experiences *(Baird, Schneier and Laird, 1983*). As adults continue to acquire newer knowledge and skills, they must integrate new learning with prior learning. When contradictions or dilemmas result, perceptions based on prior learning must be re-examined. Individuals can choose to reject the contradictory new information or revise their previous views. Transformative learning occurs when adjustments to prior learning are made (*Cranton, 1996; Pilling-Cormick, 1997)*.There are two goals in the experiential learning process. One is to learn the specifics of a particular subject matter. The other is to learn about one's own strengths and weaknesses as a learner. This understanding of learning strengths and weaknesses helps in the back-home application of what has been learned and provides a framework for continuing learning on the job. Day-to-day experience becomes a focus for testing and exploring new ideas. Learning is no longer special activity reserved for the classroom, but becomes an integral and explicit part of work itself. *(Justice and Jamieson, 1999*) To incorporate this researcher developed learners handbook based on the need assessment and extensive literature review and validated this with experts

The present study was conducted in different phases;

Phase I-Survey for need assessment was conducted using survey questionnaire (28 items) for 700 nurses from rural suburban, referral and government hospitals.

One of the most important influences in the development of Participatory research has been the work of Paulo Freire. Freire linked the process of knowing with that of learning, through an ongoing cycle of reflection and action (praxis). This learning process stimulates the growth of critical thinking, which raises critical awareness in learners of the world about them. Alongside Freire's ideas came a parallel development, that of the phenomenologist who held experience as a legitimate source of knowledge. Thus, experience was added to reflection and action, as factors that could influence practice.

In phaseII-40 nurses from different setting were elected as observers they were given to observe infection control practices Randomly selected participants were called for discussion and they were given pretest using Demographic Proforma and Knowledge Questionnaire (alpha 0.81) and observed for their infection control practices at their unit by the observers using observation checklist (r=0.9) Upon completing the pretest the learners handbook on Hospital infection control for nurses along with the video(CD) was given to them to study before attending the training program, core group nurses were participated in 2 days participatory infection control training using different participatory teaching and learning activity, organized by the participants themselves. Posttest was given to this core group nurses 1 month and 3 month after the training. During Phase III-Each of the Core group nurses trained 10 trainee group nurses from their respective units (400 trainee nurses). Pretest and posttest were given to this group at 1week interval. Phase IV-The FGD sessions were conducted at 3, 6 and 9 month at 3 months interval to assess the impact of training to improve their infection control practice. Phase V-The core group nurses also encouraged to involve infection control related practice improvement in their area with the help of their network they are encourage to share their successes and failures and get peer support during their FGD sessions. Opinion survey on administrators /supervisors (40) collected to evaluate the impact of the program in clinical area. Total sample size was 1284.

The first step of the intervention was involving core group nurses to identify the gap between current and expected infection control practice and encourage them to raise awareness from what was called *"Unconsciously incompetent to consciously competent"* among all core group members to decrease the gap using their own techniques, accessible and available to them in their own areas. The core group nurses were encouraged to involve with infection control related practice improvement along with training of other nurses. These core group nurses were formed a network and shared their problem and progress and tried to find the solutions to overcome some challenges along with researcher and some nursing administrative staff. They shared small success stories and ideas to solve infection control related problems in their work place and also the frustrations and anger towards their inability to correct most of the infection control practice related challenges.

This forum also gave them a sense of belongingness, and enhanced their capacity to communicate. The network of core group nurses helped them to share their knowledge and education materials and also helped their participation in infection control activities like surveillance and reporting at unit level .The gaps were found out using focus group discussion and analysis. The FGD was repeated every 3 months to follow up the impact of participatory infection control education and their actions to improve infection control related clinical practice.

3. Results

- Learning need assent analysis of the nurses on infection control training

Majority selected teaching methods like group discussion (83.38) demonstration (79.31), video (79.31) self study (77.03) and only16.61% selected lecture as their preferred mode of teaching and learning. There were 100% agreement with the topics like Infection transmission in the health care setting, Misconception about disease transmission, Importance of following infection control, Methods of infection control ,Standard precautions Hand washing and use of gloves, Disinfections, Aseptic technique management of sharps sterilization and waste management.

Knowledge and practice of staff nurses on hospital infection control

i. Core group nurses

The mean post-test -1 (45.55) and post test-2 (49.20) knowledge score are higher than the mean pre-test scores (23.40) of core group nurses who underwent participatory training program on infection control. The mean post-test -1 (24.75) and post test-2 (25.32) practice score are higher than the mean pre-test scores (16.87) of core group nurses who underwent participatory training program on infection control.

ii. Trainee group

The mean post-test (41.01) knowledge score are higher than the mean pretest scores (23.96). The mean post-test (25.05) practice score are higher than the mean pre-test scores (19.66) of trainee group nurses who underwent participatory training program on infection control by core group nurses.

Effectiveness of participatory training program

- Core group nurses

A repeated measures one-way ANOVA revealed that there were significant differences in the knowledge of core group nurses participated in the participatory infection control $F(1,39) = 483.89$ $p < .001$, was a relatively significant effect size (Eta-squared = 0.92). Post Hoc LSD comparisons revealed that all three means were significantly different from each other. The practice of core group nurses were significantly different between the three times of measurement, $F(1,39) = 151.628$, $p < .001$, was a relatively significant effect size (Eta-squared = 0,60). Post Hoc LSD comparisons revealed that all three means were significantly different from each other.

- Trainee group of nurses

There was a significant increase in knowledge ($t(353)= 17.05$)and the practice($t(353)= 20.20$) of trainee group who have undergone the participatory infection control training program by core group nurses. Their knowledge is independent of their age(0.85), education2.85, exposure to previous teaching (0.61) and their years of experience3.35.Their practice is also independent of the age(1.82), education(3.38), exposure to previous teaching (0.35)and their years of experience(0.52).

Clinical practice improvement

Quantitative enquiry has limitations to go in-depth for questions like; how significantly this program helps to improve infection control practice in the health care delivery system. To understand the impact of participatory infection control education, researcher aimed to reflect the opinions and experiences of the core group nurses using qualitative enquiry, which relies on inductive reasoning to interpret and structure the meanings that can be derived from the focus group discussion data. According to Bero, et al.,(1998) it is evident that no single solutions will address all barriers at many levels of health care delivery system.

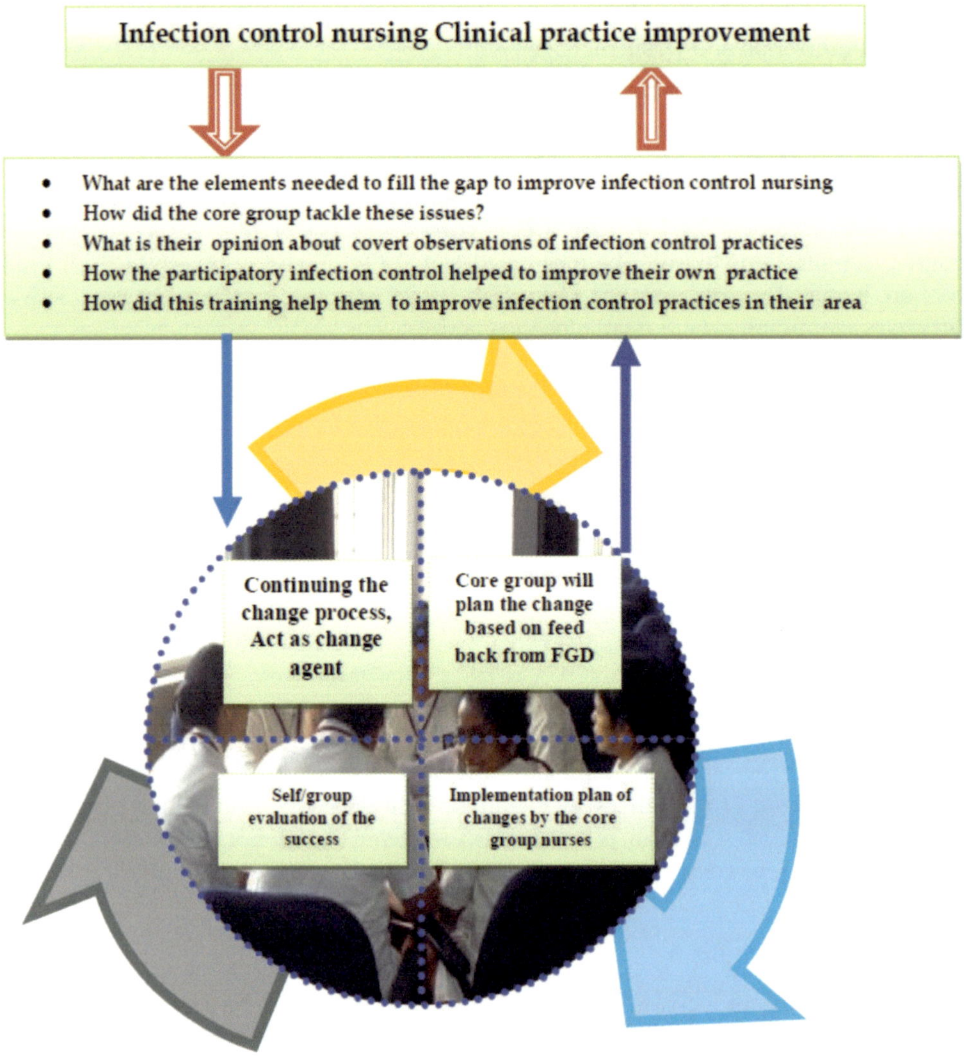

Fig. 1. Infection control nursing practice improvement model. Part of the theoretical framework was based on a strategy to change practice by Langley et al.,(1996) Institute for Healthcare Improvement, Boston

Based on the findings of Bordley, et al.,(2001) it was considered that clinical practice improvement method was bound to be effective in changing clinical practice to overcome the barriers that keep health care professionals from changing their practice and to reduce external pressures to change, such as increased workload and lack of time. The researcher utilized this model to guide the infection control practice improvement of the nurses working in the selected areas. Fundamental components for clinical practice management:

1. *Developing the knowledge and skills for understanding human performance, for minimizing and dealing with error.*
2. *The application of methods to identify measure and analyze problems with care delivery.*

3. *Action upon that information to improve both the individual and the systemic aspects of care delivery (infection control nursing).*

The researcher also analyzed the clinical practice improvement from the participatory infection control training. The results from FGD(Focus group dissuasion)II and III showed the changes in determinants of themes regarding improving infection control nursing practice were;

- Education at all levels- Increased awareness, Interested to share and monitor others practice, improved recognition, Sharing ideas, Peer support, improved communication and network
- Individual factors- Increased awareness, Interest to share and monitor others practices, Recognition, Sharing ideas, Peer support, confident, and improved communication.
- Improved participants practice , self knowledge and practice, ability to self learn, and the ability to transfer knowledge to other colleagues.
- Improved self esteem, belongingness to group and power to bring change, more assertiveness, confidence to change infection control related situation and awareness ,systematic problem solving to improve infection control related practice
- Observation /communication of observation will create awareness for a short time, this initial awareness and practice, may help to bring the change up to certain level.

Opinionaire from the key personnel after 1 year and 6moths of the participatory infection control training shows that majority of the key personnel opined that they had clear expectation of the infection control training program(22) and following participation in the program, they find their staffs performance on infection control practices is improved (23), this training helped them to communicate more effectively regarding infection control issues(25), increased their staff's involvement in infection control education and surveillance(20). Finally majority opined that their staff is effective member as they meet their expectations to prevent hospital associated infection in their respective units (24).

The core objective of the present study is to establish a sustained infection control education program for nurses in Indian settings. The results of the present study show that the core group nurses who participated in the participatory infection control training acted as change agent and were successful to enhance educational communication like procedural explanations sharing ideas ,communication to face infection control related problems, decrease negative talks and also established a network to face education related problems.

Clinical improvement process has also been considered more generally as a series of steps to help health workers and managers identify and solve problems of inadequate performance. Thus, this process shows where specific interventions fit into the larger process of managing health workers and health systems. Many of the core group nurses felt that they had improved infection control related clinical practice in their area. The group was able to identify specific issues, and instances where they felt infection control practice had been improved. For example improvement in hand washing, aseptic practices, and decrease in sharp injury, HAI rates and also improved infection control education at all level. This was attributed to the influence of the core group nurses, who had ensured that all staff understood key infection control practice. In addition, some of the core group nurses had produced education material, low cost materials/devises to improve infection control practice. The numerous examples suggest that the core group nurses have improved the quality of infection control practice. Importantly they appear to be confident in their ability to improve infection control practice. This led to influence others and empowerment, with the ultimate impact of improving quality of infection control nursing practice within the clinical area.

4. Conclusions

The following conclusions were made based on the study findings;

- Why educational programs on hospital infection control are a Herculean task to implement?

The present result showed that the core group nurses not only became change agent to cover the entire nurses' infection control education but also other staff like technical and housekeeping and also supported the educational program for doctors. They established continuing sustainable educational network without any additional cost. They developed indigenous materials and devises to improve infection control related practice. Their communication skills also improved and in one of the hospital the core group nurses are also instrumental in developing reporting network (e -surveillance).

Through participatory training mode, it is possible to train the core group nurses to have self-help by educating and empowering them and also provide education to their colleagues. Participatory training may be more effective than the other methods of education delivery, in terms of cost of mass training, sustainability and acceptance by nurses, thus empowering them to practice infection control.

A self-learning approach by participatory learning helps to develop facilitation of skills, and decision-making abilities, to increase self confidence and self-respect, and thus reduces dependency on others. This research based effort of using participatory infection control training to improve infection control related clinical practice aims to lead to improvements in the quality of care.

The present study showed that the participatory education on hospital infection control was effective in enabling participants to improve their knowledge and practice of infection control. It also facilitated their capacity to train others as change agents thereby improve the clinical practice to reduce infection in the hospital. The participatory training concept appears to offer one approach to organizations who can successfully overcome some of the barriers in implementing infection control theory into practice. However further studies are required to identify if development and empowerment influenced the clinical outcome (patient outcome).

- How to develop an effective and sustainable hospital infection control educational program to empower the nurses working in a selected hospital?

Establishing infection control teams and ongoing surveillance of hospital associated infection is required in majority of the Indian hospitals.The focus group discussion revealed that nurses in this study accomplished significant increase in knowledge of Hospital Associated Infection and were able to find solutions for the problems themselves and change their practices.

The experiences that nurses gained during this research project can be utilized as an ongoing process to introduce clinical practice improvement programs in the organization as a whole. Team effort in which the most appropriate and best-positioned people are involved in a process of participatory learning can help to bring the practice improvement. The findings can be shared with other organizations that in turn can set up their own educational programs. This experience also helped to sustain practice improvement.

- Will nurses on ward develop ownership and awareness of infection Control activities?

This is concluded by the responses of key personnel. Majority opined that their staffs are effective members as they meet their expectations to prevent hospital associated infection in their respective unit. By attending and teaching infection control classes, helping others to improve practice and participating in surveillance and reporting, they are able to achieve infection control related clinical improvement.

The result of the present study showed that there is continuing infection control education program run by the core group nurses and other nurses who participated in the training. This ongoing training is conducted on voluntary basis. The nurses also participate in surveillance and reporting activities.

- How does the culture of the clinical environment influence infection control practice?

Further, the findings of this study demonstrate that when infection control issues are not embedded in the clinical culture and infection control principles are not entrenched in clinical practice they are considered separately during care activities and easily displaced by other imperatives. Zimmerman and Peta-Anne, (2007) studied the current infection control advice applicable in low- and middle-income countries. Infection control guidelines designed for high-income countries are being utilized by Low and middle income countries, with varying degrees of success mainly because of physical, environmental, and socioeconomic factors. There is a lack of published studies exploring the implementation of comprehensive infection control advice and programs, including the minimal advice, which is designed specifically for resource-limited settings. They also concluded that this must be done in collaboration with those same health care workers who belong to low and middle income group countries. Equally, because of finance and health priorities, health care facilities should choose those interventions most relevant to the needs of their population and workers to prevent infection transmission.

Therefore, it is important to develop a positive and collaborative workplace and system culture; specifically, seek to identify the most appropriate players for each change priority and explicitly support them to learn how to function effectively as a team. Successful workplace cultures talk more about "why don't we?" and less about "why don't they" (Ancheril, 2004) the present study experience helped the core group nurses to stretch and push the professional culture congenial to infection control related clinical practice improvement .

The present study demonstrates that delivery of the programme based on participatory learning, led to confidence in the role, a belief in the importance of infection control and a feeling of legitimate empowerment. In turn, this facilitated development of empowered practice and influence at clinical level. This positively influenced clinical practice as demonstrated in the study, and led to increased ownership and motivation of the participants as described in this study.

The study provided an opportunity to think through realistic strategies for change in infection control nursing activities, especially infection control education. Whenever it is possible, researcher kept in touch with participants to offer encouragement and support. An effort is made to meet them in their work settings. The participants also created a network with their colleagues to support one another in creating change in infection control related activities in their institutions. To date this strategy has been successful in creating awareness in infection control. However to create a significant change in overall practice is still challenging and it is indisputably a collaborative effort. Most clinical practice improvement situations require that context-specific 'knowledge' be produced within the situation, in a time-bound manner. The literature in this area also points out that some of the more relevant human phenomena are not at all amenable to external observation, Most of these approaches seem to focus on creating (or improving) the situation-specific knowledge' that would improve the problem situation(Dash,1999).

Encouraging and allowing people to define their own problems, solve such problems in groups, share experiences, have critical and constructive dialogue, reflect on their own behavior and actions, adopt the inquisitive and critical mind-set, articulate positively effects change for the better, and making them change agents in the process and use their own 'local knowledge', be helpful towards each other. Such awareness and interaction in combination with the organizational support helps to bring about the required clinical practice improvement.

In the present study the information gathered during participatory infection control ranges from passive information providing to self mobilization. The results of FGD connote participant's involvement, decision making and implementing in the infection control program. It has also created an opportunity to interact with each other and generate ideas to improve infection control knowledge and practice.

There is no such thing as neutral education ... education either facilitates the integration of generations into the logic of the present system and brings conformity to it, or it becomes the 'practice of freedom', the means by which men and women deal critically and creatively with reality and discover how to participate in the transformation of their world -Freire,1972.

5. References

Ancheril, A. (2005). Evaluation of a program implemented to reduce surgical wound infection in an acute care hospital in India : A clinical practice improvement project. Unpublished PhD, UTS, Sydney.

Aboelela, S. W., Stonea, P. W. Larson, E. L. (2007). Effectiveness of bundled behavioural interventions to control healthcare-associated infections: systematic review of the literature. Journal of Hospital Infection, 66(2), 91.

Baird,L. S., Laird, D. Amherst, M. A. (1983). The training and development sourcebook.: Human Resource Development Press.

Bero, L., Grilli, R., Grimshaw, J. (1998). Effective Practice and Organization of Care Review Closing the gap between research and practice: an overview of systematic reviews of interventions to promote the implementation of research. BMJ Publishing, 317, 465-468.

Bordley, W., Margolis, P. A., Stuart, J., Lannon, C. Keyes, L. (2001). Improving preventive service delivery through office systems. Pediatrics (41), 108

Brigham, C. J., Foster, S. L., Hudson, K. E. (1991). A participatory learning module: Asepsis and universal precautions.16 (1), from www.cte.usf.edu/bibs/active_learn/nurse/bib_nurse.html.

Chandra, P. N., Milind, K. (2001). Lapses in measures recommended for preventing hospital-acquired infection. Journal of Hospital Infection,, 47(3),218-222.

Cranton, P. (1996). Professional development as transformative learning: New perspectives for teachers of adults. San Francisco: Jossey-Bass.

Dash, D. P. (1999). Current debates in action research. Systemic Practice and Action Research. Retrieved 5, 12, fromhttp://www.wkap.nl/journalhome.htm/1094-429X

Dubbert, P., Dolce, J., Richter, W., Miller, M., & Chapman, S. (1990). Increasing ICU staff hand washing effects of education and group feedback. Infection Control and Hospital Epidemiology, (11,), 191-193.

Freire, P. (1972). Pedagogy of the Oppressed. Harmondsworth: Penguin.

Gallagher, R. (2000). Infection control: public health, clinical effectiveness andeducation. Br Journal of Nursing, Dec 9- Jan.

Goetz, A. M., Kedzuf, S., Wagener, M., Muder, R.R. (1999). Feedback to nursing staff as an intervention to reduce catheter-associated urinary tract

Hoffman, K. K. (1997). The modern infection control practitioner in Prevention And Control Of Nosocomial Infections,Baltimore :Williams and Wilkins.

Justice, T., Jamieson, D. W. (1999). The Facilitator's Field book: Step-by-StepProcedures: AMACON,.

Kiessling. (2004). Participatory learning: a Swedish perspective. Heart.(90), 113-116.

Kim, L. E., Evanoff, B-A., Parks, R-L., Jeffe, D-B., Mutha, S., Haase, C., Fraser, V. (1999). Compliance with Universal Precautions among emergency department personnel: Implications for prevention programs. American Journal of Infection Control, 2 7(5), 453-455.

Larson E., A. A. (2006). Systematic risk assessment methods for the infection control professional. Am J Infection Control, 34:323-32 6.

Mukherjee, V. (2001). Hospital associated infection in India, Dangerous proportions., from http://www.inpharm.com/intelligence/frost

Pilling-Cormick, J. (1997).Transformative self-directed learning in practice. New Directions For Adult and Continuing Education,74, 69-77.

RAO, C. S. (1997). Participatory Irrigation Management Programme in Andhra Pradesh: New Delhi, India: Water & Power Consultancy Services (India)Ltd.

Rowe, A. K. d. S., D.; Lanata, C.F.; Victoria, C.G. (2005). How can we achieve and maintain high-quality performance of health workers in low-resource settings. The Lancet., 36(05).

Scheckler, W. E., Brimhall, D., Buck, A. S., Farr, B. M., Friedman, C., Garibaldi, R. A., Gross, P. A., Harris, J. A., Hierholzer, W. J., Martone, W. J., McDonald, L. L., Solomon, S. L. (1998). 'Requirements of Infrastructure and Essential Activities of Infection Control and Epidemiology in Hospitals: A Consensus Panel Report'. Infection Control and Hospital Epidemiology, 19, 114-124.

Shaheen, R. (2002). Hospital Infection Control Programme: An Overview. Indian Journal for the Practicing Doctor, Vol. 2, (3).

Sudhaker, C., Jain, A. G. (2007).Participatory training program on prevention of HIV/AIDS, with agent exposure, among Anganwadi workers for training young village women. Indian J Community Med, 32: 230-231.

Zimmerman, P. (2007). Current infection control advice applicable in low- and middle income countries. Infection control guidelines. American Journal of Infection control

8

Infectious Disease and Personal Protection Techniques for Infection Control in Dentistry

Bahadır Kan[1] and Mehmet Ali Altay[2]
[1]Oral & Maxillofacial Surgeon, Gulhane Military Medical Academy
Turkish Armed Forces Rehabilitation Centre, Dental Unit, Bilkent-Ankara
[2]Hacettepe University, Faculty of Dentistry
Department of Oral & Maxillofacial Surgery, Sihhiye-Ankara
Turkey

1. Introduction

Progressively gaining importance, "Infection control" is an important subject in dentistry, on which many researches have been performed in recent years. Both dentists' and the societies' sensibility rapidly enhances the amount of efforts made in creating a "perfect" infection control.

Dental team workers are members of a "high risk" group when dealing with patients in terms of cross infections. When the part of the body dentists mainly work on and the procedures performed are taken into account, contamination via blood and saliva can be clearly identified as a high risk. It should be kept in mind that other body fluids can also act as contamination risk factors.

For an infection to emerge, microorganisms of adequate count and a disease causing potential must contaminate the host thru a proper path. These contamination paths are specified (Esen 2007);

- Body fluids' direct contact with the wound site during operation,
- Injuries of the skin and the mucosa with sharp objects.
- Body fluids' and contaminated materials' contact with eyes.
- Aerosols arise during the operation with air turbined and ultrasonic devices. Contamination via droplet infection
- Surgical smoke formed during electro-cautery or laser applications.

2. Infectious diseases of concern in dentistry

A number of infectious diseases can and should be of concern in dental procedures.

2.1 Viral infections

Herpes Simplex Virus, one of the most common types of Herpes Virus family. Among major signs of the primary infection are fewer, malaise lymphadenopathy and ulcerative gingivostomatitis. Recurrent infections in the form of herpes labialis can also occur. A herpes simplex virus infection of the fingers (herpetic whitlow) is usually caused by direct contact with a herpetic lesion or infected saliva (Malik 2008).

Transmission occurs by direct contact of the affected part of the skin. Mucosa lesions and secretions can also be responsible for the transmission. Lesion in general is characterized by vesicles and sequent crusting. When the processor symptoms are present, acyclovir can be used for treatment or at least avoiding the worsening of the symptoms. Wearing gloves when treating patients with Herpes lesions provides adequate protection for the clinician.

Varicella Zoster Virus*,* causative agent of both chickenpox (primary disease) shingles (secondary disease) caused by the reactivation of the latent virus residing in sensory ganglia. Mild form is chickenpox mainly encountered in children. Shingles on the other hand can be very painful.

Chickenpox is considered highly contagious and spreads via-airborne route. The non-immune dental staff may contact the disease via inhalation of aerosols from a patient who is incubating the disease. Even though masks and gloves offer some level of protection they are usually not adequate for absolute protection of the healthcare professionals.

Epstein-Barr Virus causes infectious mononucleosis and can remain latent in epithelial tissues. Can be transmitted by skin contact or blood and the virus is present in saliva, thus members of the dental team are considered in the low risk group of EBV infection.

Human Herpes Virus 6 (HHV6)*,* A relatively new member of the Herpes Family. Generalized rash is encountered frequently in patients. The virus is present in the saliva but medical or dental staff is considered as members of the low-risk group.

Influenza, Rhino and Adenoviruses*,* Commonly cause respiratory tract infections. Transmission route is droplet infection members of the dental team are at risk of these infections but wearing masks and gloves offer adequate amount of protection.

Rubella (German Measles) is a toga virus capable of affecting developing foetus causing cataract, deafness etc. Route of transmission is droplets. Female members of the dental team should be warned of possible dangers because at risk are non-immune females of childbearing age. Combined vaccine applications of MMR should be administered to the members of the dental staff.

Coxsackie Virus, causative agent of herpangina and hand-foot and mouth disease. Considered as significant in dentistry due to presence of oral lesions and possibility of spreading in dental office. The virus is present in saliva and can pread via direct contact or aerosols. Gloves and masks offer adequate protection.

Human T-Lymphotropic Virus, is a retrovirus and plays a key role adult T Cell Leukemia and spastic paraparesis. Route of transmission is blood, sexual transmission and IV drug use. In dental practice, can spread via sharp instruments oriented injuries.

Hepatitis B Virus (HBV)*,* A DNA virus causative of acute hepatitis. Hepatitis B surface antigen (HbsAg) is identified by serological tests as the main indicator of active infection. HbeAg on the other hand indicates continuing activity of the virus present in the liver and its higher levels correlates with higher levels of infectivity.

The routes of transmission are, sexual intercourse, blood transfusion, contaminated material injuries and perinatal way.

All members of the dental team should be vaccinated against Hepatitis B and maintain this vaccination schedule.

Hepatitis C Virus (HCV), is a RNA virus, causative of non-A and non-B Hepatitis. Route of transmission is similar to HBV. Following the primary infection, which is usually asymptomatic, majority of the infected individuals become persistent carriers of the virus and there is a long-term risk of chronic liver disease with cirrhosis and hepatocellular carcinoma.

Human Immunodeficiency Virus (HIV), is a RNA retrovirus and is capable of infecting various cellular components of the immune system, T-Helper cells in particular. Route of transmission is similar to HBV, through sexual intercourse, blood borne and perinatal ways. HIV infections have oral manifestations, which can be helpful for the diagnosis of the disease. Among these oral manifestations are;

- Oral Candidiasis
- Oral Hairy Leukoplakia
- Oral Necrotising Ulcerative gingivitis
- Oral Kaposi's Sarcoma

2.2 Bacterial infections

Tuberculosis, caused by M. Tuberculosis is transmitted by inhalation, ingestion and inoculation. Cervical lymphadenitis and pulmonary infections are usually encountered. Immunization with BCG vaccine adequately covers dental team members. Gloves and masks on the side must be utilized. It should be kept in mind that M. Tuberculosis is highly resistant to chemicals and heat and disinfection protocols should be strictly followed.

Legionellosis caused by Gram-negative bacteria, which usually reside in warm and stagnant water reservoirs. Is capable of causing life threatening pneumonias in elder people? Since the organism is water-borne, it can easily be transmitted via aerosols formed during routine dental procedures. There have been reports about Legionella proliferations in dental unit water systems, thus systems, which remain unused for long periods of time should be regularly checked for legionella presence. The members of the dental team should be informed about the long term risk of legionellosis.

Syphilis, caused by T.pallidum. wearing gloves offer adequate protection.

3. Personal protection methods

Dental team professionals must adapt a series of precautions in order to avoid these infections.

The priority in infection control in dentistry is laid on the enhancement of awareness levels of dentists and other team members on infection control and personal protection techniques. An education emphasizing the importance of sensibility in this subject undoubtedly is the first and the most important step of precautions (Atac & Turgut 2007).

Personal protection techniques comprise of a series of applications that aim to reduce contaminations risks. It is not a realistic option to check all patients in terms of contagious diseases and dental professionals are exposed to these sorts of risks countless times everyday. Thus the main principle in infection control is to treat every patient as if he/she is an infected patient and to apply standard protection techniques properly is a "must" in a perfect infection control (Kulekci 2000).

3.1 Routine procedure

A proper medical and dental history should be obtained for all patients at the first visit and updated regularly. On the form, inclusion of patient views about the place cleanliness where they had received medical and dental treatment is useful.

The history and examination may not reveal asymptomatic infectious disease. This means operator must obey the same infection control rules for all patients.

3.2 Immunization

Dentists and other dental team workers who are members of "the high risk group" must be vaccinated against Hepatitis B by means of personal protection (Kohn 2003). 3 doses of vaccination is required. Vaccination must be started in ten days after onset of practice and must be carried on during practice. Individuals who have been vaccinated before the onset of their practice must check their levels of immunity sufficiency against Hepatitis B (Thomas 2008). All dental health care personnel are also strongly urged to receive the following vaccinations: influenza, measles (live-virus), mumps (live-virus), rubella (live-virus), and varicella-zoster (live-virus). Besides, women who have pregnancy uncertainty are strongly recommended to be vaccinated against rubella (Molinari 2005). Vaccination against influenza may also be beneficial for professionals of dental health who are under risk of contamination with droplet infections in terms of close working distance with patients. Updates of Centre for Disease Control (CDC) must be checked and paid attention in this subject.

3.3 Hand hygiene

Providing and maintaining a certain level of hand hygiene is of great importance in protection techniques. All member of the dental team must adapt the habit of maintaining providing hand hygiene. The idea and the practice of washing the hands with antiseptics date back to 19th century. In 1846, Semmelweis reported a lower rate of infection and mortality in obstetric clinics performed by students and physicians who have the habit of washing hands with chlorine when compared with midwifes who had lower levels of hand washing habits (Semmelweis 1983).

In 1961, the U.S. Public Health Service produced a training film that demonstrated hand washing techniques recommended for use by health-care workers (HCWs)(Coppage 1961). At the time, recommendations directed that personnel wash their hands with soap and water for 1-2 minutes before and after patient contact. Rinsing hands with an antiseptic agent was believed to be less effective than hand washing and was recommended only in emergencies or in areas where sinks were unavailable (Boyce & Pittet 2002). CDC published a "how to" guideline for washing hands in 1975 and 1985 and according to these publications hands must be washed with antimicrobial soaps before and after invasive procedures performed on patients. At times when washing hands is not an option, application of water-free antiseptics is recommended.

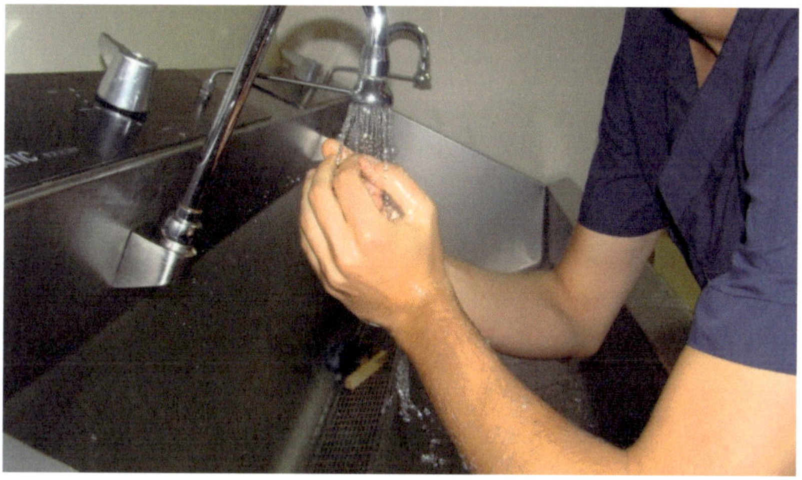

Fig. 1. Hands should be washed before and after all procedure.

It should be kept in mind that using gloves is not an alternative to washing hands. For routine procedures other than surgical ones, normal or antibacterial soaps are appropriate (Kohn 2004). When an obvious stain is not present, alcohol-containing (% 60-95 ethanol or isopropanol) hand cleaning agents can be utilized (Garner & Favero 1986; Steere & Mallison 1975). And also, alcohol-containing agents are very affective and preferable between the procedures when hand washing facility located far away from the dental unit. Cold water must be of choice when washing hands de to the fact that exposure of the skin to hot water repeatedly may increase the risk of dermatitis. Application of liquid soaps when washing hands for a minimum duration of 15 seconds and disposable paper towels for drying hands is recommended (Figure 1). Reducing numbers of pathogen microorganisms in hand washing before surgical procedures is of great importance. This is why application of antibacterial soaps and a detailed cleaning (arms, nails etc.) followed with alcohol containing liquids are recommended (Esen 2007). Despite the fact that antibacterial effects of alcohol containing cleansers arise rapidly, they do not last long and for a longer effect, antiseptics such as trichlosane, quarterner amonnium compounds, chlorehexidine and octenidine must be included (Boyce & Pittet 2002). Rings, watches and other accessories must be taken off before surgical hand washing and no nail polishes or other artificial (acrylics) must be present (Kohn 2004). After the washing, hands must be dried with sterile towels and other surfaces must not be contacted until wearing sterile gloves. Following the procedure, after taking the gloves off, it is highly recommended to wash hands once again with regular soaps.

3.4 Single use (disposable) items

Equipment described by manufacturer as "single use", should be preferred and used whenever possible. "Single use" means that a device can be used on a patient during one treatment session and then discarded (Thomas 2008). These items are local anaesthetic needles and cartridges, scalpel blades, suction tubes, matrix bands, impression trays, surgery burs, patient gown, working area covers.

3.5 Barrier techniques

Dental team members must utilize personal protective equipment during applications in order to protect themselves and avoid cross infections. Hardships and limitations when using these equipment must be known and valued and when using new ones, detailed information about these protects must be gained. Guidelines for using these products must be kept under record and updated under contemporary data.

3.5.1 Masks, eyewear and face shields

Contact of blood and saliva of patients with dentists' eyes and airways and contamination with aerosols formed during dental procedures is inevitable if proper precautions are not taken. A mask and a protective eyewear must be used during all applications (Figure 2, Figure 3).

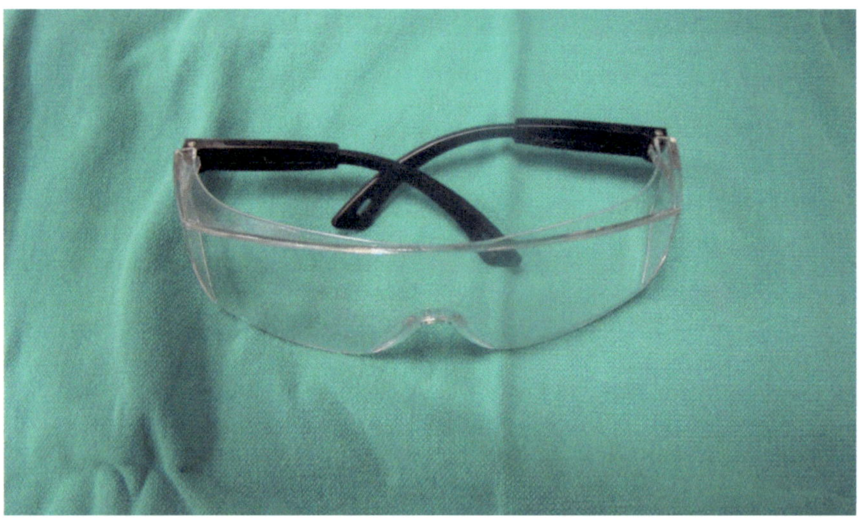

Fig. 2. Protective eyewear should be worn during the procedure

Even though masks were first thought to be used by patient, today masks are mostly utilized for healthcare professionals. Dental masks must have the capacity to block 95% of all bacteria of 3-5 μm diameter and other particles (Esen 2007; Thomas 2008). If the masks get wet when dealing with a patient, they must be changed or thoroughly cleaned before using them for another patient's application.

Sides and upper edges of the protective eyewear must adapt the face well and provide protection against all kinds of infection agents (Thomas 2008). Face shields are more practical then protective glasses for dentists who also have to wear medical glasses and also a lower level of misting is experienced when using. However, wearing and keeping them at place appear to be troublesome which is why they are more often avoided by clinicians (Bebermayer 2005; Esen 2007).

3.5.2 Gloves

Gloves were first used in medical procedures by William Halstead a century ago for avoiding nurses' hands from harsh antiseptics (Randers-Pehrson 1960). Identification of diseases and their contamination routes resulting from viruses such as Hepatitis B and HIV, using gloves has been more and more popular in recent years (Field 1997). The Expert Group on Hepatitis in Dentistry suggested the use of non-sterile gloves for the first time in 1979, when dealing with patients infected with Hepatitis B and as HIV on the side spread around the world, non-sterile gloves have been concluded to be used for all patients routinely (Burke & Wilson 1989; EGHD 1979).

During all kinds of procedure in dentistry, it is impossible to avoid contact of hands with blood and saliva. This is why all clinicians must wear protective hand gloves before they perform any kind of procedure on their patients. It is strongly recommended for dental professionals to use protective gloves both in America and all over Europe (Field 1994; Molinari 2005). Gloves are mainly produced of latex or vinyl and aside from the non-sterile ones, which are appropriate for regular dental procedures, less permeable sterile ones for surgical approaches offered in sterile packs are also available on the market. However, due to the fact that using sterile gloves during routine dental procedures increase costs and seen as an economical burden, clinicians most commonly prefer non-sterile ones instead.

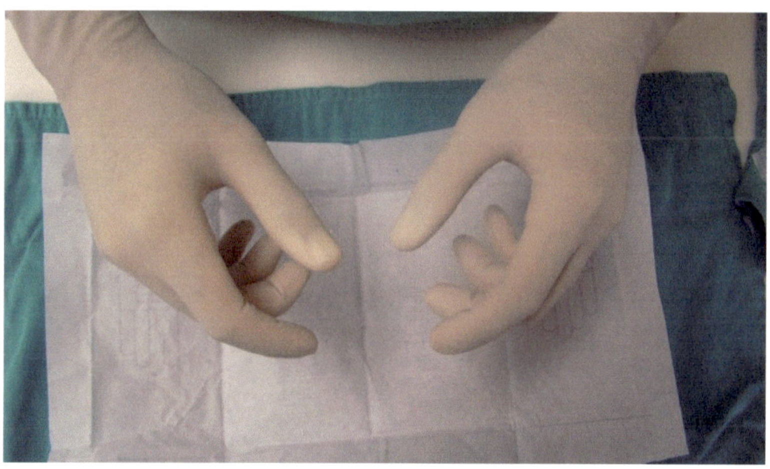

Fig. 3. Gloves must be worn during the operation by all working team.

A separate pair of gloves must be used for every patient and contact with surfaces when with gloves must be avoided to prevent cross infections. Not only the dentist but also other members of the dental team must put on gloves during dental procedures. When cleaning dental appliances and instruments more durable gloves than regular non-sterile ones must be utilized to prevent injuries.

Gloves are powdered to make them easier to put on. However, the powder present inside the gloves are reported to cause skin irritations (Field 1997). Wilson and Garach further reported that this powder could cause starch granulomas on surgical sites among which oral cavity is mentioned (Wilson & Garach 1981). Powder-free gloves are produced and available in the market today and they should be used when such reactions are experienced.

Allergies and contact dermatitis due to latex can be encountered in some people. Dental team members should be warned about this subject. Allergic symptoms may include local ones such as itching, redness, rash, dryness, fissures/cracking, hyperkeratosis and swelling and at times, systemic ones such as sneezing, wheezing, urticarial and red watered eyes can emerge. In such a situation latex gloves should be avoided and a medical consultation should be obtained. Latex-free gloves are also available for allergic individuals.

3.5.3 Protective clothing

Protective clothing should be utilized instead of daily clothing (Figure 4). Whenever the clinician is to deal with patients with contagious diseases, he/she should prefer long-sleeved protective clothing. This way, contact of pathogens with skin can be avoided. In case the clothing gets wet, they should be changed immediately with new ones and should be taken off when the clinician is to leave the operation area.

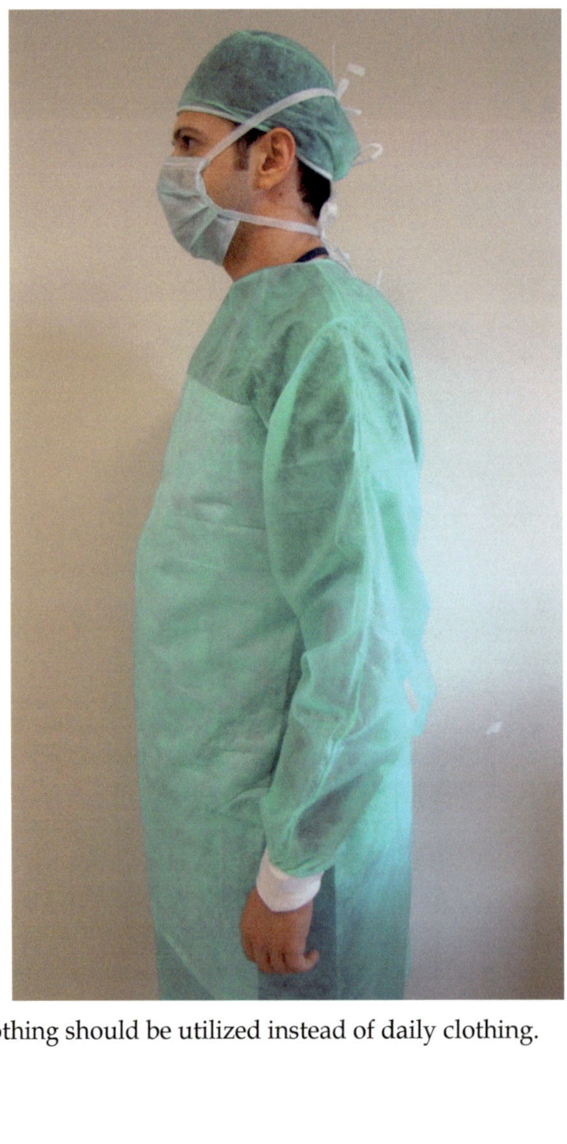

Fig. 4. Protective clothing should be utilized instead of daily clothing.

3.5.4 Operation room protection

a. Floor
   - The floor covering should be impervious and non-slip. Carpeting must be avoided.
   - The floor covering should be seam free; where seams are present, they should be sealed.
   - The junctions between floor and wall and the floor and cabinetry should cove or be sealed to prevent inaccessible areas where cleaning might be difficult (BDA 2003).

b. Work Surface
   - Work surfaces should be easy to clean and disinfection.
   - Work surface joins should be sealed to retention of contaminated matter.
   - All work surface junctions should be rounded or coved to aid cleaning (BDA 2003).

3.6 Post-exposure protocol

In case skin gets injured with contaminated instruments or open wounds come in contact with body fluids of the patient, procedure should be imeediately intercepted and injured area should be rinsed with ample amount of soap and water and mucosa if involved, water should be used for flushing. If another member of the dental team gets injured, he/she should inform the dentist. According to Control Disease Center (CDC)'s recommendations, following injuries with contaminated material or contact with certain body fluids;

- Injury's date and time
- How and with what sort of instrument injury occurred,
- With which body fluid exposure occurred
- Details about the exposure source (information regarding the presence of any contagious disease)
- Detailed medical information of the injured,
- Precautions followed before and during the injury should be recorded in detail (CDC 2009).

If an injury with contaminated materials utilized in HIV, HBV or HCV infected patients occurs, patient's detailed medical history should be questioned and tested should be carried out for certain markers if required. CDC's post-exposure management publication regarding this subject should be referred as the guideline and necessary precautions should be taken (CDC 2001).

4. Referances

Atac, A., & Turgut, D. (2007). Infection Control Management in Dentistry. *Turkish journal of Hospital Infections, 11*(3), 179-186.

BDA. (2003). Infection control in dentistry. *British Dental Association Advice Sheet*(A12).

Bebermayer, R., Dickinson, S., & Thomas, L. (2005). Personnel health elements of infection conrol in the dental health care setting--a review. *Tex Dent J, 122*(10), 1028-1035.

Boyce, J. M., & Pittet, D. (2002). Guideline for Hand Hygiene in Health-Care Settings: recommendations of the Healthcare Infection Control Practices Advisory Committee and the HICPAC/SHEA/APIC/IDSA Hand Hygiene Task Force. [Guideline

Research Support, Non-U.S. Gov't]. *Infection control and hospital epidemiology: the official journal of the Society of Hospital Epidemiologists of America, 23*(12 Suppl), S3-40.
Burke, F. J. T., & Wilson, N. H. F. (1989). Non-sterile glove use: a review. *Am J Dent, 2*, 255-261.
CDC. (2001). Updated U.S. Public Health Service Guidalines for the Management of Occupational Exposures to HBV, HCV, and HIV and Recommendations for Postexposure Prophylaxis. *MMWR. Recommendations and reports / Centers for Disease Control, 50(RR11)*, 1-42
CDC. (2009). Infection Contrl in Dental Settings. Bloodborne Pathogens - Occupational Exposure
Coppage, C. (1961). *Hand Washing in Patient Care [Motion picture]*. Washington, DC: US Public Health Service.
EGHD. (1979). *(Expert Group on Hepatitis in Dentistry) A Guide to Blood-borne Viruses* HMSO.
Esen, E. (2007). Personnel protective measures for infection control in dental health care settings. *Turkish journal of Hospital Infections, 11*(2), 143-146.
Field, E. A. (1994). Hand hygiene, hand care and hand protection for clinical dental practise. *Br Dent J, 176*, 129-134.
Field, E. A. (1997). The use of powdered gloves in dental practise: a cause for concern? . *journal of Dentistry, 25*(Nos 3-4), 209-214.
Garner, J. S., & Favero, M. S. (1986). CDC guidelines for the prevention and control of nosocomial infections. Guideline for handwashing and hospital environmental control, 1985. Supersedes guideline for hospital environmental control published in 1981. *American journal of infection control, 14*(3), 110-129.
Kohn, W. G., Collins, A. S., Cleveland, J. L., Harte, J. A., Eklund, K. J., & Malvitz, D. M. (2003). Guidelines for infection control in dental health-care settings--2003. [Guideline]. *MMWR. Recommendations and reports: Morbidity and mortality weekly report. Recommendations and reports / Centers for Disease Control, 52*(RR-17), 1-61.
Kohn, W. G., Harte, J. A., Malvitz, D. M., Collins, A. S., Cleveland, J. L., & Eklund, K. J. (2004). ADA Division of Science. Guidelines for infection control in dental health care settings-2003. *J Am Dent Assoc, 135*, 33-47.
Kulekci, G., Cintan, S., & Dulger, O. (2000). Infection control from the point of dentistry, infection control in dentistry. *Journal of Turkish Dental Association, Special Volume 58*, 91-93.
Malik, N. A. (2008). *Textbook of Oral and Maxillofacial Surgery* (2 ed.). New Delhi: Jaypee Brothers Medical Publisher.
Molinari, J. A. (2005). Updated CDC infection control guidelines for dental health care settings: 1 year later. *Compendium of continuing education in dentistry, 26*(3), 192, 194, 196.
Randers-Pehrson, J. (1960). *The Surgeons Glove.* Springfield, Illinois.
Semmelweis, I. (1983). *Etiology, Concept, and Prophylaxis of Childbed Fever.* (1st ed.). Madison, WI: The University of Wisconsin Press.
Steere, A. C., & Mallison, G. F. (1975). Handwashing practices for the prevention of nosocomial infections. *Annals of internal medicine, 83*(5), 683-690.
Thomas, M. V., Jarboe, G., & Frazer, R. Q. (2008). Infection control in the dental office. *Dental clinics of North America, 52*(3), 609-628, x.
Wilson, D. F., & Garach, V. (1981). Surgical glove starch granulomas. *Oral Surg, 51*, 342-345.

9

Skin Irritation Caused by Alcohol-Based Hand Rubs

Nobuyuki Yamamoto
NOF Corporation
Japan

1. Introduction

In the late 1990s and early part of the 21st century, alcohol-based hand rubs started to gain popularity. Today, alcohol-based hand rubs are widely used for infection control in clinical practice. However, many healthcare workers complain about unacceptable skin irritation caused by alcohol-based hand rubs. In spite of the complaint, when the irritant effect of alcohol on the skin has been evaluated, most authors found low toxicity (Boyce et al., 2000; de Haan et al., 1996; Lübbe et al., 2001; Winnefeld et al., 2000).

Kownatzki has pointed out that the skin irritation of healthcare workers is not simply caused by alcohol antisepsis but by combined damage resulting from the alcohol antisepsis dissolving lipids in the stratum corneum, the removal of lipids from the skin surface by detergent washing, and the skin becoming over-hydrated from wearing gloves.

To reduce the adverse effects of alcohol-based hand rubs, it is known that adding emollients or humectants is efficacious (Many studies are reviewed in Boyce & Pittet, 2002).

By contrast, addition of a certain type of chemical compound such as cationic antiseptics may cause irritation (Tsuji et al., 1993).

Thus, so-called "alcohol-based hand rubs" include wide variations of alcohol formulations. When we discuss the skin irritancy of alcohol-based hand rubs, we need to note the formulation of each testing sample and the type and concentrations of the alcohols, emollients, and antiseptic compounds contained.

To evaluate the skin irritancy of alcohol-based hand rubs in human, animal experiments such as Draize rabbit tests are quite useful. However, using experimental animals requires special techniques and facilities, and also have problem in animal protection.

Hence, alternatives to animal experiments have been developed in last decades. To predict the skin irritancy in human, *in vitro* skin irritation tests using three-dimensional human skin models are quite useful. The EU has accepted the *in vitro* skin irritation test using a human skin model as stand-alone test to determine the skin irritation potential of a substance (OECD TG 439). However, the *in vitro* skin irritation tests using human skin models cannot be used for high alcohol-content solutions, such as alcohol-based hand rubs. To overcome this problem, the author has developed a novel *in vitro* evaluation method named "Skin model blowing method (SMBM)" (Yamamoto et al., 2010).

The first objective of this review is to summarize the structure and barrier function of the skin, the mechanism and evaluation methods of skin irritation, and the irritancy of alcohol-based hand rubs. The second objective is to implement the novel *in vitro* evaluation method "SMBM" for assessing the skin irritation caused by alcohol-based hand rubs, and show the evaluation results of some of the alcohol-based hand rubs used in Japan.

2. Structure and barrier function of the skin

2.1 Structure of the skin

The skin is the largest human organ and consists of two main layers: epidermis and dermis (Fig.1). One major task of the skin is to protect the organism from water loss and mechanical, chemical, microbial, and physical influences. The protective properties are provided by the outermost layer of the skin, the epidermis. The epidermis is approximately 100 to 150 micrometers thick, has no blood flow and includes the superficial layer known as the stratum corneum (Fig.2).

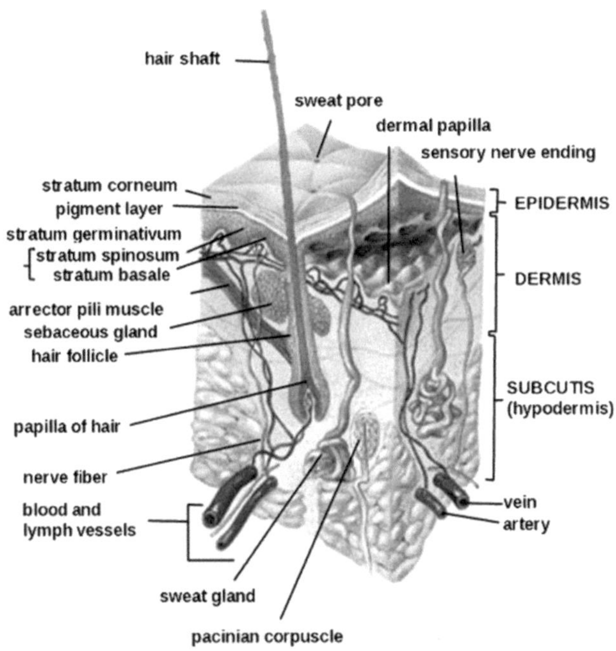

Fig. 1. Histological structure of the human skin[1]

The stratum corneum consists of slabs of flat, platelike dead cells called corneocytes. The corneocytes, which are anucleated cells derived from keratinocytes, have no viable function and are called "dead" cells. They are continuously being sloughed off and then replaced in cycles of 3 to 4 weeks. The cells are pushed up from the living layer just lying below. The corneocytes are embedded in the intercellular lipid matrix, thus the structure of the stratum corneum can be roughly described by a "brick and mortar" model (Elias, 1983).

---

1. U.S. National Cancer Institute, In: *Anatomy of the Skin*, Available from http://training.seer.cancer.gov/melanoma/anatomy/

2.2 Barrier function of the skin

The major factor that keeps the skin moist and pliable is the presence of intercellular lipids. These form a lamellar (stacked bilayers) structure surrounding the corneocytes and incorporate water into the stratum corneum. The lipids are derived from lamellar granules, which are released into extracellular spaces from degrading cells in the granular cell layer; and the membranes of these cells also release lipids, including cholesterol, free fatty acids and sphingolipids. Ceramide, a type of sphingolipid, is mainly responsible for generating the stacked lipid structures that trap water molecules in their hydrophilic region.

These lamellar lipids surround the corneocytes and form a semi-permeable barrier that prevents water and natural moisturizing factors (NMF) from moving out from the surface layers of the skin.

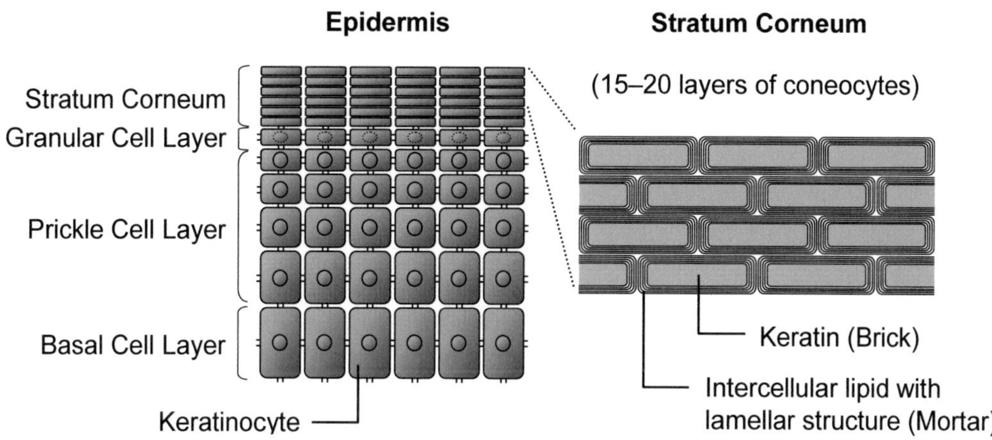

Fig. 2. Schematic diagrams of the epidermis and stratum corneum based on the "brick and mortar" model (Elias, 1983)

2.3 Measurement of the skin barrier function

2.3.1 Transepidermal water loss (TEWL)

The measurement of transepidermal water loss (TEWL) is an important non-invasive method for assessing the barrier function of the stratum corneum. As a consequence, TEWL has been found to be a very useful index for studying skin irritation induced by various physical and chemical effects. Exposure of the skin to chemicals (detergents) and physical conditions (occlusion and stripping) generally results in an increase of TEWL (Barel & Clarys, 1995).

Several TEWL measuring instruments such as Evaporimeter EP-2 (ServoMed, Sweden), Tewameter TM 300 (Courage+Khazaka electronic GmbH, Germany) and VapoMeter (Delfin Technologies, Finland) are commercially available. Evaporimeter and Tewameter are based on the open chamber system with two humidity and temperature sensors for measuring the water evaporation gradient at the surface of the skin.

By contrast, VapoMeter is based on the closed chamber system, and is easier to use than the open chamber device. However, its tendency to become saturated under high water loss conditions could be a disadvantage when assessing dynamic TEWL (Cohen et al., 2009). Tewameter is able to detect significantly smaller differences than VapoMeter (de Paepe et al., 2005).

2.3.2 Electrical characteristics of skin surface

Deterioration of the skin barrier function leads to reduced hydration levels of the skin surface. To determine the hydration level of the skin surface, Corneometer CM 825 (Courage+Khazaka electronic GmbH, Germany) and SKICON-200EX (I.B.S Co., Ltd., Japan) are widely used. Corneometer CM 825 measures the changes in the dielectric constant caused by skin surface hydration by measuring changes in capacitance with a precision capacitor. SKICON-200EX measures high frequency conductance of the skin, which is sensitively correlated to the skin surface water content.

3. Mechanism of skin irritation

3.1 Inflammatory response

Foreign materials (e.g., micro-organisms, surfactants, etc.) that have penetrated the stratum corneum barrier encounter living epidermal cells. Interactions with keratinocyte surface molecules or membrane lipids activate the cells. Cytokines are released, emitting signals requesting assistance to blood vessels and white blood cells. Activation of Langerhans cells initiates an immune response, which is particularly effective when a given foreign material is encountered repeatedly. When these responses exceed a certain level, inflammatory symptoms are elicited (Gallin et al., 1992).

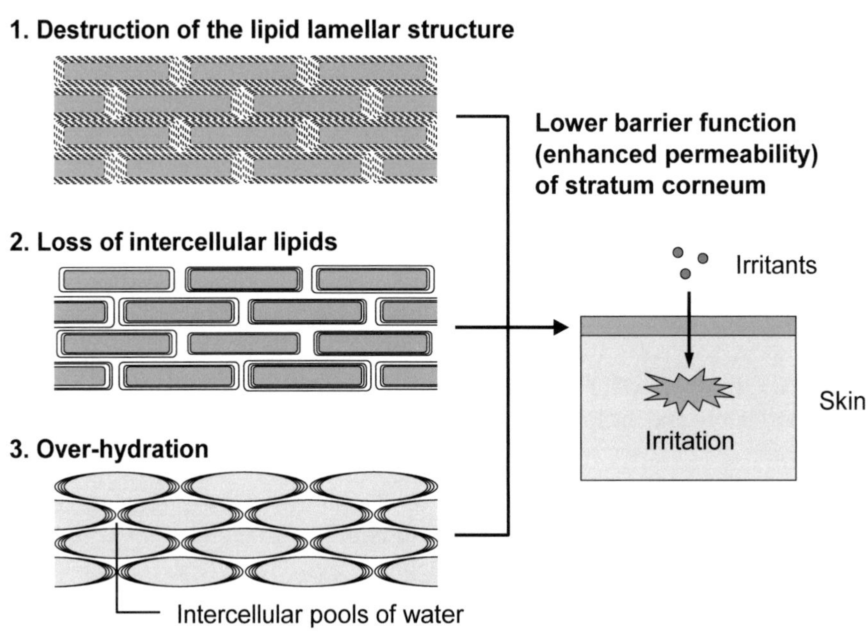

Fig. 3. Diagrams of structurally altered stratum corneum. Due to the deterioration of the barrier function (enhanced permeability) of epidermis, irritants can penetrate through the stratum corneum.

3.2 Hand hygiene and skin barrier function

The mechanism of skin barrier damage in healthcare workers was summarized by Kownatzki (Kownatzki, 2003). The main concern in hygiene-dependent risks to the skin's health is damage to the lipid barrier. The lipid barrier is jeopardized on three occasions: when the lipid lamellar structure is destroyed, the intercellular lipid is lost, and the skin is over-hydrated. In healthcare settings, these phenomena usually occur in a concerted situation of alcohol antisepsis, detergent cleaning, and glove work.

Destruction of the lipid lamellar structure

Antiseptic alcohols, which are organic solvents, are capable of dissolving stratum corneum lipids and destroying the barrier. Alcohol remaining on the skin evaporates leaving the lipids on the skin, but the lipids do not reassume the original structure and arrangement of the barrier and do lose the sealing function.

Loss of intercellular lipids

Detergents clean surfaces by removing lipids, together with any adhering contaminants. Sebum lipids on the skin surface, which are encountered and emulsified first by detergents, may provide protection for the underlying barrier lipids. Repeated detergent washes and progressive removal of surface lipids reduce the lipid-dependent cleaning efficiency and allow the detergent molecules to penetrate deep in the stratum corneum. In individuals with less supply of sebum lipids, this occurs more quickly.

Over-hydration

There is a high rate of hand problems among professions whose hands have frequent contact with water or wet objects such as food workers and hair dressers. Also the gloves worn by healthcare workers create a wet environment as they do not allow the sweat to evaporate. Extended water exposure leads to extensive disruption of stratum corneum intercellular lipid lamellae. The hydration induces disruption of the intercellular lipid lamellae, forms large pools of water in the intercellular space and creates corneocyte separations (Warner et al., 2003).

4. *In vivo* and *in vitro* evaluation of skin irritation

Human patch testing is commonly used to evaluate the skin irritation caused by a substance. Animal and *in vitro* testing is also utilized to predict the skin irritancy in human.

4.1 Human testing (single-application patch test)

Widely used method for assessing skin irritation include single-application patch testing, cumulative irritation test, chamber scarification test and immersion tests (Levin & Maibach, 2004). Especially, many variations of single-application patch test have been developed. Testing is often performed on undiseased skin (Skog, 1960) of the dorsal upper arm or back. The required test area is small, and up to ten materials can be tested simultaneously and compared. A reference irritant substance is often included to interpret variability in test responses. In general, screening of new materials involves open application on the back or dorsal upper arm for a short time (30 min to 1 hr) to minimize potential adverse events in the subjects.

The National Academy of Sciences (National Academy of Sciences and Committee for the Revision of NAS Publication 1138, 1977) recommended a 4-hr single-application patch test protocol for routine testing of skin irritation in humans. In general, patches are occluded onto the dorsal upper arm or back skin of patients. The degree of occlusion varies according to the type of occlusive device; the Hilltop or Duhring chambers or an occlusive tape will enhance percutaneous penetration as compared to a non-occlusive tape or cotton bandage (Patil et al., 1996). Potentially volatile materials should always be tested with a non-occlusive tape.

Exposure time to the putative irritant varies greatly, and is often customized by the investigator. Volatile chemicals are generally applied for 30 min to 1 hr while some chemicals have been applied for more than 24 hr.

Following patch removal, the skin is rinsed with water to remove the residue. Skin responses are evaluated 30 min to 1 hr following patch removal in order to allow hydration and pressure effects of the patch to subside. Another evaluation is performed 24 hr following the patch removal. The animal Draize scale is used to analyze test results (see Table 1). The Draize scale does not include papular, vesicular, or bullous responses; and other scales have been developed to address these needs.

Single-application patch tests generally heal within one week. Depigmentation at the test site results in some subjects.

Erythema		
	No erythema	0
	Slight erythema	1
	Well-defined erythema	2
	Moderate or severe erythema	3
	Severe erythema or slight eschar formation (injuries in depth)	4
Edema		
	No edema	0
	Very slight edema	1
	Slight edema (well-defined edges)	2
	Moderate edema (raised >1 mm)	3
	Severe edema (raised >1 mm and extending beyond the area of	4

Table 1. Draize scoring system

4.2 Animal testing (Draize rabbit test)

In order to evaluate the skin irritation, Draize rabbit test, guinea pig immersion test and mouse ear test are utilized as animal models. Especially, the Draize scores are most accurate when compared to related compounds with a record of human exposure (Levin & Maibach, 2004).

The Draize rabbit test was developed in 1944, and has since been adopted in the US Federal Hazardous Substance Act (Patrick & Maibach, 1989). The test involves two (1 square inch) test sites on the dorsal skin of six albino rabbits. One site is abraded (through use of a hypodermic needle across the rabbit skin) and the other site remains intact. The stratum corneum is broken on the abraded site, without loss of blood. The undiluted "irritant" materials (0.5 g for solids or 0.5 ml for liquids) are placed on a patch and applied to the test sites. They are secured with two layers of surgical gauze (1 square inch) and tape. The animal is wrapped in cloth so that the patches are secure for a 24-hr period. Assessment of erythema and edema, utilizing the scale noted in Table 1, takes place 24 hr and 72 hr following patch application. Severe reactions are again assessed on days 7 or 14. Radiolabeled tracers or biochemical techniques to monitor skin healing is also utilized by some investigators. Other investigators supplement with histological evaluation of skin tissue (Mezei et al., 1966; Murphy et al., 1979).

The Draize test ultimately quantifies irritation with the primary irritation index (PII), which averages the erythema and edema scores of each test site and then adds the averages together. Materials producing a PII of <2 are considered nonirritating, 2–5 mildly irritating, and >5 severely irritating and require precautionary labelling. Subsequent studies have demonstrated that the PII is somewhat subjective because the scoring of erythema and edema require clinical judgment (Patil et al., 1998).

Main critics of the Draize test oppose the harsh treatment of animals. They argue that the Draize test is unreliable at distinguishing between mild and moderate irritants. Furthermore, they believe the Draize is not an accurate predictor of skin irritancy as it does not include vesiculation, severe eschar formation or ulceration in evaluating the PII. Finally, they argue that the Draize procedure is not reproducible (Weil & Scala, 1971) and they question its relevance with regard to human experience (Edwards, 1972; Nixon et al., 1975; Shillaker et al., 1989). Proponents of the Draize test point out that the test is somewhat inaccurate but it generally overpredicts the severity of skin damage produced by chemicals, and thereby errs on the side of safety for the consumer (Patil et al., 1996). This topic is still being hotly debated. For the meantime, the Draize assays are recommended by regulatory bodies.

4.3 *In vitro* testing (human skin models)

4.3.1 Overview of human skin models

Animal experiments such as Draize rabbit tests are quite useful for determining the skin irritancy in human. However, using experimental animals requires special techniques and facilities, and also have problem in animal protection. Three-dimensional human skin models and cultured human skin models, which have been proposed for therapeutic purpose of a full thickness skin defect resulting from burn or trauma, can be used to replace animal-based irritative studies. The human skin models have been developed during the last decades (Green et al., 1979; Bell et al., 1981; Asselineau et al., 1985). The first skin model was proposed by Green et al. in 1979, who made an artificial epidermis from human epidermal keratinocytes. This type of human skin model is called "reconstructed human epidermis (RhE)". The skin model consisting of dermis and epidermis which resembled the real human skin was reported by Bell et al. in 1981. Various human skin models have been developed thereafter and are commercially available today (Table 2).

Product Name	Structure	Manufacturer
EpiDerm	Epidermis	MatTek Corp.
EpiDermFT	Epidermis on dermis	MatTek Corp.
EPISKIN	Epidermis on collagen gel	SkinEthic Laboratories
SkinEthic RHE	Epidermis	SkinEthic Laboratories
EST-1000	Epidermis	CellSystems Biotechnologie Vertrieb GmbH
TESTSKIN	Epidermis on dermis with collagen gel	TOYOBO Co., Ltd.
Vitrolife-Skin	Epidermis on dermis with collagen sponge	GUNZE Ltd.
LabCyte EPI-MODEL	Epidermis	Japan Tissue Engineering Co., Ltd.

Table 2. Commercially available human skin models

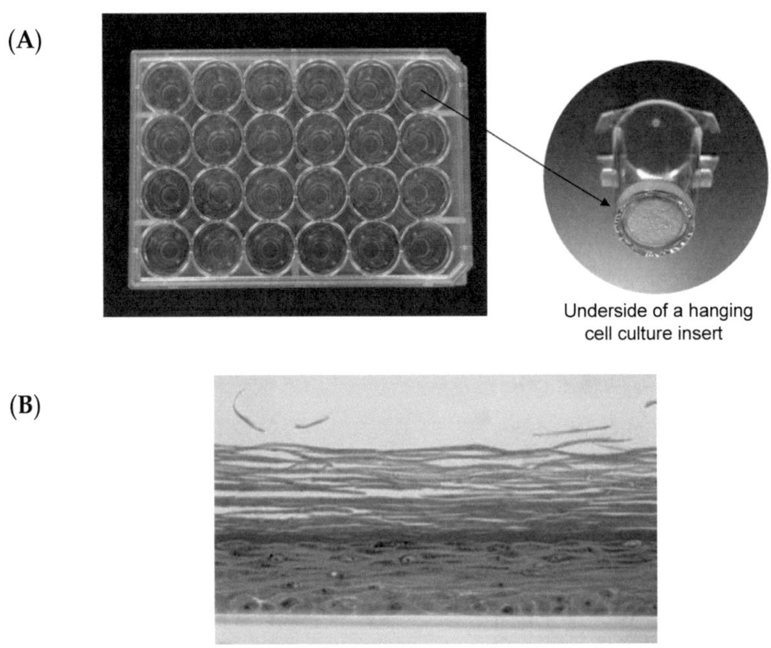

Fig. 4. An example of human skin model (LabCyte EPI-MODEL 24).[2] (A) Appearance of the skin model in hanging cell culture insert in 24-well microplate. (B) Histological cross-sectional view of the skin model with H&E staining. Epidermal cells were located on a microporous membrane.

2. Photographs by courtesy of Japan Tissue Engineering Co., Ltd.

4.3.2 *In vitro* evaluation of skin irritation by using human skin models

To evaluate and predict the skin irritancy in human, *in vitro* skin irritation tests using human skin models have been developed. During the development processes, appropriate endpoints for skin irritancy evaluation have been determined. Triglia et al. compared four endpoints on their dermal model: 1) cell viability determination with neutral red (NR), 2) cell viability determination with 3-(4,5-dimethyl-2-thiazolyl)-2,5-diphenyl-2H tetrazolium bromide (MTT), 3) release of prostaglandine E_2 (PGE_2), and 4) release of lactate dehydrogenase (LDH) (Triglia et al., 1991). They tested 13 chemicals, but there were no significant differences among the results of the four endpoints. Morota et al. compared six endpoints: 1) cell viability with MTT, 2) cell viability with NR, 3) release of PGE_2, 4) LDH, 5) interleukin-1α (IL-1α), and 6) interleukin-8 (IL-8) (Morota et al., 1999). They concluded that cell viability assays revealed good correlations with animal testing (Draize score of skin irritancy) and were advantageous to the other endpoints as they were easier to use and less costly. Recently, the EU has accepted the *in vitro* skin irritation test using RhE as stand-alone test to determine the skin irritation potential of a substance (OECD TG 439). In this guideline, cell viability assay with MTT is adopted.

However, *in vitro* skin irritation tests using human skin models have some limitations. For example, they cannot be used for samples containing high concentrations of ethanol. It is because most skin models are more sensitive to alcohols than the skin *in vivo*. Instead of the low irritation scores demonstrated in Draize rabbit skin tests, ethanol showed high toxicity in human skin model tests. In a dose-response test, higher concentration of ethanol resulted in lower cell viability (Genno et al., 1998; Li et al., 1991). It was found that ethanol concentrations above 30% affected the skin model, but had minimal effects on the rabbit skin.

Cytotoxicity of ethanol in human skin models are affected not only by the concentration of ethanol but also by the time of exposure. From the time course change of cytotoxicity test, it was shown that cell viability was not affected by short time exposure to ethanol (Nagasawa et al., 2002). Cell viability was found to be negligible when the skin was exposed to 76.9–81.4 vol% of ethanol for a period shorter than 1 minute (Yamamoto et al., 2010).

5. Irritancy and antimicrobial activity of alcohol-based hand rubs

Most alcohol-based hand rubs contain either ethanol, isopropanol or n-propanol, or a combination of two of them. Assessments of alcohol effects on the skin have involved evaluating the effects of individual alcohol at various concentrations, combinations of two or more alcohols, and alcohol solutions containing thickening agents, foaming agents, and/or small amounts of antiseptics.

5.1 Irritancy of alcohol

Most irritancy assessments of alcohol have shown that alcohols are little toxic to the skin (Boyce et al., 2000; de Haan et al., 1996; Lübbe et al., 2001; Winnefeld et al., 2000). However, many healthcare workers complain about unacceptable skin irritation caused by alcohol-based hand rubs. Even in the Guideline for Hand Hygiene in Healthcare Settings of the Centers for Disease Control (Boyce et al., 2002), skin tolerability of alcohol-based hand rubs is stated as potentially problematic: 'Although alcohols are among the safest antiseptics available, they can cause dryness and irritation'.

According to the well-designed patch testing with alcohols and sodium lauryl sulphate (SLS) as a model detergent, it was found that alcohols lead to only minor skin barrier changes and cause no changes in erythema independent of the concentration tested (Löffler et al., 2007). Compared to alcohols, the detergent SLS induced a much stronger barrier disruption and a pronounced skin hydration decrease.

Kownatzki has pointed out that the skin irritation of healthcare workers is not simply caused by alcohol antisepsis but by combined damage resulting from the alcohol antisepsis dissolving stratum corneum lipids, the removal of lipids from the skin surface by detergent washing, and the skin becoming over-hydrated from wearing gloves.

5.2 Basic formulation of alcohol-based hand rubs

Antimicrobial activity of alcohols results from their ability to denature proteins. Alcohol solutions containing 60–80% alcohol are most effective, with higher concentrations being less potent (Price, 1938; Harrington & Walker, 1903). This paradox results from the fact that proteins are not denatured easily in the absence of water (Larson & Morton, 1991). The alcohol content of solutions may be expressed as a percentage by weight, which is not affected by temperature or other variables, or as a percentage by volume, which may be affected by temperature, specific gravity and reaction concentration. For example, 70% alcohol by weight is equivalent to 76.8% by volume if prepared at 15°C, and 80.5% if prepared at 25°C (Price, 1938). In the Japanese Pharmacopoeia, ethanol solution for disinfection is defined as the concentration of 76.9–81.4% by volume.

5.3 Gel and foam formulations

Alcohol-based hand rubs intended for use in hospitals are available as low viscosity rinses, gels, and foams. For example, thickening agents such as polyacrylic acid or cellulose derivatives are commonly formulated in alcohol gels to increase the viscosity of alcohol solutions.

Limited data are available regarding the relative efficacy of various formulations. One field trial demonstrated that an ethanol gel was slightly more effective than a comparable ethanol solution in reducing bacterial counts on the hands of healthcare workers (Ojajärvi, 1991). However, a more recent study indicated that rinses reduced more bacterial counts on the hands than the gels tested (Kramer et al., 2002). Further studies are warranted to determine the relative efficacy of alcohol-based rinses and gels in reducing transmission of healthcare-associated pathogens.

In prospective trials, alcohol-based gels containing humectants caused significantly less skin irritation and dryness than the soaps or antimicrobial detergents tested (Boyce et al., 2000; Newman & Seitz, 1990).

5.4 Antiseptics formulation

Some alcohol-based hand rubs contain antiseptics in order to provide persistent (residual) activity. Addition of antiseptics (e.g., chlorhexidine or quaternary ammonium compounds) to alcohol-based formulations can result in persistent activity (Rotter, 1999).

Chlorhexidine, a cationic bisbiguanide, was developed in the United Kingdom in the early 1950s. It is effective against grampositive bacteria and has substantial residual activity.

Chlorhexidine base is barely soluble in water, and thus the water-soluble digluconate form (CHG) is widely used. Addition of low concentrations (0.5–1%) of chlorhexidine to alcohol-based preparations results in significantly greater residual activity than alcohol alone (Aly & Maibach, 1979; Lowbury et al., 1974).

Quaternary ammonium compounds are composed of a nitrogen atom linked directly to four alkyl groups, which may vary considerably in their structure and complexity (Merianos, 1991). Among this large group of compounds, alkyl benzalkonium chlorides (BAC) are the most widely used as antiseptics.

In Japan, alcohol-based hand rubs containing CHG or BAC are widely used in healthcare settings. For example, WELPAS (0.2% w/v BAC, 70% ethanol solution) and WELLUP (0.2% w/v CHG, 70% ethanol solution) are recommended for hand hygiene in the Guideline for the prevention of healthcare-associated infection in urological practice in Japan (Hamasuna et al., 2011).

Compared with CHG, BAC shows stronger activity to various microorganisms (Jono et al., 1985; Shimizu et al., 2002). However, alcohol-based hand rubs containing CHG are less irritative to the skin than those containing BAC (Tsuji et al., 1993). The skin irritancy level of alcohol-based hand rubs containing antiseptics correlates with the irritancy of the antiseptic compound contained (Tsuji et al., 1996).

It is known that alcohols may enhance skin permeation. For example, the enhancement ability of ethanol is maximized at the concentration of 50–70% (Kim et al., 1996; Watkinson et al., 2009). Hence the irritancy of antiseptic compounds may be amplified in alcohols-based hand rubs.

6. Reduction of skin irritancy

In prospective trials, alcohol-based hand rubs containing humectants caused significantly less skin irritation and dryness than the soaps or antimicrobial detergents tested. These results suggest that addition of humectants can minimize the skin irritation and dryness.

6.1 Humectants

Most alcohols-based hand rub formulations contain humectants (or emollients). The drying effect of alcohol can be reduced or eliminated by adding 1%–3% glycerol or other skin-conditioning agents (Many studies are reviewed in Boyce & Pittet, 2002). Moreover, in several recent prospective trials, alcohol-based rinses or gels containing emollients caused substantially less skin irritation and dryness than the soaps or antimicrobial detergents tested (Winnefeld et al., 2000; Boyce et al., 2000; Larson et al., 2001a, 2001b).

These studies, which were conducted in clinical settings, used various subjective and objective methods for assessing skin irritation and dryness. Further studies are warranted to know whether products with different formulations would yield similar results or not.

6.2 Skin barrier stabilizers

Lamellar structures of intercellular lipid in the stratum corneum are quite important to maintain the barrier property of the skin. It is known that some kind of compounds can stabilize the lamellar structures.

Ceramide

Ceramides are characteristic components of intercellular lipids in the stratum corneum. The lamellar structures of intercellular lipids are stabilized by long-chain ceramides. Alcohol-based hand rubs containing synthetic pseudo-ceramide are less likely to roughen the skin of the hands in comparison with hand rubs containing no emollient (Tsuboi et al., 2006).

MPC polymers (Lipidure®)

MPC polymers are novel phospholipid-like synthetic polymers composed of 2-methacryloyloxyethyl phosphorylcholine (MPC). They are biomimetic materials which have excellent biocompatiblity as its structure closely resembles that of cell membrane phospholipids (Iwasaki & Ishihara, 2005). Recently, unique functions of the MPC polymers have been reported.

MPC homo-polymer can protect the barrier property of the stratum corneum by preventing the intercellular lipid bilayer (ILB) structure from being disrupted by extensive skin hydration (Lee, 2004). It helps maintain the barrier property of the skin by preventing disruption of the ILB structure, and functions as a barrier-like membrane to prevent toxic substances from penetrating into the skin.

The effects of MPC/n-butyl methacrylate (BMA) co-polymer on the water barrier function and water-holding capacity of the stratum corneum were examined by measuring transepidermal water loss (TEWL) and electrical conductance of the skin surface (Kanekura et al., 2002). The MPC/BMA co-polymer reduced TEWL in laboratory mice significantly compared with the control. Human skin treated with this polymer showed significantly greater ability to retain water at all time points.

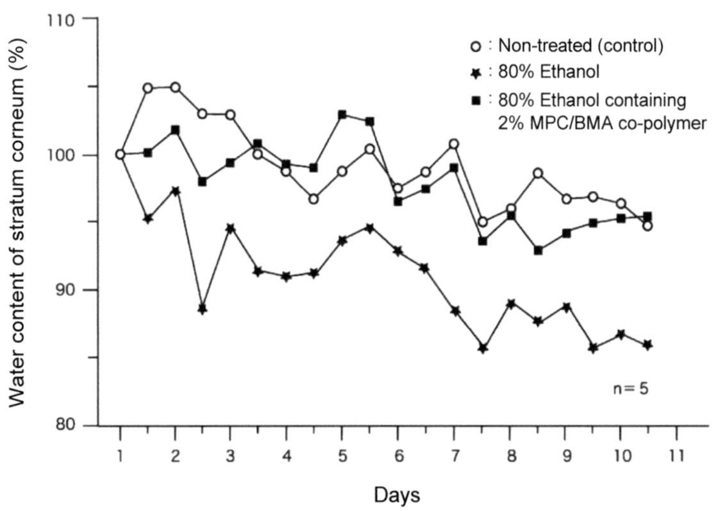

Fig. 5. Water content in the stratum corneum of hairless mice. A 100 μL solution (80% ethanol or 80% ethanol + 2% MPC/BMA co-polymer) was applied on the back skin of hairless mice twice a day for 10 days. (Figure modified from Andoh et al., 2008)

The skincare function of the MPC/BMA co-polymer was also determined by Andoh. As shown in Fig. 5, both the control and the ethanol solution containing MPC/BMA co-polymer showed the same tendency. By contrast, applying ethanol solution without MPC/BMA co-polymer decreased the water content of the stratum corneum. In addition, the presence or absence of MPC/BMA co-polymer had no relation to the bactericidal activity of the ethanol solutions (Andoh et al., 2008).

Recently, the unique function of MPC/stearyl methacrylate (SMA) co-polymer has been reported. It was found that the MPC/SMA co-polymer forms a self-assembled mosaic lamellar structure, which is structurally similar to ILB, by simple drying process. It is considered that the MPC/SMA co-polymer has a potential to act as an artificial intercellular lipid for damaged skin (Yamamoto et al., 2007).

Commercially available MPC polymers for skincare products are shown in Table 3.

Chemical Structure	Product Name
MPC* homo-polymer	Lipidure®-HM
MPC/BMA** co-polymer	Lipidure-PMB®
MPC/SMA*** co-polymer	Lipidure®-S
Polyol solution of MPC/SMA co-polymer	Lipidure®-NR

Note: *MPC: 2-methacryloyloxyethyl phosphorylcholine. **BMA: n-Butyl methacrylate. ***SMA: Stearyl methacrylate.

Table 3. Commercially available MPC polymers for skincare products[3]

7. *In vitro* evaluation of skin irritation caused by alcohol-based hand rubs

Animal experiments are quite useful for estimating the skin irritation potential in human. However, using experimental animals requires special techniques and facilities, and also has problem in animal protection. Thus development of an alternative to animal experiments is important not only from the viewpoint of ethical aspects but also for efficient research and development. The *in vitro* reconstructed human epidermis (RhE) has been applied for evaluating the skin irritancy of various substances. However, RhE has not been used for the evaluation of alcohol-based hand rubs because of the high skin permeability and cytotoxicity of alcohols. Recently, the author has developed a novel *in vitro* experimental method named "Skin model blowing method" (SMBM), which mimics the actual usage of alcohol-based hand rubs: putting on, spreading, rubbing into the skin, and drying. The skin irritation potential of alcohol-based hand rubs could be estimated by using SMBM. In this section, details of SMBM and evaluation results of some of alcohol-based hand rubs used in Japan are described.

7.1 Development of *in vitro* evaluation method using RhE

7.1.1 Experimental

Alcohol-based hand rubs used in this study

The alcohol-based hand rubs used in this study are summarized in Table 4.

---

[3] http://www.nof.co.jp/business/life/lipidure/english/
Lipidure and Lipidure-PMB are registered trademarks of NOF Corporation in the U.S., and are registered trademarks or trademarks in other countries. All other product names are registered trademarks or trademarks of each company.

Code	Product Name	Antiseptics**	Supplier***
a	Ethanol for disinfection*	-	Kozakai
b	ISODINE PALM	PVP-I 0.5%	Meiji
c	WELLUP	CHG 0.2%	Maruishi
d	WELPAS	BAC 0.2%	Maruishi

Note: *Complying with the Japanese Pharmacopoeia (76.9–81.4 vol% of ethanol). **Antiseptics: Povidone iodine (PVP-I), Chlorhexidine gluconate (CHG), Benzalkonium chloride (BAC). ***Supplier: Kozakai Pharmaceutical Co., Ltd., Meiji Seika Pharma, Ltd., Maruishi Pharmaceutical Co., Ltd.

Table 4. Alcohol-based hand rubs (76.9–81.4 vol% of ethanol) used for studies

Reconstructed human epidermis (RhE)

The RhE kit LabCyte EPI-MODEL was purchased from Japan Tissue Engineering Co., Ltd.

Blowing equipment

Blowing equipment consisting of an air pump (exhaust volume: 1.3 L/min), tube and 4-channel nozzle (VACUBOY adapter, Integra Bioscience AG) was assembled in house.

(A)

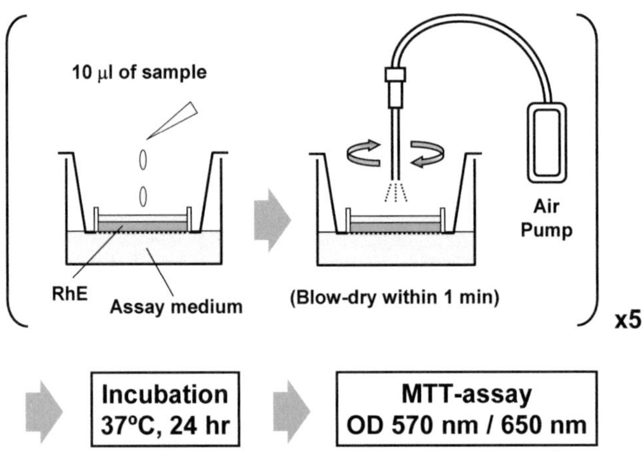

(B)

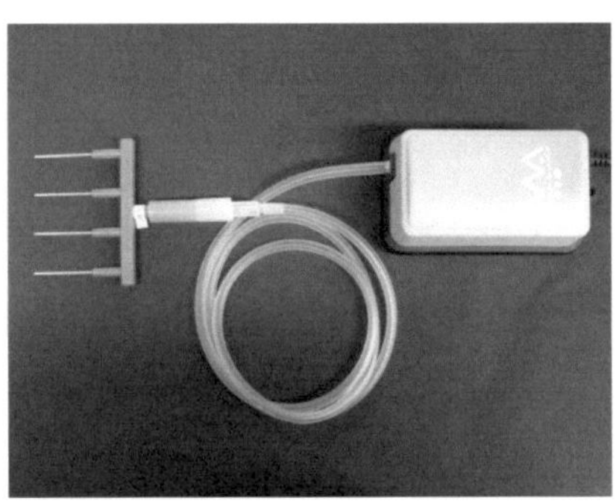

Fig. 6. Testing protocol and the blowing equipment. (A) Schematic illustration of testing protocol named "Skin model blowing method". (B) Blowing equipment consisting of an air pump (exhaust volume: 1.3 L/min), tube and 4-channel nozzle. The 4-channel nozzle corresponds to the tandem 4 epidermis models in 24-well microplate.

In vitro evaluation of skin irritancy, "Skin model blowing method" (SMBM)

Ten μL each of alcohol-based hand rub was applied to the surface of RhE, and blow-dried within 1 minute by using blowing equipment. This operation was repeated 5 times. As a control, only blow-drying was applied. After the operation, the RhE was incubated in an assay medium for 24 hr at 37°C in 5% CO_2 atmosphere. Then the RhE were further incubated in a MTT medium (0.5 mg of 3-(4,5-dimethyl-2-thiazolyl)-2,5-diphenyl-2H tetrazolium bromide in assay medium) for 3 hr at 37°C in 5% CO_2 atmosphere. Living cells were dyed with purple formazan. The dyed RhE was put into microtube; then 200 μL of isopropyl alcohol was added to extract purple formazan. The extracts were measured for the absorbance at 570 nm (reference wavelength 650 nm) using a microplate reader (SpectraMax 250, Molecular Devices). Three RhE were used per group (n=3).

Comparative analysis between *in vivo* and *in vitro* experiments

The cell viability values obtained from SMBM and the integrated scores of irritation index of skin in rabbit (Tsuji et al., 1993) was compared. The integrate scores of **primary** irritation index were a: 1.2, b: 1.7, c: 5.7, and d: 58.3. The integrate scores of **cumulative** irritation index were a: 7.0, b: 6.5, c: 22.5, and d: 104.0.

Statistical analysis

Values were represented in means ± SD. Experimental groups were compared with the control using Student's t-test. $P < 0.05$ and $P < 0.01$ were taken to be the level of statistical significance.

7.1.2 Results

In vitro evaluation of skin irritancy by SMBM

The cell viability of the RhE exposed to alcohol-based hand rub was determined by MTT-assay. The order of cell viability was as follows: Ethanol for disinfection = ISODINE PALM > WELLUP > WELPAS (Fig. 7). The RhE exposed to ISODINE PALM was stained with povidone iodine, but the stain disappeared after the incubation and did not affect the MTT-assay.

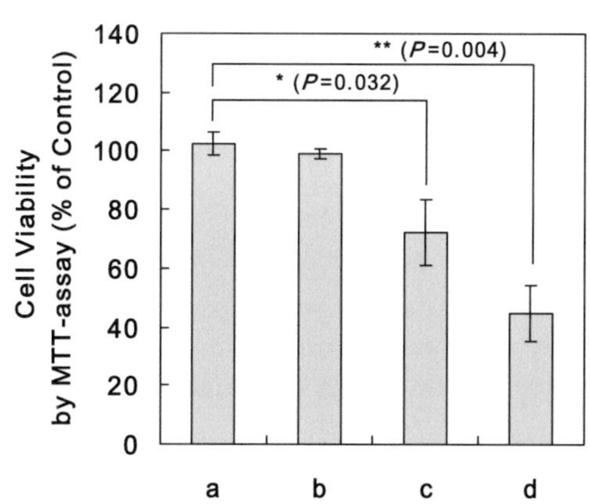

Fig. 7. Cell viability determined by MTT-assay; a: ethanol for disinfection, b: ISODINE PALM, c: WELLUP, d: WELPAS. The cell viability of RhE exposed to alcohol-based hand rub is expressed as a percentage relative to untreated one (negative control). Data are presented as means ± SD (n=3). $^{*}P < 0.05$ and $^{**}P < 0.01$ compared with ethanol for disinfection.

Comparative analysis between *in vivo* and *in vitro* experiments

The cell viabilities obtained from SMBM (this study) and the skin irritation index obtained from Draize rabbit tests (previous study: Tsuji et al., 1993) were examined. Fig. 8 shows a high correlation between the cell viability and skin irritation index.

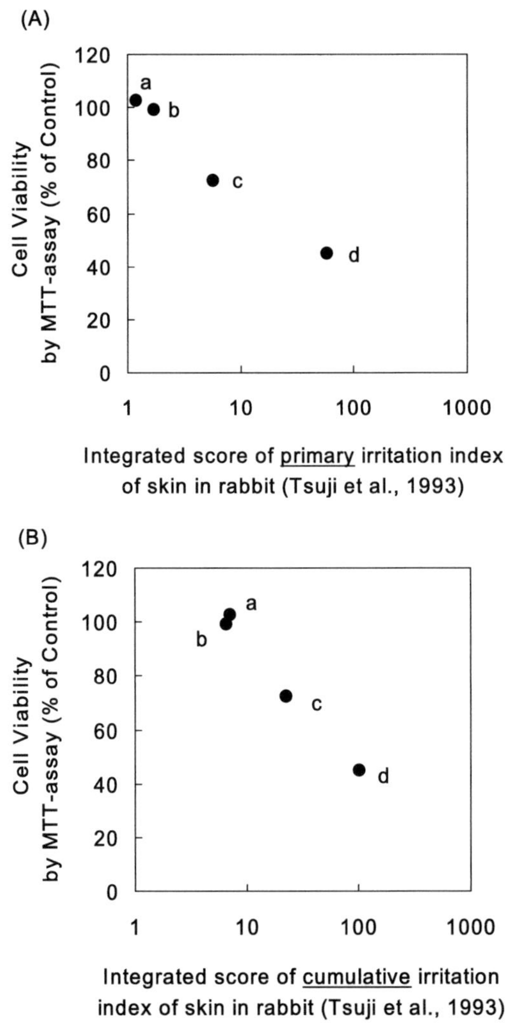

Fig. 8. Comparative analysis of *in vivo* and *in vitro* experiments. (A) Correlation of integrated score of primary irritation index of skin in rabbit and mean cell viability. (B) Correlation of integrated score of cumulative irritation index of skin in rabbit and mean cell viability.

7.1.3 Discussion

As already mentioned in Section 5.4, alcohols may enhance skin permeation, thus the irritancy of alcohol-based hand rubs containing antiseptics should be evaluated for the whole formulation, not for each component. In this study, a novel *in vitro* experimental method named SMBM was developed. SMBM mimics the actual usage of alcohol-based hand rubs: putting on, spreading, rubbing into the skin and drying. As described in Section 4.3.2, cytotoxicity of ethanol in RhE is negligible for exposure shorter than 1 minute (Yamamoto et al., 2010). The results of the SMBM showed that the method can evaluate the overall irritation potential of the whole formulation of alcohol-based hand rubs containing antiseptics.

From the comparative analysis between *in vivo* and *in vitro* experiments, it was found that there was a high correlation between cell viability and skin irritation index. Therefore, SMBS is effective for quantitatively estimating the skin irritation potential of alcohol-based hand rubs containing antiseptics.

7.2 Evaluation of alcohol-based hand rubs containing cationic antiseptics by SMBM

7.2.1 Experimental

Alcohol-based hand rubs containing cationic antiseptics used in this study

The alcohol-based hand rubs used in this study are summarized in Table 5.

Code	Product Name	Antiseptics	Other components	Supplier*
A	Hibiscohol A	CHG 0.2%	Diisobutyl adipate, Allantoin, PEG glyceryl cocoate	Saraya
B	WELLUP	CHG 0.2%	Isopropyl myristate, 4 Non-disclosed components	Maruishi
C	WELLUP Hand Lotion 0.5%	CHG 0.5%	HM-HPMC**, 1,3-Butylene glycol, Glycyrrhetinic acid, Diisopropyl adipate, Glycerine fatty acid ester, Buffering agent	Maruishi
D	WELPAS	BAC 0.2%	Propylene glycol, Isopropyl myristate, 4 Non-disclosed components	Maruishi
E	RABINET	BAC 0.2%	Urea, Glycerin, Tocopherol acetate, Allantoin, PCA ethyl cocoyl arginate	Kenei
F	Puremist	BAC 0.2%	Lipidure-PMB®***, Isopropyl myristate, Glycerin, 2 Non-disclosed components	Johnson & Johnson

Note: *Supplier: Saraya Co., Ltd., Maruishi Pharmaceutical Co., Ltd., Kenei Pharmaceutical Co., Ltd., Johnson & Johnson K.K. **HM-HPMC: Hydrophobically-modified hydroxypropyl methylcellulose. ***Lipidure-PMB®: Poly(2-methacryloyloxyethyl phosphorylcholine-co-n-butyl methacrylate).

Table 5. Alcohol-based hand rubs (76.9–81.4 vol% of ethanol) containing cationic antiseptics

Other materials and methods

Reconstructed human epidermis (RhE) and blowing equipment were prepared; and *in vitro* evaluation of skin irritancy and statistical analysis were carried out as previously described in Section 7.1.1.

7.2.2 Results

The mean cell viability of the 0.5% CHG formulation was slightly lower than that of 0.2% CHG formulations, but there were no significant differences in statistical analysis. On the other hand, the three 0.2% BAC formulations showed differences in cell viability (Fig. 9).

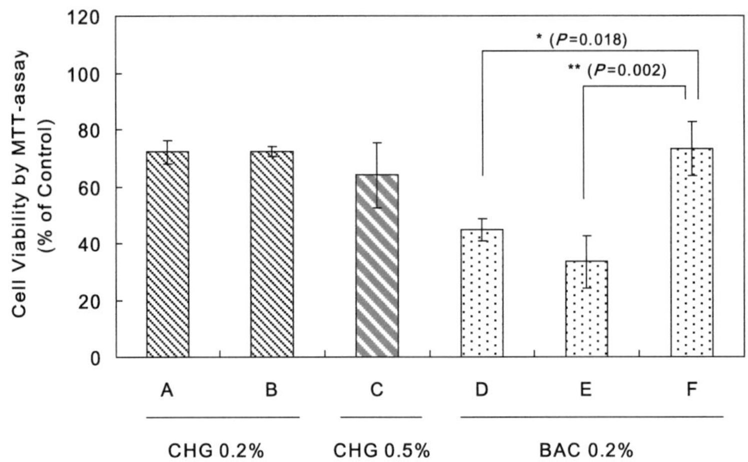

Fig. 9. Means ± SD of cell viability of commercially available alcohol-based hand rubs determined by using SMBM

7.2.3 Discussion

Tested samples containing 0.2% or 0.5% CHG showed 64–72% cell viability, and therefore, their skin irritation potential was likely to be mild. The difference in CHG concentration did not significantly affect cell viability.

By contrast, in the case of BAC, the cell viability differed depending on formulation although the BAC concentration was the same. Of these, code F (Puremist) showed especially high cell viability (73% of cell viability). It was suggested that some components other than BAC may have reduced the skin irritation potential. Since isopropyl myristate and glycerin are also formulated in the other products (code D and E), they were unlikely to be the factor regulating the phenomenon. It is noteworthy that Lipidure-PMB® (MPC/BMA co-polymer) is contained in Puremist. As already mentioned in Section 6.2, MPC polymers stabilize the skin barrier. The results of this study suggest that the MPC polymers are possibly capable of reducing the cytotoxicity of alcohol-based hand rubs containing antiseptics.

8. Conclusion

In this review, the author summarized the structure and barrier function of the skin, the mechanism and evaluation methods of skin irritation, and the irritancy of alcohol-based hand rubs. It also described a novel *in vitro* evaluation method for assessing the skin irritation caused by alcohol-based hand rubs. The newly developed *in vitro* evaluation method "SMBM" has several advantages including 1) replacing animal experiments, 2) enabling multiple substances to be tested at once, 3) easy quantitative estimation because it is based on simple cytotoxicity test. The author believes that this new approach is quite efficient and useful for developing less irritating alcohol-based hand rub products.

9. References

Aly, R. & Maibach, H.I. (1979). Comparative study on the antimicrobial effect of 0.5% chlorhexidine gluconate and 70% isopropyl alcohol on the normal flora of hands. *Applied and environmental microbiology*, Vol. 37, pp. 610–613.

Andoh, N.; Obi, N.; Miyazaki, T. & Ochiai, H. (2008). Antibacterial and skin protective effects of polyquaternium-51-containing ethanol, *Japanese Journal of Environmental Infections*, Vol. 23, pp. 35–40.

Asselineau, D.; Bernhard, B.; Bailly, C. & Darmon, M. (1985). Epidermal morphogenesis and induction of the 67 kD keratin polypeptide by culture of human keratinocytes at the liquid-air interface, *Experimental cell research*, Vol. 159, pp. 536–539.

Barel, A.O. & Clarys, P. (1995). Study of the stratum corneum barrier function by transepidermal water loss measurements: comparison between two commercial instruments: Evaporimeter and Tewameter, *Skin pharmacology*, Vol. 8, No. 4, pp. 186–195.

Bell, E.; Ehrlich, H.; Buttle, D. & Nakatsuji, T. (1981). Living tissue formed *in vitro* and accepted as skin-equivalent tissue of full thickness, *Science*, Vol. 211, pp. 1052–1054.

Boyce, J.M., Kelliher, S. & Vallande, N. (2000). Skin irritation and dryness associated with two hand-hygiene regimens: soap-and-water hand washing versus hand antisepsis with an alcoholic hand gel, *Infection control and hospital epidemiology*, Vol. 21, pp. 442–448.

Boyce, J.M. & Pittet, D. (2002). Guideline for Hand Hygiene in Health-Care Settings. Recommendations of the Healthcare Infection Control Practices Advisory Committee and the HIPAC/SHEA/APIC/IDSA Hand Hygiene Task Force, *American journal of infection control*, Vol. 30, pp. S1–46.

Cohen, J.C.; Hartman, D.G.; Garofalo, M.J.; Basehoar, A.; Raynor, B.; Ashbrenner, E. & Akin, F.J. (2009). Comparison of closed chamber and open chamber evaporimetry, *Skin research and technology*, Vol. 15, No. 1, pp. 51–54.

de Haan, P.; Meester, H.H.M. & Bruynzeel, D.P. (1996). Irritancy of alcohol, In: *The Irritant Contact Dermatitis Syndrome*, Van der Valk, P.G. & Maibach, H.I. (Ed.), pp 65–70, CRC Press Inc., Boca Raton, FL.

de Paepe, K.; Houben, E.; Adam, R.; Wiesemann, F. & Rogiers, V. (2005). Validation of the VapoMeter, a closed unventilated chamber system to assess transepidermal water loss vs. the open chamber Tewameter. *Skin research and technology*, Vol. 11, No. 1, pp. 61–69.

Edwards, C.C. (1972). Hazardous substances. Proposed revision of test for primary skin irritants, *Federal Register*, Vol. 37, 27635–27636.

Gallin, J.I.; Goldstein, I.M. & Snyderman, R. (Ed.). (1992). Inflammation: Basic Principles and Clinical Correlates, 2nd Ed., Ravan Press, New York, NY.

Genno, M.; Yamamoto, R. & Kojima, H. (1998). Evaluation of a New Alternative to Primary Draize Skin Irritation Testing Using the EpiDerm™ Skin Model. *AATEX (Alternatives to animal testing and eperimentation)*, Vol. 5, pp. 195–200.

Green, H.; Kehinde, O. & Thomas, J. (1979). Growth of cultured human epidermal cells into multiple epithelia suitable for grafting. *Proceedings of the National Academy of Sciences of the United States of America*, Vol. 76, No. 11, pp. 5665-5668.

Hamasuna, R.; Takahashi, S.; Yamamoto, S.; Arakawa, S.; Yanaihara, H.; Ishikawa, S. & Matsumoto, T. (2011). Guideline for the prevention of health care-associated infection in urological practice in Japan. *International journal of urology*, Vol. 18, pp. 495-502.

Harrington, C. & Walker, H. (1903). The germicidal action of alcohol. *Boston Medical and Surgical Journal*, Vol. 148, pp. 548-552.

Iwasaki, Y. & Ishihara, K. (2005). Phosphorylcholine-containing polymers for biomedical applications. *Analytical and bioanalytical chemistry*, Vol. 381, No. 3, pp. 534-546.

Jono, K.; Uemura, T.; Kuno, M. & Higashide, E. (1985). Bactericidal activity and killing rate of benzalkonium chloride and chlorhexidine gluconate, *YAKUGAKU ZASSHI (Journal of the Pharmaceutical Society of Japan)*, Vol. 105, pp. 751-759.

Kim, D.D.; Kim, J.L. & Chien, Y.W. (1996). Mutual hairless rat skin permeation-enhancing effect of ethanol/water system and oleic acid, *Journal of pharmaceutical sciences*, Vol. 85, pp. 1191-1195.

Kanekura, T.; Nagata, Y.; Miyoshi, H.; Ishihara, K.; Nakabayashi, N. & Kanzaki, T. (2002). Beneficial effects of synthetic phospholipid polymer, poly(2-methacryloyloxyethyl phosphorylcholine-co-n-butyl methacrylate), on stratum corneum function, *Clinical and Experimental Dermatology*, Vol. 27, pp. 230-234.

Kownatzki, E. (2003). Hand hygiene and skin health. *The Journal of hospital infection*, Vol. 55, pp. 239-245.

Kramer, A.; Rudolph, P.; Kampf, G. & Pittet, D. (2002). Limited efficacy of alcohol-based hand gels, *Lancet*, Vol. 359, pp. 1489-1490.

Larson, E.L.; Aiello, A.E.; Bastyr, J.; Lyle, C.; Stahl, J.; Cronquist, A.; Lai, L. & Della-Latta, P. (2001a). Assessment of two hand hygiene regimens for intensive care unit personnel, *Critical care medicine*, Vol. 29, pp. 944-951.

Larson, E.L.; Aiello, A.E.; Heilman, J.M.; Lyle, C.T.; Cronquist, A.; Stahl, J.B. & Della-Latta , P. (2001b). Comparison of different regimens for surgical hand preparation, *Association of Operating Room Nurses Journal*, Vol. 73, pp. 412-418.

Larson, E.L. & Morton, H.E. (1991). Alcohols, In: *Disinfection, sterilization and preservation, 4th ed.*, Block, S.S., (Ed.), pp. 191-203, Lea & Febiger, Philadelphia, PA.

Lee, A-R.C. (2004). Phospholipid polymer, 2-methacryloyloxyethyl phosphorylcholine and its skin barrier function, *Archives of pharmacal research*, Vol. 27, pp. 1177-1182.

Levin, C. & Maibach, H.I. (2004). Animal, human and *in vitro* test methods for predicting skin irritation, In: *Dermatotoxicology, Sixth Edition*, Zhai, H. & Maibach, H.I. (Ed.), pp. 678-690, CRC Press Inc., Boca Raton, FL.

Li, L.N.; Margolis, L.B. & Hoffman, R.M. (1991). Skin toxicity determined *in vitro* by three-dimensional, native-state histoculture. *Proceedings of the National Academy of Sciences of the United States of America*, Vol. 88, pp. 1908-1912.

Lowbury, E.J.; Lilly, H.A. & Ayliffe, G.A. (1974). Preoperative disinfection of surgeons' hands: use of alcoholic solutions and effects of gloves on skin flora. *British medical journal*, Vol. 4, pp. 369-372.

Löffler, H.; Kampf, G.; Schmermund, D. & Maibach, H.I. (2007). How irritant is alcohol?, *The British journal of dermatology*, Vol. 157, pp. 74-81.

Löffler, H. & Happle, R. (2003). Profile of irritant patch testing with detergents: sodium lauryl sulfate, sodium laureth sulfate and alkyl polyglucoside, *Contact Dermatitis*, Vol. 48, pp. 26–32.

Lübbe, J.; Ruffieux, C.; van Melle, G. & Perrenoud, D. (2001). Irritancy of the skin disinfectant n-propanol, *Contact dermatitis*, Vol. 45, pp. 226-231.

Merianos, J.J. (1991). Quaternary ammonium antimicrobial compounds. In: *Disinfection, sterilization, and preservation, 4th ed.*, Block, S.S. (Ed.), pp. 225–255, Lea & Febiger, Philadelphia, PA.

Mezei, M.; Sager, R.W.; Stewart, W.D. & DeRuyter, A.L. (1966). Dermatitic effect of nonionic surfactants. I. Gross, microscopic, and metabolic changes in rabbit skin treated with nonionic surface-active agents, *Journal of Pharmaceutical Sciences*, Vol. 55, pp. 584–590.

Morota, K.; Morikawa, N.; Morita, S.; Kojima, H. & Konishi, H. (1999). Alternative to primary Draize skin irritation test using cultured human skin model: Comparison of six endpoints, *AATEX (Alternatives to animal testing and eperimentation)*, Vol. 6, pp. 41–51.

Murphy, J.C.; Watson, E.S.; Wirth, P.W.; Skierkowski, P.; Folk, R.M. & Peck, G. (1979). Cutaneous irritation in the topical application of 30 antineoplastic agents to New Zealand white rabbits, *Toxicology*, Vol. 14, pp. 117–130.

Nagasawa, M.; Hayashi, H. & Nakayoshi, T. (2002). *In vitro* evaluation of skin sensitivity of povidone-iodine and other antiseptics using a three-dimensional human skin model, *Dermatology*, Vol. 204, pp. 109–113.

National Academy of Sciences and Committee for the Revision of NAS Publication 1138. (1977). Principles and procedures for evaluating the toxicity of household substances, pp. 23–59, National Academy of Sciences, Washington DC.

Nixon, G.A.; Tyson, C.A. & Wertz, W.C. (1975). Interspecies comparisons of skin irritancy, *Toxicology and Applied Pharmacology*, Vol. 31, pp. 481–490.

Newman, J.L. & Seitz, J.C. (1990). Intermittent use of an antimicrobial hand gel for reducing soap-induced irritation of health care personnel, *American journal of infection control*, Vol. 18, pp. 194–200.

Ojajärvi, J. (1991). Handwashing in Finland, *Journal of Hospital Infection*, Vol. 18(suppl B), pp. 35–40.

Patil, S.M.; Patrick, E. & Maibach, H.I. (1996). Animal, human and *in vitro* test methods for predicting skin irritation, In: *Dermatotoxicology*, Fifth Edition, Marzulli, F.N. & Maibach, H.I. (Ed.), pp. 411–436, Taylor and Francis, Washington DC.

Patil, S.M.; Patrick, E. & Maibach, H.I. (1998). Animal, human and *in vitro* test methods for predicting skin irritation, In: *Dermatotoxicology methods: the laboratory worker's vade mecum*, Marzulli, F.N. & Maibach, H.I. (Ed.), pp. 89–104, Taylor and Francis, Washington DC.

Patrick, E. & Maibach, H.I. (1989). Comparison of the time course, dose response and mediators of chemically induced skin irritation in three species. In: *Current Topics in Contact Dermatitis*, Frosch, P., Dooms-Goossens, A., Lachapelle, J.M., Rrcroft, R.J.G. & Scheper, R.J. (Ed.), pp. 399–402, Springer-Verlag, New York.

Price, P.B. (1938). New studies in surgical bacteriology and surgical technic. *The Journal of the American Medical Association*, Vol. 111, pp. 1993–1996.

Rotter, M. (1999). Hand washing and hand disinfection. In: *Hospital epidemiology and infection control, 2nd ed.*, Mayhall, C.G., (Ed.) , pp. 1339–1355, Lippincott Williams & Wilkins, Philadelphia, PA.

Shillaker, R.O.; Bell, G.M.; Hodgson, J.T. & Padgham, M.D. (1989). Guinea pig maximization test for skin sensitisation: The use of fewer test animals, *Archives of Toxicology*, Vol. 63, pp. 283–288.

Shimizu, M.; Okuzumi, K.; Yoneyama, A.; Kunisada, T.; Araake, M.; Ogawa, H. & Kimura, S. (2002). *In vitro* antiseptic susceptibility of clinical isolates from nosocomial infections, *Dermatology*, Vol. 204, pp. 21–27.

Skog, E. (1960). Primary irritant and allergic eczematous reactions in patients with different dermatoses, *Acta dermato-venereologica*, Vol. 40, pp. 307–312.

Triglia, D.; Sherard Braa, S.; Yonan, C. & Naughton, G.K. (1991). Cytotoxicity testing using neutral red and MTT assays on a three-dimensional human skin substrate. *Toxicology in vitro*, Vol. 5, pp. 573–578.

Tsuboi, R.; Arai, K.; Sumida, H.; Nishio, M.; Hasebe, K.; Hioki, Y. & Okuda, M. (2006). Efficacy of an alcohol-based hand rub containing synthetic pseudo-ceramide for reducing skin roughness of the hand, *Japanese Journal of Environmental Infections*, Vol. 21, No. 2, pp. 73–80.

Tsuji, A.; Nakayoshi, T.; Sannomiya, F.; Yashiro, J. & Goto, S. (1993). Rabbit skin irritation of alcoholic solutions for hand disinfection, *Japanese Journal of Environmental Infections*, Vol. 8, No. 2, pp. 33–41.

Tsuji, A.; Sannomiya, F.; Yashiro, J.; Nakajima, S. & Goto, S. (1996). Skin irritation study of anticeptics with rabbit, *Japanese Journal of Environmental Infections*, Vol. 11, No. 3, pp. 207–220.

Warner, R.R.; Stone, K.J. & Boissy Y.L. (2003). Hydration disrupts human stratum corneum ultrastructure, *The Journal of investigative dermatology*, Vol. 120, pp. 275–284.

Watkinson, R.M.; Herkenne, C.; Guy, R.H.; Hadgraft, J.; Oliveira, G. & Lane, M.E. (2009). Influence of ethanol on the solubility, ionization and permeation characteristics of ibuprofen in silicone and human skin, *Skin pharmacology and physiology*, Vol. 22, pp. 15–21.

Weil, C.S. & Scala, R.A. (1971). Study of intra- and interlaboratory variability in the results of rabbit eye and skin irritation tests. *Toxicology and Applied Pharmacology*, Vol. 19, pp. 276–360.

Winnefeld, M.; Richard, M.A.; Drancourt, M. & Grob, J.J. (2000). Skin tolerance and effectiveness of two hand decontamination procedures in everyday hospital use. *The British journal of dermatology*, Vol. 143, pp. 546–550.

World Health Organization (2009). WHO Guidelines on Hand Hygiene in Health Care.

Yamamoto, N.; Miyamoto, K. & Katoh, M. (2010). Development of alternative to animal experiment in evaluation of skin irritation caused by alcohol-based hand rubs. *YAKUGAKU ZASSHI (Journal of the Pharmaceutical Society of Japan)*, Vol. 130, pp. 1069–1073.

Yamamoto, N.; Shuto, K.; Yamagishi, T. & Nakamoto, Y. (2007). Self-assembled mosaic lamellar structures in hydrophobic phospholipid polymer films. *KOBUNSHI RONBUNSHU (Japanese Journal of Polymer Science and Technology)*, Vol. 64, pp. 115–118.

Part 4

Emerging Trends

10

Heteroresistance

Meletis Georgios
Clinical Microbiologist, Research Assistant
Aristotle University of Thessaloniki, School of Medicine
Greece

1. Introduction

The emergence of clinical infection due to methicillin resistant *Staphylococcus aureus* (MRSA) with decreased susceptibility to vancomycin and the frequent isolations in some countries of multidrug-resistant (resistant to three or more classes of antimicrobials), extensively drug resistant (resistant to all but one or two classes) or even pandrug-resistant (resistant to all available classes) Gram negative nosocomial pathogens are causing great concern worldwide. In an era of increasing antimicrobial resistance many recent studies have focused on the heteroresistance phenomenon that is considered to be a precursor stage, which may or may not lead to the emergence of a resistant strain.

The term heteroresistance has been mostly used to describe hetero-vancomycin intermediate Staphylococcus aureus (hVISA) that spontaneously produces VISA cells within its cell population at a frequency of 10^{-6} or above (Neoh et al., 2008). In a broader sense though, heteroresistance may be understood as mixed populations of drug-resistant and drug-sensitive cells in a single clinical specimen or isolate where the proportion of resistant organisms may not be explicable by the natural "background" mutation rate alone (Rinder, 2001); and even more precisely, heteroresistance can be defined as resistance to certain antibiotics expressed by a subset of a microbial population that is generally considered to be susceptible to these antibiotics according to traditional *in-vitro* susceptibility testing (Falagas et al., 2008). The frequency of these resistant organisms is about one sub-clone in every 10^5-10^6 colonies, which roughly equals the normal rate of mutation.

2. Heteroresistance in *Staphylococcus aureus*

S. aureus is the species in which the phenomenon has been reported more often and studied more in detail. Heteroresistance to methicillin (Ryffel et al., 1994) and oxacillin (Cimolai et al., 1997; H. Liu et al., 1990; Wannet, 2002) is dependent on the *mecA* gene that codes for a lower-affinity penicillin-binding protein conferring strain-specific variable resistance from borderline to elevated resistance to beta-lactam antibiotics. It has been shown that in addition to this resistance, chromosomal mutations not related to *mecA* may generate a small proportion of highly methicillin-resistant subclones (Strandén et al., 1996).

The first reports of VISA (Hiramatsu et al., 1997a) and hVISA (Hiramatsu et al., 1997b) were made from Japanese hospitals in 1997 and inspired further research because vancomycin has been the drug of choice for infections due to MRSA. Mu 3 was the first MRSA strain heteroresistant to vancomycin and it is used since then as a control strain in different methodologies for the detection of vancomycin heteroresistance in MRSA. Several later studies from various parts of the world (Borg et al., 2005; Chesneau et al., 2000; Howe et al., 1999; M.N. Kim et al., 2002; Marchese et al., 2000; Reverdy et al., 2001; Wang et al., 2004) have proved that heteroresistance to vancomycin among MRSA was maybe ignored or underestimated but not absent. Furthermore, since early VISA isolates in the USA were resistant to teicoplanin too (Appelbaum, 2007), and reduced susceptibility (Park et al., 2000) or heterogeneous resistance (Nunes et al., 2007) to this drug were also reported, the term glycopeptide-intermediate *S. aureus* (GISA) has been added to indicate a broader resistance profile.

Reduced vancomycin susceptibility of hVISA and VISA strains is not linked to the *vanA* gene, which causes the high-level vancomycin resistance of certain enterococcal species and has been found rarely in vancomycin-resistant MRSA (VRSA) (Cui et al., 2006; Howden et al., 2008) but is rather a consequence of several phenotypic changes (Rong & Leonard, 2010). Among those suggested, the thickened bacterial cell wall is the most frequently observed (Kim et al., 2000). This cell wall change could probably explain also the cross-heteroresistance between vancomycin and daptomycin- a relatively large molecule that has to access relevant binding regions on the bacterial cell membrane in order to act (Sakoulas et al., 2006).

3. Heteroresistance among Gram negative nosocomial pathogens

Carbapenems are the most effective antimicrobial agents against Gram negative bacteria. Furthermore, they are stable to the hydrolytic activity of extended spectrum beta-lactamases and therefore they have been used widely for treating infections caused by multidrug resistant isolates. The extended use however of these compounds has led to the emergence of carbapenem resistance mechanisms mainly in members of the Enterobacteriaceae family, in *Pseudomonas aeruginosa* and *Acinetobacter baumanii*. Carbapenem heteroresistance among *A. baumanii* strains has been reported in a preliminary (Pournaras et al., 2005) and a complete study (Ikonomidis et al., 2009) from Greece where Pournaras et al. found also meropenem heteroresistant subpopulations in six apparently meropenem-susceptible, carbapenemase (KPC)-producing *Klebsiella pneumoniae* (KPC-KP) clinical isolates (Pournaras et al., 2010).

Colistin is among the last-resort therapy for treating infections caused by carbapenem resistant pathogens but resistance to this drug is emerging in multidrug-resistant Gram negative bacteria (Kontopoulou et al., 2010). Heteroresistance to colistin was initially described among clinical *A. baumannii* (Li et al., 2006; C.H. Tan et al., 2007; Yau et al., 2009) and *Enterobacter cloacae* isolates (Lo-Ten-Foe et al., 2007). Intrestingly, in *A. baumannii*, this heteroresistance was documented to be related to previous colistin therapy (Hawley et al., 2008). Heteroresistance to colistin has been reported in *K. pneumoniae* isolates collected from 16 medical centers in various countries (Poudial et al., 2008) and among carbapenemase-producing *K. pneumoniae* (KPC or VIM-1) regardless prior colistin therapy in a Greek hospital where resistant rates to colistin in carbapenemase-producing *K. pneumoniae* rose from 0% in 2007 to 24.3% in 2009 (Meletis et al., 2011).

4. Heteroresistance in other species

Heteroresistance to glycopeptides is not limited in *S. aureus* but has been described for *Enterococcus faecium* (Alam et al., 2001; Qu et al., 2009) and coagulase-negative staphylococci as well, including *S. epidermidis, S. auricularis, S. capitis, S. haemolyticus, S. simulans* and *S.*

warneri (Nunes et al., 2006; Wong et al., 1999). Heteroresistance to penicillin has been reported in *Streptococcus pneumoniae* (Morand & Muhlemann, 2007), heteroresistance to fluconazole and other azoles in *Cryptococcus neoformans* (Mondon et al., 1999; Yamazumi et al., 2003) while metronidazole heteroresistance in *Gardnerella vaginalis* has been blamed for therapeutic failures (Altrichter et al., 1994).

The heteroresistance phenomenon is present even in clinical tuberculosis. It is not rare and not restricted to a particular resistance gene, but is obscured by cultivation as well as by some, culture-independent resistance prediction tests (Rinder et al., 2001). In fact, heteroresistant subpopulations are frequent in *Mycobacterium tuberculosis* although they seem to be well hidden. This observation may be explained by studies showing that acquisition of resistance results in an- at least temporary- decrease in growth rate (Billington et al., 1999; Gillespie et al., 2001).

It will be very interesting to find out if heteroresistance exists even among other species or concerns more antimicrobial agents. It is conceivable that there is more to be found and further research may provide new insight in this field.

5. Detection methods

Detection of heteroresistance is difficult and labor-intensive. Disc diffusion method or commercial automated systems may fail to detect most heteroresistant isolates (Lo-Ten-Foe et al., 2007; Tenover, 1999), and E-test results depend on the medium used (T.Y. Tan & Ng., 2007). Gradient plates, Disc-agar Method, E-test GRD (Glycopeptide Resistance Detection), Vancomycin-containig plates and E-test Macrodilution have all been explored for the detection of hGISA and GISA staphylococci but Population Analyses Profiles remains to date the most reliable method to detect heteroresistant subpopulations in Gram positive as well as in Gram negative bacteria. Growth of resistant subcolonies within a clear E-test inhibition zone and Population Screening Plates can be used for screening purposes, therefore, these two techniques are also described in this chapter.

Various studies used Population Analysis Profiles-Area Under the Curve (PAP-AUC) (Wooton et al., 2001) as the gold standard in order to evaluate the sensitivity and specificity of some of the other methods. Walsh et al. evaluated seven methods in 2001 among which, E-test Macrodilution appeared to perform better (sensitivity 96%, specificity 97%) for the detection of *Staphylococcus* strains with reduced susceptibilities to vancomycin (SRSV) (a term that contains both GISA and hGISA) (Walsh et al., 2001). In 2007, Wootton et al. performed a large-scale multicenter study involving 3 different methods of GISA and hGISA detection (brain-heart infusion agar with 6 mg/L vancomycin (BHIA6V), Mueller-Hinton agar with 5 mg/L teicoplanin (MHA5T), and E-test Macrodilution. Among them, BHIA6V had a very low sensitivity for hGISA (11.47%) whereas MHA5T and E-test Macrodilution performed both well. MHA5T though, gave twice as many false-positive results compared to E-test Macrodilution which moreover, resulted in significantly less variation between laboratories (Wooton et al., 2007). In 2011, Satola et al. evaluated the E-test Macrodilution method, E-test GRD and BHI screen agar plates containing 4 mg/L vancomycin and 16 g/L casein using 0.5 and 2.0 McFarland inocula. E-test Macrodilution was 57% sensitive and 96% specific, E-test GRD was 57% sensitive and 97% specific, and BHI screen agar was 90% sensitive and 95% specific with a 0.5 McFarland inoculum and 100% sensitive and 68% specific with a 2.0 McFarland inoculums (Satola et al., 2011). In the same year, van Hal et al. screened 458 MRSA bloodstream isolates to determine the most accurate testing strategy to detect the presence of heteroresistance. Compared to PAP-AUC, the sensitivities and specificities of E-test Macrodilution, E-test GRD, vancomycin broth microdilution (using a MIC cutoff of ≥ 2 mg/L), and standard vancomycin E-test (using a MIC cutoff of ≥ 2 mg/L) were 89 and 55%, 71 and 94%, 82 and 97%, and 71 and 94%, respectively (van Hal et al., 2011).

Research for the most effective method to detect SRSV is still going on but reports of heteroresistance even among other clinically important species worldwide highlight the need for the development of a reliable and easy-to-use susceptibility testing method that can be used in the everyday laboratory practice.

5.1 Population analysis profiles

Step 1: Prepare agar plates containing varied antibiotic concentrations, for example 0, 0.5, 1, 2, 3, 4, 5, 6, 8… mg/L.

Step 2: Culture bacteria overnight in tryptone soya broth (TSB).

Step 3: Prepare a cell suspension of approximately 10^8 CFU/ml (OD 0.3 at 578 nm or 2:3 dilution of a 0.5 McFarland suspension).

Step 4: Make 10-fold serial dilutions of the cell suspension and spread 50µl from each dilution onto a complete series of antibiotic-containing plates. (Fig. 1)

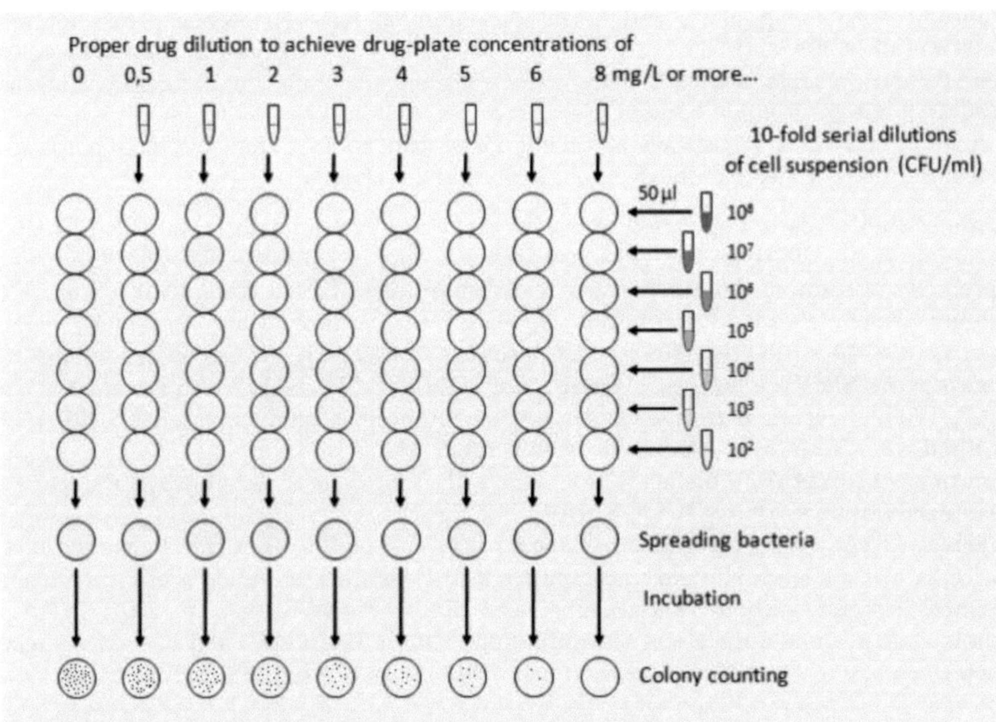

Fig. 1. Meletis, G 2011, 'Population analysis profiles method', in possession of the author.

Step 5: Incubate at 35-37 °C for 48h.

Step 6: Count the number of colonies grown on each plate (Table 1).

		Drug concentration (mg/L)							
		0,5	1	2	3	4	5	6	8
CFU/ml	10^8								
	10^7								
	10^6								
	10^5								
	10^4								
	10^3								
	10^2								

Table 1. Colony counting table.

Step 7: Plot the colony counts on a semi-logarithmic graph with colony counts on the vertical axis and drug concentration on the horizontal axis (Fig 2).

Step 8: Calculate the frequency of resistant subpopulations at the highest drug concentration by dividing the number of colonies grown on an antibiotic containing plate by the colony counts from the same bacterial inoculum plated onto antibiotic-free plates.

Step 9: Determine the MIC of the resistant subpopulations and reassess it after serial daily subcultures on antibiotic-free medium for 7-14 days in order to evaluate whether the resistance is stable.

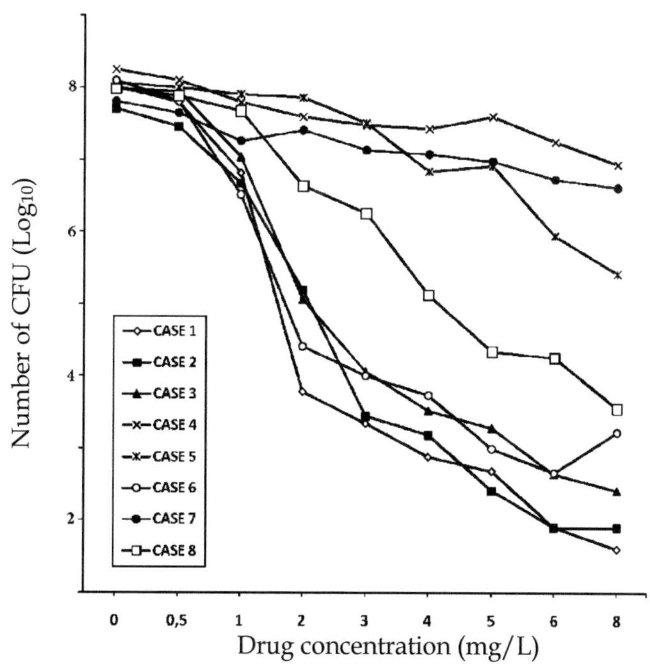

Fig. 2. Colony counts plotting of eight *K. pneumoniae* strains tested for heteroresistance to colistin on a semi-logarithmic graph. Strains 4, 5 and 7 are resistant.

5.2 Modified population analysis profiles-AUC (area under the curve)

Modified PAP-AUC was proposed by Wooton et al. for the detection of heteroresistance to vancomycin among *S. aureus* strains and is considered to date the gold standard for hGISA detection (Wooton et al., 2001). It is based upon the calculation of the ratio of the test strain's AUC divided by the corresponding Mu 3 AUC. After 24h incubation in TSB, cultures are diluted in saline to 10^{-3} and 10^{-6} and plated onto BHIA plates containing 0.5, 1, 2, 2.5 and 4 mg/L vancomycin. Colonies are counted after 48h incubation at 37 °C and the viable count is plotted against vancomycin concentration. The AUC of the study strain and Mu 3 are calculated and their ratio is evaluated as follows: <0.9, GSSA; 0.9-1.29, hGISA; ≥ 1.3, GISA (Wooton et al., 2005).

5.3 Gradient plates

Step 1: Culture Mu 3 and test strains overnight in TSB.

Step 2: Pour 25 ml of BHIA containing 4 mg/L vancomycin in a 10 cm square Petri dish at an angle of 12° and keep solidified for 30 min in room temperature (Fig. 3).

Step 3: Overlay 25 ml of BHIA and leave to set horizontally. Keep the solidified agar at room temperature for 120 min.

Step 4: Adjust each culture to a turbidity equal to 0.5 McFarland and streak the Mu 3 and test strains onto the gradient agar plate with a cotton swab.

Step 5: Measure the growth distance of the bacteria after 48h incubation at 37 °C and divide it with the distance grown by Mu 3 on the same plate. A ratio of ≥ 1 denotes an hGISA (Wooton et al., 2001).

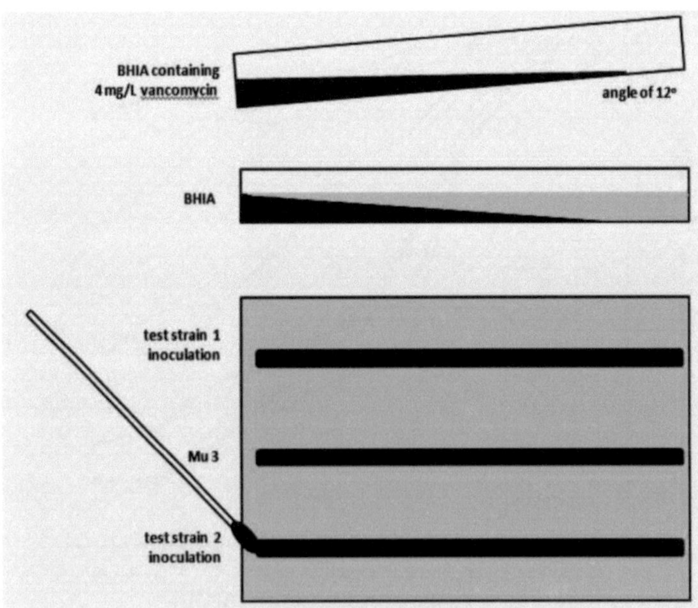

Fig. 3. Meletis, G 2011, 'Gradient plates preparation and inoculation', in possession of the author.

5.4 E-test macrodilution

Bolmström et al. proposed that the use of a dense inoculum, rich medium and a 48h incubation period can optimize the detection of VISA and hVISA (Bolmström et al., 1999).

Step 1: Spread 250 μl of a 2 McFarland suspension onto BHI agar plates and put one vancomycin and one teicoplanin E-test for each strain (Fig. 4).

Step 2: Incubate at 35-37 °C for 48h.

Step 3: Interpretation (hVISA when vancomycin MIC and teicoplanin MIC ≥ 8 or when teicoplanin MIC ≥ 12 and vancomycin MIC <4).

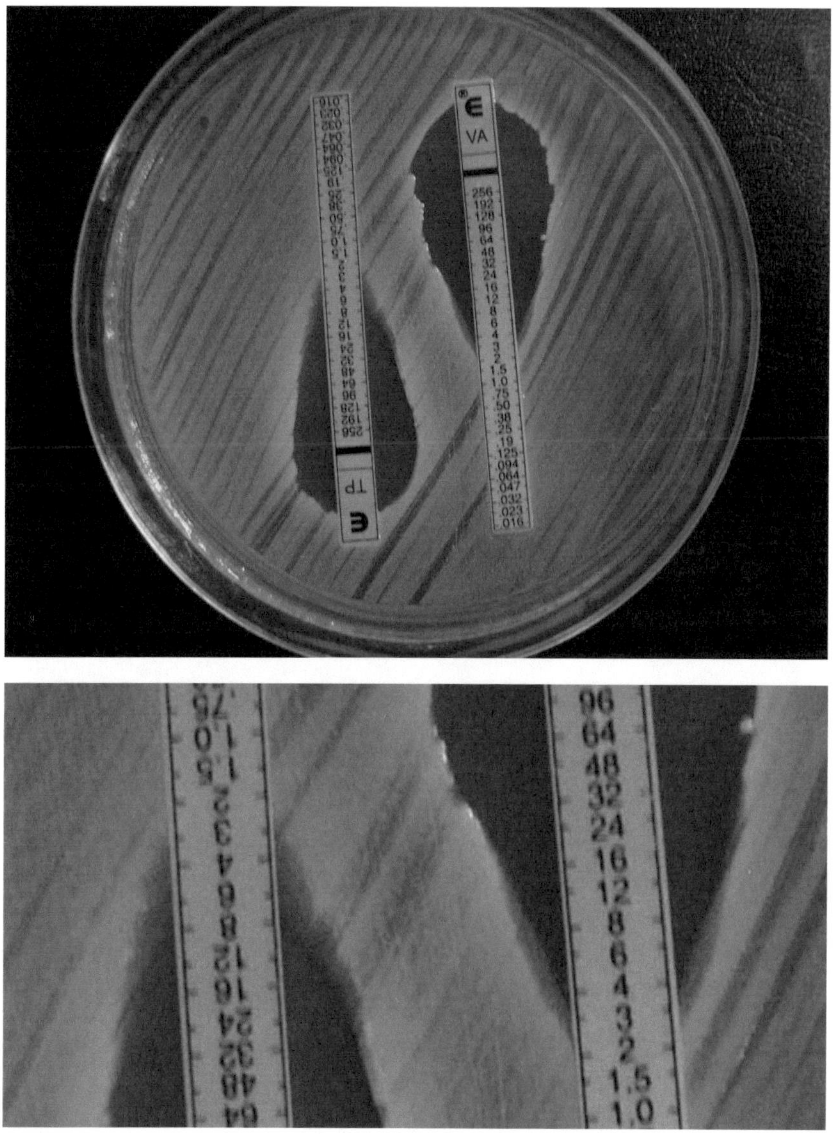

Fig. 4. E-test Macrodilution. Photo courtesy of Dr. Tzampaz Egki.

5.5 Disc-agar method

The disc-agar method has been used to demonstrate both the presence of potential intermediate vancomycin resistant staphylococci and staphylococci with heteroresistance to vancomycin on the same plate. It is based upon the observation that beta-lactam antibiotics (Aritaka et al., 2001; Y.S. Kim et al., 2003) and higher salinity can induce the phenotypic expression of vancomycin resistance and for this purpose aztreonam is preferred over other beta-lactam antibiotics because it has no inhibitory effect on Gram positive bacteria (Fig. 5).

Wong et al. performed a preliminary study of the disc-agar method using different beta-lactams including penicillins, oxacillin, cephalosporin and carbapenems. Although sometimes sattelitism could be seen around other beta-lactam discs, the results were less consistent than they were with aztreonam, and some strains had a large zone of inhibition around the disc (Wong et al., 1999).

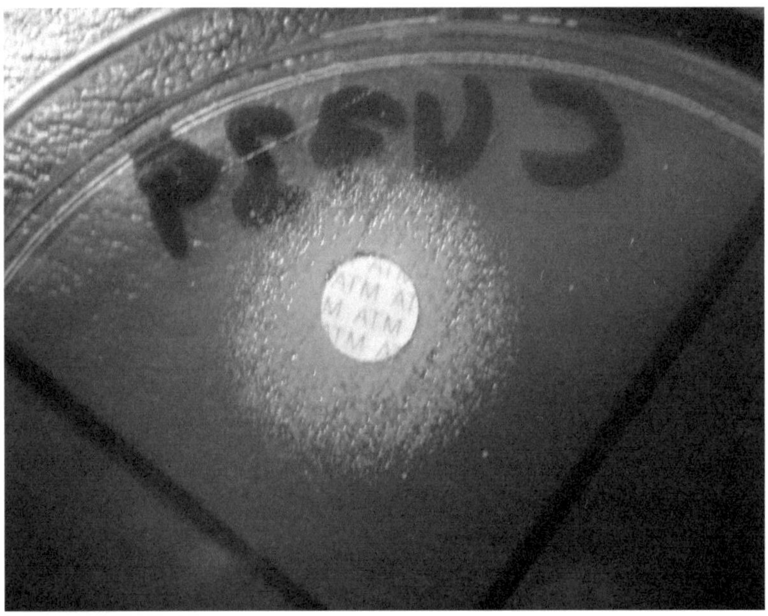

Fig. 5. Bacterial growth around aztreonam disc. Photo courtesy of Dr. Tzampaz Egki.

Step 1: Prepare vancomycin-salt agar plates by incorporating 4 mg/L vancomycin and 4% NaCl into MHA.

Step 2: Make a 1 McFarland bacterial suspension.

Step 3: Inoculate with a sterile cotton swab and place a 30 μg aztreonam disc 5 minutes afterwards.

Step 4: Incubate at 37 °C for 48h.

Step 5: Suspect heteroresistance if bacterial growth is observed around the disc. The colonies may be homogeneous or heterogeneous in size (Fig. 6).

Note: In any case further testing by population analysis profiles is recommended for the characterization of the strain's resistance profile.

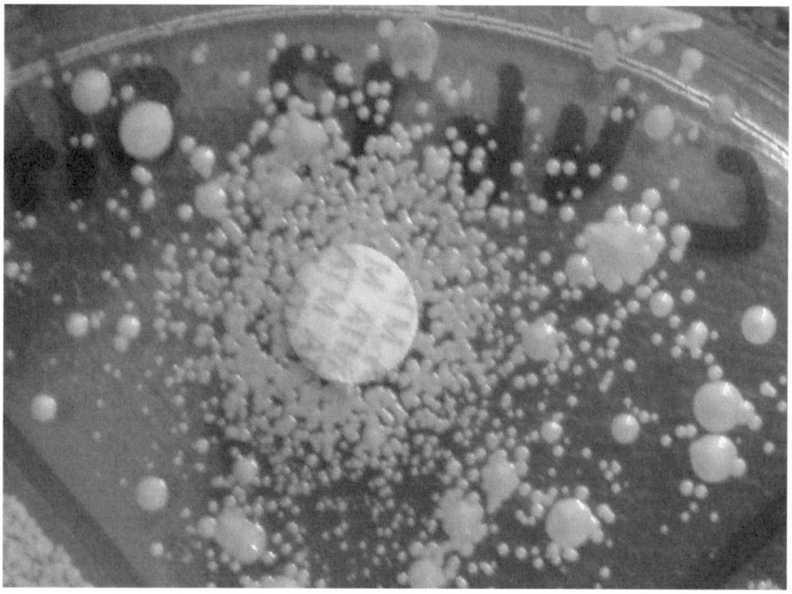

Fig. 6. Different size colonies around aztreonam disc. Photo courtesy of Dr. Tzampaz Egki.

5.6 E-test GRD (glycopeptide resistance detection)

The E-test GRD strip consists of a double-sided gradient of vancomycin and teicoplanin on a calibrated plastic strip. This double-sided predetermined gradient of vancomycin and teicoplanin is used exclusively for the detection of GISA or hGISA phenotypes.

Strains that give a positive E-test GRD result (vancomycin or teicoplanin ≥ 8) should be send to a reference laboratory for further investigation by population analysis profiles (Fig. 7 and 8).

Note: The endpoints read from the E-test GRD strips should not be regarded as true MICs, but rather as modified results with interpretive cutoffs defined for the phenotypic detection of glycopeptides resistance phenotypes in *S. aureus* (Yusof et al., 2007).

Step 1: Determine the MIC of the study strain.

Step 2: Use standard inoculum (0.5 McFarland) onto Mueller Hinton + 5% blood agar plates and add the GRD strip. Ensure that the whole length of the strip is in complete contact with the agar surface. If necessary, remove air pockets by pressing gently on the strip with forceps, always moving from the lowest concentration upwards. Small bubbles under the strip will not affect the results.

Note: Once applied, the strip cannot be moved because the antibiotic is instantaneously released into the agar.

Step 3: Incubation at 35-37 °C for 24 and 48h.

Step 4: Results interpretation according to manufacturer's instructions (GISA: positive E-test GRD and vancomycin MIC ≥ 4 mg/L, hGISA: positive E-test GRD and vancomycin MIC < 4 mg/L). When mutant colonies are present in the inhibition eclipse, read the result where these colonies are completely inhibited.

Note: Although the procedure is straightforward, proper use of the test requires the judgment of skilled personnel trained in microbiology and antimicrobial susceptibility testing.

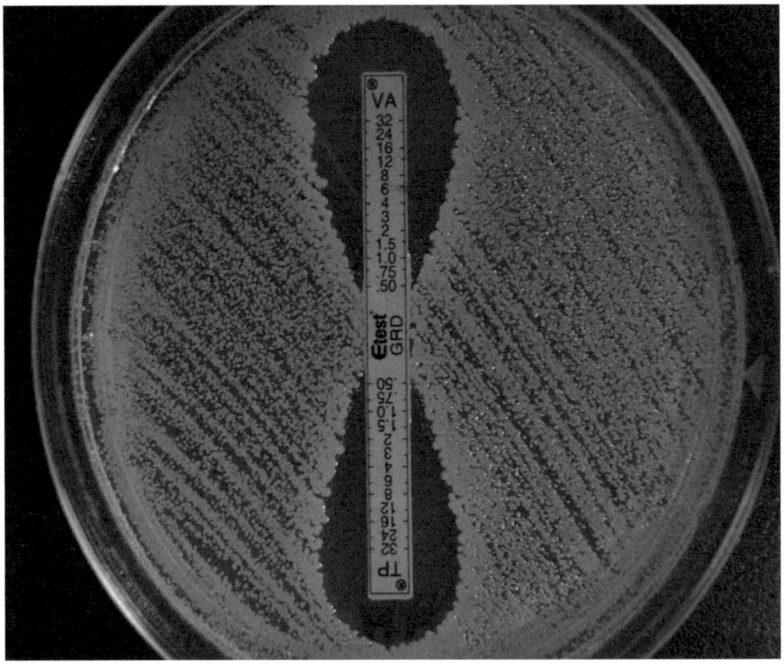

Fig. 7. Negative E-test GRD. Photo courtesy of Dr. Tzampaz Egki.

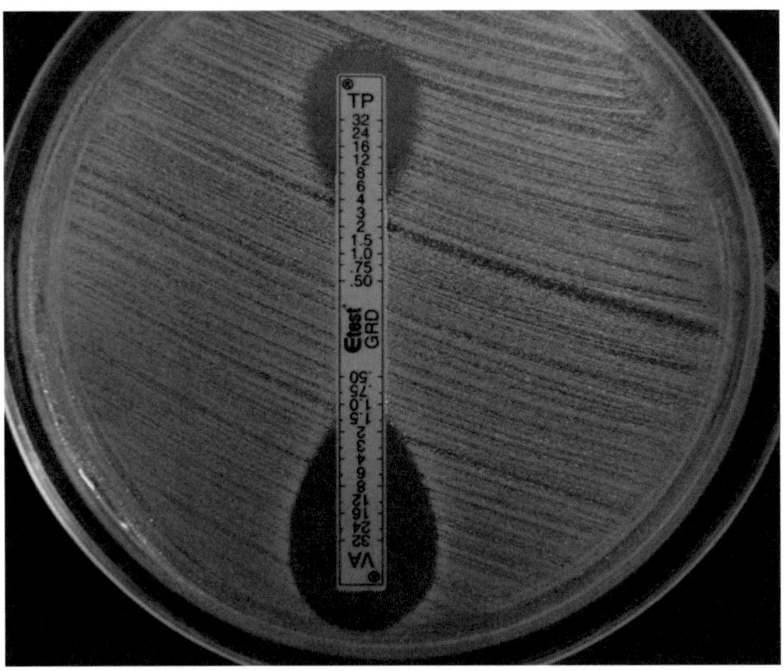

Fig. 8. Positive E-test GRD. Photo courtesy of Dr. Tzampaz Egki.

5.7 Standard E-test

The presence of resistant subcolonies within a clear inhibition zone (Fig. 9) can potentially indicate for a heteroresistant isolate and in such cases, population analysis profiles is suggested.

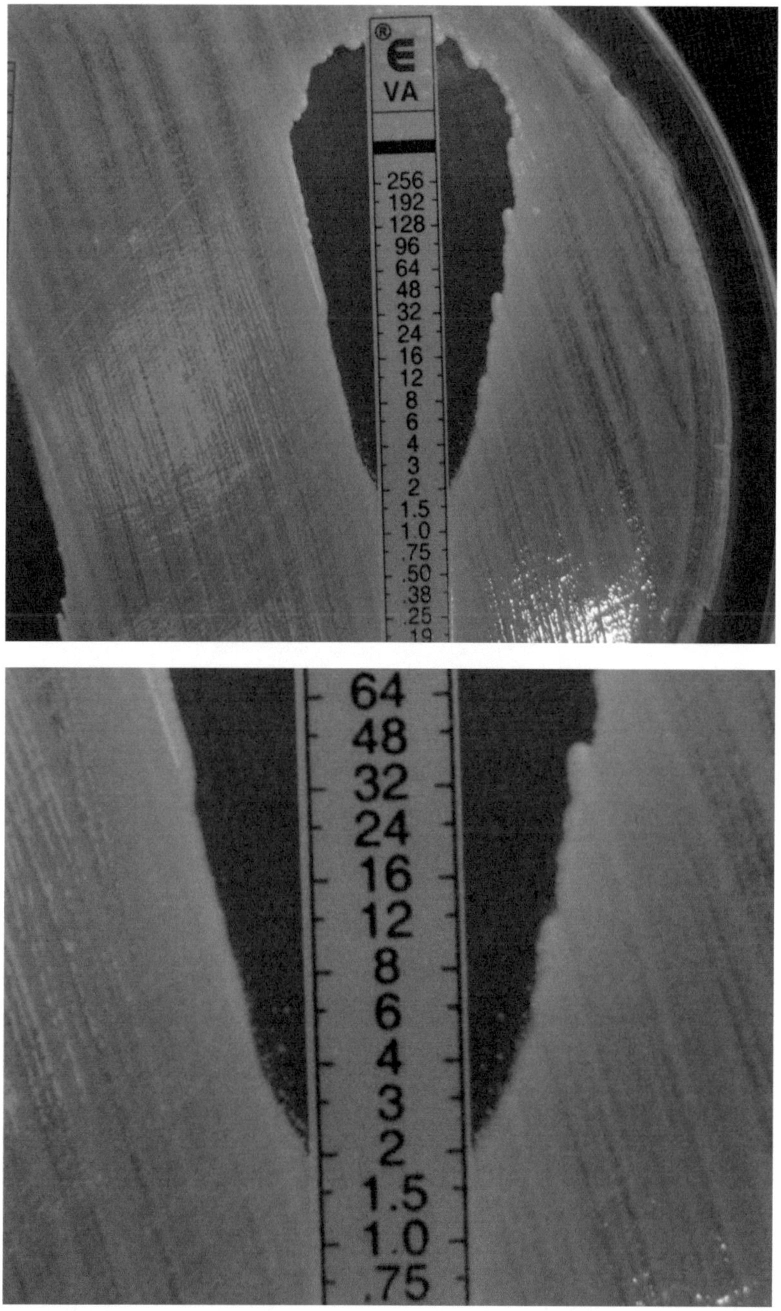

Fig. 9. Subpopulations grown within the inhibition zone. Photo courtesy of Dr. Tzampaz Egki.

5.8 Population screening plates

Screening for potential vancomycin resistance can be performed using BHIA plates with 4 mg/L vancomycin. 10 µl of a bacterial suspension from an overnight culture adjusted to 0.5 McFarland standard is spread on the plate and bacterial growth after incubation at 37 °C for 24 and 48h is observed. Growth at 24h may be deemed to be of the GISA phenotype and growth occurring between 24 and 48h may be deemed to be an hGISA strain (Walsh et al., 2001).

6. Conclusion

Many studies have tried to associate hGISA with failure of vancomycin therapy but this is still up for debate as results are controversial (van Hal & Paterson, 2011; C. Liu & Chambers., 2003; Neoh et al., 2007; Rong & Leonard, 2010). A further research problem is that such studies are difficult to perform because of the serious nature and high mortality rate among patients infected by MRSA.

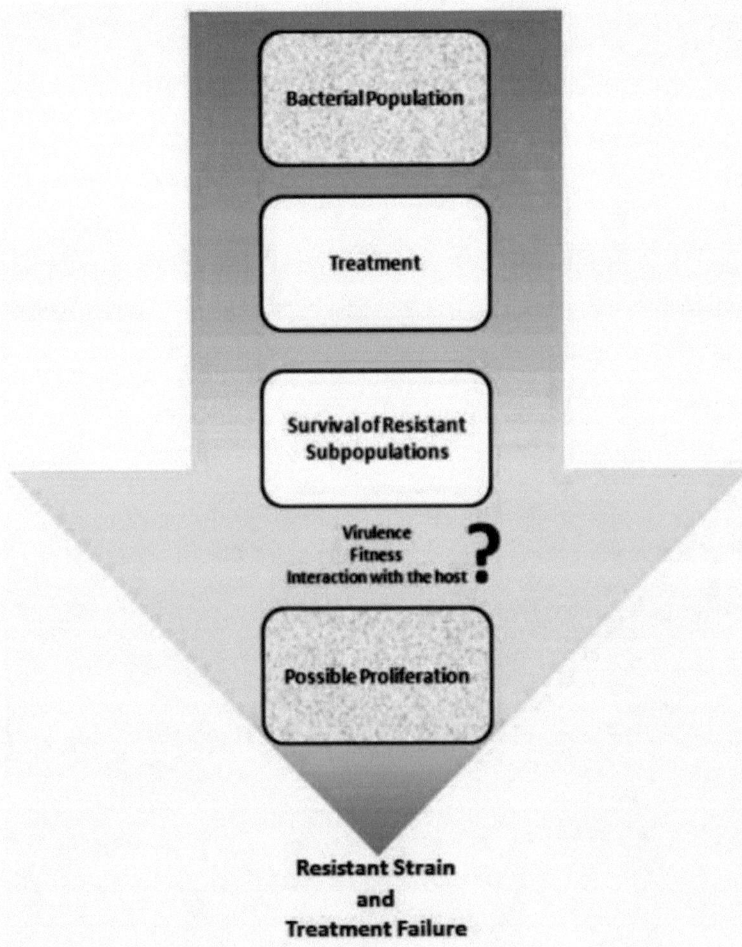

Fig. 10. Meletis, G 2011, 'Natural evolution to drug resistance due to heteroresistance', in possession of the author.

However, heteroresistance could very possibly be a tool for natural evolution to drug resistance, since it provides bacteria with an opportunity to explore the possibility of growth in the presence of antibiotics (Morand & Muhlemann, 2007). The resistant subpopulations may proliferate readily in the absence of competition by the inhibited susceptible cells, thereby giving rise to a new resistant population (Falagas et al., 2008). On the other hand, the emergence of resistant strains *in vitro* may not necessarily have therapeutic implications (Johnson, 1998) mainly because acquisition of resistance in some cases may be accompanied by loss of virulence (Fig. 10).

Nevertheless, heteroresistant strains have been deemed to be responsible for treatment failures (Moore et al., 2003; Wong et al., 1999) and difficulties to detect heteroresistant isolates could already be contributing to a hidden spread of these strains within hospital facilities (Falagas et al., 2008). Therefore, more research is needed to determine the true clinical impact of heteroresistance and its role in the development of fully-resistant bacterial populations.

7. Acknowledgements

The author is most indebted to Dr. Maria Bagkeri, Dr. Egki Tzampaz, Dr. Effrosyni Sianou, and Dr. Danai Sofianou for their help and support in research over the last three years and especially during the study of the heteroresistance phenomenon.

8. References

Alam, M.; Donabedian, S.; Brown, W.; et al. (2001). Heteroresistance to vancomycin in Enterococcus faecium. In: *J Clin Microbiol*, Vol: 39. 3379–81. ISSN: 0095-1137.

Altrichter, T. & Heizmann, W.R. (1994). Gardnerella vaginalis: transport, microscopy, testing resistance. In: *Geburtshilfe Frauenheilkd*, Vol: 54. 606-11. ISSN: 0016-5751.

Appelbaum PC. (2007). Reduced glycopeptide susceptibility in methicillin-resistant Staphylococcus aureus (MRSA). In: *Int J Antimicrob Agents*, Vol: 30. 398-408. ISSN: 0924-8579.

Aritaka, N.; Hanaki, H.; Cui, L.; Hiramatsu, K. (2001). Combination effect of vancomycin and beta-lactams against a Staphylococcus aureus strain, Mu3, with heterogeneous resistance to vancomycin. In: *Antimicrob Agents Chemother*, Vol: 45. 1292–4. ISSN: 0066-4804.

Billington, O.J.; McHugh, T.D.; Gillespie, S.H. (1999). Physiological Cost of Rifampin Resistance Induced In Vitro in Mycobacterium tuberculosis. In: *Antimicrob Agents Chemother*, Vol: 43. 1866-9. ISSN:0066-4804.

Bolmström, A.; Karlsson, A. & Wong, P. (1999). Macro-method conditions are optimal for detection of low level glycopeptides resistance in staphylococci. In: *Clin Microbiol Infect*, Vol: 5(S3). 113. ISSN: 1198-743X.

Borg, M.A.; Zerafa, R.; Morrison, D.; et al. (2005). Incidence of glycopeptide hetero-intermediate Staphylococcus aureus strains in Maltese hospitals. In: *Clin Microbiol Infect*, Vol: 11. 405-7.ISSN: 1198-743X.

Chesneau, O.; Morvan, A. & Solh, N.E. (2000). Retrospective screening for heterogeneous vancomycin resistance in diverse Staphylococcus aureus clones disseminated in French hospitals. In: *J Antimicrob Chemother,* Vol:45. 887-90. ISSN: 0305-7453.

Cimolai, N.; Trombley, C. & Zaher, A. (1997). Oxacillin susceptibility of coagulase-negative staphylococci: role for mecA genotyping and E-test susceptibility testing. In: *Int J Antimicrob Agents,* Vol: 8. 121-5. ISSN: 0924-8579.

Cui, L.; Iwamoto, A.; Lian, J.Q.; et al. (2006). Novel mechanism of antibiotic resistance originating in vancomycin-intermediate Staphylococcus aureus. In: *Antimicrob Agents Chemother,* Vol: 50. 428-38. ISSN: 0066-4804.

Falagas, M.E.; Makris, G.C.; Dimopoulos, G.; et al. (2008).Heteroresistance: a concern of increasing clinical significance? In: *Clin Microbiol Infect,* Vol: 14. 101–4. ISSN: 1198-743X.

Gillespie, S.H. (2001). Antibiotic resistance in the absence of selective pressure. In: *Int J Antimicrob Agents,* Vol: 17. 171-6. ISSN: 0924-8579.

van Hal, S.J.; Wehrhahn, M.C.; Barbagiannakos, T.; et al. (2011). Performance of various testing methodologies for detection of heteroresistant vancomycin-intermediate Staphylococcus aureus in bloodstream isolates. In: *J Clin Microbiol,* Vol: 49. 1489-94. ISSN: 0095-1137.

van Hal, S.J. & Paterson, D.L. (2011). Systematic Review and Meta-Analysis of the Significance of Heterogeneous Vancomycin-Intermediate Staphylococcus aureus Isolates. In: *Antimicrob Agents Chemother,* Vol: 55. 405-10. ISSN: 0066-4804.

Hawley, J.S.; Murray, C.K, & Jorgensen, J.H. (2008). Colistin heteroresistance in Acinetobacter and its association with previous colistin therapy. In: *Antimicrob Agents Chemother,* Vol: 52. 351-2. ISSN: 0066-4804.

Hiramatsu, K.; Hanaki, H.; Ino, T.; et al. (1997a). Methicillin-resistant Staphylococcus aureus clinical strain with reduced vancomycin susceptibility. In: *J Antimicrob Chemother,* Vol: 40. 135–6. ISSN: 0305-7453.

Hiramatsu, K.; Aritaka, N.; Hanaki, H.; et al. (1997b). Dissemination in Japanese hospitals of strains of Staphylococcus aureus heterogeneously resistant to vancomycin. In: *Lancet,* Vol: 350. 1670–3. ISSN: 0140-6736.

Howden, B.P.; Stinear, T.P.; Allen, D.L.; et al. (2008). Genomic analysis reveals a point mutation in the two-component sensor gene graS that leads to intermediate vancomycin resistance in clinical Staphylococcus aureus. In: *Antimicrob Agents Chemother,* Vol: 52. 3755-62. ISSN: 0066-4804.

Howe, R.A.; Wooten, M.; Walsh, T.R., et al. (1999). Expression and detection of hetero-vancomycin resistance in Staphylococcus aureus. In: *J Antimicrob Chemother,* Vol: 44. 675–8. ISSN: 0305-7453.

Ikonomidis, A.; Neou, E.; Gogou, V.; et al. (2009). Heteroresistance to Meropenem in Carbapenem-Susceptible Acinetobacter baumannii. In: *J Clin Microbiol,* Vol: 47. 4055-9. ISSN: 0095-1137.

Johnson, AP. (1998). Intermediate vancomycin resistance in Staphylococcus aureus: a major threat or a minor inconvenience? In: *J Antimicrob Chemother,* Vol: 42. 289-91. ISSN: 0305-7453.

Kim, M.N.; Pai, C.H.; Woo, J.H.; et al. (2000). Vancomycin-intermediate Staphylococcus aureus in Korea. *J Clin Microbiol,* Vol: 38. 3879-81. ISSN: 0095-1137.

Kim, M.N.; Hwang, S.H.; Pyo, Y.J.; et al. (2002). Clonal spread of Staphylococcus aureus heterogeneously resistant to vancomycin in a university hospital in Korea. In: *J Clin Microbiol,* Vol: 40. 1376–80. ISSN: 0095-1137.

Kim, Y.S.; Kiem, S.; Yun, H.J.; et al. (2003). Efficacy of vancomycin-β-lactam combinations against Heterogeneously Vancomycin-Resistant Staphylococcus aureus (hetero-VRSA). In: *J Korean Med Sci,* Vol: 18. 319-24. ISSN: 1011-8934

Kontopoulou, K.; Protonotariou, E.; Vasilakos, K.; et al. (2010). Hospital outbreak caused by Klebsiella pneumoniae producing KPC-2 b-lactamase resistant to colistin. In: *J Hosp Infect,* Vol: 76. 70–3.ISSN: 0195-6701.

Li, J.; Rayner, C.R.; Nation, R.L.; et al. (2006). Heteroresistance to colistin in multidrug-resistant Acinetobacter baumannii. In: *Antimicrob Agents Chemother,* Vol: 50. 2946-50. ISSN: 0066-4804.

Liu, C. & Chambers, H.F. (2003). Staphylococcus aureus with heterogeneous resistance to vancomycin: epidemiology, clinical significance, and critical assessment of diagnostic methods. In: *Antimicrob Agents Chemother,* Vol: 47. 3040–5. ISSN: 0066-4804.

Liu, H.; Buescher, G.; Lewis, N.; et al. (1990). Detection of borderline oxacillin-resistant Staphylococcus aureus and differentiation from methicillin-resistant strains. In: *Eur J Clin Microbiol Infect Dis,* Vol: 9. 717-24. ISSN: 0934-9723.

Lo-Ten-Foe, J.R.; de Smet, A.M.; Diederen, B.M.; et al. (2007). Comparative evaluation of the VITEK 2, disk diffusion, etest, broth microdilution, and agar dilution susceptibility testing methods for colistin in clinical isolates, including heteroresistant Enterobacter cloacae and Acinetobacter baumannii strains. In: *Antimicrob Agents Chemother,* Vol: 51. 3726-30. ISSN: 0066-4804.

Marchese, A.; Balistreri, G.; Tonoli, E.; et al. (2000). Heterogeneous vancomycin resistance in methicillin resistant Staphylococcus aureus strains isolated in a large Italian hospital. In: *J Clin Microbiol,* Vol: 38. 866–9. ISSN: 0095-1137.

Meletis, G.; Tzampaz, E.; Sianou, E.; et al. (2011). Colistin heteroresistance in carbapenemase-producing Klebsiella pneumoniae. In: *J Antimicrob Chemother,* Vol: 66. 946-947. ISSN: 0305-7453.

Mondon, P.; Petter, R.; Amalfitano, G.; et al. (1999). Heteroresistance to Fluconazole and Voriconazole in Cryptococcus neoformans. In: *Antimicrob Agents Chemother,* Vol: 43. 1856-61. ISSN: 0066-4804.

Moore, M.R.; Perdreau-Remington, F. & Chambers, H.F. (2003). Vancomycin treatment failure associated with heterogeneous vancomycin-intermediate Staphylococcus aureus in a patient with endocarditis and in the rabbit model of endocarditis. In: *Antimicrob Agents Chemother,* Vol:47. 1262–6. ISSN: 0066-4804.

Morand, B. & Muhlemann, K. (2007). Heteroresistance to penicillin in Streptococcus pneumonia. In: *Proc Natl Acad Sci USA,* Vol: 104. 14098–103. ISSN: 1091-6490.

Neoh, H.; Hori, S.; Komatsu, M.; et al. (2007). Impact of reduced vancomycin susceptibility on the therapeutic outcome of MRSA bloodstream infections. In: *Annals of Clinical Microbiology and Antimicrobials,* Vol: 6. 13. ISSN: 1476-0711.

Neoh, H.; Cui, L.; Yuzawa, H.; et al. (2008). Mutated Response Regulator graR Is Responsible for Phenotypic Conversion of Staphylococcus aureus from Heterogeneous Vancomycin-Intermediate Resistance to Vancomycin-Intermediate Resistance. In: *Antimicrob Agents Chemother,* Vol: 52. 45-53. ISSN: 0066-4804.

Nunes, A.; Teixeira, L.M.; Pontes Iorio, N.L.; et al. (2006). Heterogeneous resistance to vancomycin in Staphylococcus epidermidis, Staphylococcus haemolyticus and Staphylococcus warneri clinical strains: characterisation of glycopeptide susceptibility profiles and cell wall thickening. In: *Int J Antimicrob Agents,* Vol: 27. 307–15. ISSN: 0924-8579.

Nunes, A.; Schuenck, R.P.; Bastos, C.R.; et al. (2007). Heterogeneous resistance to vancomycin and Teicoplanin Among Staphylococcus spp. Isolated from Bacteremia. In: *Brazilian J Infect Dis,* Vol: 11. 345-50. ISSN: 1413-8670.

Park, Y.J.; Kim, M.; Oh, E.J.; et al. (2000). Screening method for detecting staphylococci with reduced susceptibility to teicoplanin. In: *J Microbiol Methods,* Vol: 40. 193-8. ISSN: 0167-7012.

Poudyal, A.; Howden, P.B.; Bell, J.M.; et al. (2008). In vitro pharmacodynamics of colistin against multidrug-resistant Klebsiella pneumoniae. In: *J Antimicrob Chemother,* Vol: 62. 1311–8. ISSN: 0305-7453.

Pournaras, S.; Ikonomidis, A.; Markogiannakis, A.; et al. (2005). Heteroresistence to carbapenems in Acinetobacter baumannii. In: *J Antimicrob Chemother,* Vol: 55. 1055–6. ISSN: 0305-7453.

Pournaras, S.; Kristo, I.; Vrioni, G.; et al. (2010). Characteristics of Meropenem Heteroresistance in Klebsiella pneumonia Carbapenemase (KPC)-Producing Clinical Isolates of K. pneumoniae. In: *J Clin Microbiol,* Vol: 48. 2601-4. ISSN: 0095-1137.

Qu, T.; Zhang, J.; Zhou, Z.; et al. (2009). Heteroresistance to Teicoplanin in Enterococcus faecium Harboring the vanA Gene. In: *J Clin Microbiol,* Vol: 47. 4194-6. ISSN: 0095-1137.

Reverdy, M.E.; Jarraud, S.; Bobin-Dubreux, S.; et al. (2001). Incidence of Staphylococcus aureus with reduced susceptibility to glycopeptides in two French hospitals. In: *Clin Microbiol Infect,* Vol: 7.267-72. ISSN: 1198-743X.

Rinder, H. (2001). Hetero-resistance: an under-recognised confounder in diagnosis and therapy? In: *J Med Microbiol,* Vol: 50. 1018-20. ISSN: 0022-2615.

Rinder, H.; Mieskes, K.T. & Loscher, T. (2001). Heteroresistance in Mycobacterium tuberculosis. In: *Int J Tuberc Lung Dis,* Vol: 5. 339–45. ISSN: 1027-3719.

Rong, S.L. & Leonard, S.N. (2010). Heterogeneous vancomycin resistance in Staphylococcus aureus: a review of epidemiology, diagnosis, and clinical significance. In: *Ann Pharmacother,* Vol: 44. 844-50. ISSN: 1060-0280.

Ryffel, C.; Strassle, A.; Kayser, F.H.; et al. (1994). Mechanisms of Heteroresistance in Methicillin-Resistant Staphylococcus aureus. In: *Antimicrob Agents Chemother,* Vol: 38. 724-8. ISSN:0066-4804.

Sakoulas, G.; Alder, J.; Thauvin-Eliopoulos, C.; et al. (2006). Induction of daptomycin heterogeneous susceptibility in Staphylococcus aureus by exposure to vancomycin. In: *Antimicrob Agents Chemother,* Vol: 50. 1581–5. ISSN: 0066-4804.

Satola, S.W.; Farley, M.M.; Andrerson, K.F.; et al. (2011). Comparison of Detection Methods for Heteroresistant Vancomycin-Intermediate Staphylococcus aureus, with the Population Analysis Profile Method as the Reference Method. In: *J Clin Microbiol,* Vol: 49. 177-83. ISSN: 0095-1137.

Strandén, A.M.; Roos, M. & Berger-Bächi, B. (1996). Glutamine synthetase and heteroresistance in methicillin-resistant Staphylococcus aureus. In: *Microb Drug Resist,* Vol: 2. 201-7. ISSN: 1076-6294.

Tan, C.H.; Li, J. & Nation, R.L. (2007). Activity of colistin against heteroresistant Acinetobacter baumannii and emergence of resistance in an in vitro pharmacokinetic/pharmacodynamic model. In: *Antimicrob Agents Chemother,* Vol: 51. 3413-5. ISSN: 0066-4804.

Tan, T.Y. & Ng, S.Y. (2007). Comparison of Etest, Vitek and agar dilution for susceptibility testing of colistin. In: *Clin Microbiol Infect,* Vol: 13. 541–4. ISSN: 1198-743X.

Tenover, F.C. (1999). Implications of vancomycin-resistant Staphylococcus aureus. In: *J Hosp Infect,* Vol:43 Suppl: S3-7. ISSN: 0195-6701.

Walsh, T.R.; Bolmström, A.; Quarnstrom, A.; et al. (2001). Evaluation of current methods of detecting vancomycin resistance and hetero-resistance in Staphylococcus aureus and other staphylococci. In: *J Clin Microbiol,* Vol: 39. 2439–44. ISSN: 0095-1137.

Wang, J.L.; Tseng, S.P.; Hsueh, P.R.; et al. (2004).Vancomycin heteroresistance in methicillin-resistant Staphylococcus aureus, Taiwan. In: *Emerg Infect Dis,* Vol: 10. 1702-4. ISSN: 1080-6040.

Wannet, W. (2002). Spread of an MRSA clone with heteroresistance to oxacillin in the Netherlands. In: *Eurosurveillance* Vol: 5. 73–4. ISSN: 1560-7917.

Wong, S.; Ho, P.L.; Woo, P.C.; et al. (1999). Bacteremia caused by staphylococci with inducible vancomycin heteroresistance. In: *Clin Infect Dis,* Vol: 29. 760–7. ISSN: 1058-4838.

Wootton, M.; Howe, R.A.; Hillman, R.; et al. (2001). A modified population analysis method (PAP) to detect heteroresistance to vancomycin in Staphylococcus aureus in a UK hospital. In: *J Antimicrob Chemother,* Vol: 47. 399–403. ISSN: 0305-7453.

Wootton, M.; Bennett, P.M.; MacGowan, A.P.; et al. (2005). Reduced expression of the atl autolysin gene and susceptibility to autolysis in clinical heterogeneous glycopeptide-intermediate Staphylococcus aureus (hGISA) and GISA strains. In: *J Antimicrob Chemother,* Vol: 56: 944–7.ISSN: 0305-7453.

Wooton, M.; MacGowan, A.P.; Walsh, T.R.; et al. (2007). A Multicenter Study Evaluating the Current Strategies for Isolating Staphylococcus aureus Strains with Reduced Susceptibility to Glycopeptides. In: *J Clin Microbiol,* Vol: 45. 329-32. ISSN: 0095-1137.

Yamazumi, T.; Pfaller, M.A.; Messer, S.A.; et al. (2003). Characterization of heteroresistance to fluconazole among clinical isolates of Cryptococcus neoformans. In: *J Clin Microbiol,* Vol: 41. 267–72. ISSN: 0095-1137.

Yau, W.; Owen, R.J.; Poudyal, A.; et al. (2009). Colistin hetero-resistance in multidrug-resistant Acinetobacter baumannii clinical isolates from the Western Pacific region in the SENTRY antimicrobial surveillance programme. In: *J Inf,* Vol: 58. 138-44. ISSN: 0163-4453.

Yusof, A.; Engelhardt, A.; Karlsson, A.; et al. (2008). Evaluation of a New Etest Vancomycin-Teicoplanin Strip for Detection of Glycopeptide-Intermediate Staphylococcus aureus (GISA), in Particular, Heterogeneous GISA. In: *J Clin Microbiol,* Vol: 46. 3042-7. ISSN: 0095-1137.

11

Pseudomonas Aeruginosa and Newer β-Lactamases: An Emerging Resistance Threat

Silpi Basak, Ruchita O. Attal and Monali N. Rajurkar
Jawaharlal Nehru Medical College, Datta Meghe Institute of Medical Sciences, Wardha (M.S.)
India

1. Introduction

The discovery of penicillin, the Magic bullet in 1928 and its clinical use in 1941 led the people to think that mankind has won the war against microbes. With a short span of seventy years, antimicrobial discovery from Penicillin to Tigecycline, mankind is facing the problem with some hospital strains resistant to almost all antimicrobials, and is busy in writing the obituary for antimicrobials.

Infact, the rising trend of developing resistance to multiple antibiotics in microbes, leading to therapeutic failure is a serious problem of global magnitude. P.aeruginosa, Methicillin Resistant Staphylococcus aureus (MRSA), Vancomycin resistant Enterococci(VRE), Glycopeptide Intermediate Staphylococcus aureus (GISA), Glycopeptide Resistant Staphylococcus aureus (GRSA), Acinetobacter baumani, Stenotrophomonas maltophila etc. need special attention as they are commonly isolated from Health Care Associated Infections(HAI) and belong to Multidrug resistant Organism (MDRO) i.e. they are resistant to one or more classes of antibiotics (Harrison & Lederberg, 1998). P. aeruginosa is responsible for 10-15% of nosocomial infections worldwide. The β-lactam group of antibiotics which include Penicillins, Cephalosporins, Monobactams and Carbapenems are mainly used to treat infections caused by Gram negative bacteria. The widespread use of antibiotics put tremendous selective pressure on bacteria which develop new mechanisms to escape the lethal action of the antibiotics. These infections are difficult to treat because of emergence of newer β-lactamases such as Extended Spectum β-lactamases (ESBL), AmpCβ-lactamases and Carbapenemases. The β-lactamases inactivate β-lactam antibiotics by cleaving the structural β-lactam ring. Failure to detect these enzymes producing strains has contributed to their uncontrolled spread in Health Care setup and therapeutic failure.

Major mechanisms causing resistance to the β-lactam antibiotics in P.aeruginosa are the production of β-lactamases, reduced outer membrane permeability and altered affinity of targetPenicillin binding proteins. (Washington et al, 2006; Pitt, 1990).

1.1 Classification of β-lactamases

β-lactamase can be classified according to Functional or Bush Jacoby Mederious classification (Bush et al, 1995), into group 1, 2a, 2be, 2br, 2c, 2d, 2e, 2f and according to molecular or Ambler classification (Ambler, 1980) into Ambler class A,B,C and D. Detection of β-lactamase production has been achieved in the past by measuring the production of penicilloic acid, which is produced when benzyl penicillin is hydrolysed. The acid production can be detected by acidometric method, iodometric method and chromogenic cephalosporin (nitrocephin) method (Miles & Amyes, 2008). The first plasmid mediated β-lactamase was described in early 1960. The TEM1 enzyme was named after the patient Temoniera from whom it was originally found in isolated strains of E.coli, (Medeiros, 1984) whereas β-lactamase SHV-1 (Sulphydryl variable) is chromosomally encoded in most isolates of Klebsiella pneumoniae but is usually plsmid mediated in E.coli (Tz-ouvelekis, 1999).

1.1.1 Extended spectrum β-lactamases (ESBL)

ESBLs were first reported in 1983 in Klebsiella pneumoniae from Germany. Typically ESBLs are mutant plasmid mediated β-lactamases derived from older broad-spectrum β-lactamases. The mutations alter the amino acid configuration around active site of β-lactamases (Thomson, 2001). The first ESBL to be described in 1983 was actually TEM3 (Soughakoff et al, 1980) and now over 130 additional TEMs have been isolated. ESBLs have an extended substrate profile that cause hydrolysis of cephalosporins, penicillins and aztreonam and are inhibited by β-lactamase inhibitors, such as clavulanate, tazobactam and sulbactam. ESBLs are commonly produced by Klebsiella species and Escherichia coli; but also occur in other Gram negative bacteria, including Enterobacter, Salmonella, Proteus, Serratia marcescens, Pseudomonas aeruginosa, Burkholderia, Acinetobacter species, etc.

1.1.2 AmpC β-lactamases

Molecular class C or AmpC primarily hydrolyses cephems (cephalosporins and cephamycins) but also hydrolyze penicillins and aztreonam. These enzymes are resistant to the currently available β-lactamase inhibitors such as clavulanate, tazobactam and sulbactam (Philippon et al, 2002). With rare exceptions, the hydrolysis of cephamycins, such as cefotetan and cefoxitin, is a property that can help to distinguish AmpCs from ESBLs. Genes encoding inducible chromosomal AmpC β-lactamases are part of the genomes of many Gram negative bacteria specially P.aeruginosa. High level production of AmpC may cause resistance to the first, second and third-generation cephalosporins and cephamycins, penicillins and β-lactamase inhibitor combination. Higher level AmpC production may occur as a consequence of mutation or when the organism is exposed to an inducing agent. Cephamycins (e.g. cefoxitin and cefotetan), ampicillin, and carbapenem are good inducer (Moland et al, 2008). AmpC β-lactamases producing organisms are on rise and leads to therapeutic failure if 3rd Generation cephalosporins are given empirically or not tested in the laboratory for AmpC β-lactamases production (Basak et al, 2009). The chromosomally mediated AmpC β-lactamases are only inducible.

1.1.3 Carbapenemases

These include β-lactamases which cause carbapenem hydrolysis, with elevated carbapenem MICs and they belonged to molecular classes A, B and D. Molecular classes A, C and D include the β-lactamases with serine at their active site, whereas class B β-lactamases are all metalloenzymes with an active site zinc (Queenan & Bush, 2007).

Metallobetalactamases - They belong to molecular class B β-lactamases, and have 3 characteristics -

1. Hydrolyze carbapenems
2. Resistant to clinically used β-lactamase inhibitors and
3. Inhibited by EDTA, a metal ion chelator.

Other MBL inhibitors used are 2-mercaptoethanol, sodium mercapto acetic acid (SMA), 2-mercaptopropionic acid, copper chloride and ferric chloride (Arkawa et al, 2000). MBLs have a broad substrate spectrum and in addition to carbapenems, they can hydrolyze cephalosporin and penicillins but cannot hydrolyse aztreonam. Interestingly, not all of the MBLs readily hydrolyze nitrocefin. The first MBL detected were chromosomally encoded and was detected in Bacillus cereus (Lim et al, 1988). Since then there has been a dramatic increase in detection and spread of acquired or transferable families of these MBLs. There are 5 major families of acquired MBLs (IMP, VIM, SPM, GIM and SIM) (Toleman et al, 2007). In 1990, IMP-1, the 1st MBL encoded on plasmid, was discovered in Japan (Watanabe et al, 1991). The MBLs are located on integrons and are incorporated as gene cassettes.When these integrons become associated with plasmids or transposons, transfer between bacteria is facilitated.

Classification of MBLS

MBLS are classified into 3 subclasses—B1,B2 and B3. Subclass B1 and B3 are divided by aminoacid homology, bind 2 zinc atoms for optimal hydrolysis and have broad hydrolysis spectrum. Subclass B2 are inhibited when a second zinc atom is bound and preferentially hydrolyse carbapenem (Free et al, 2005).

Molecular class A carbapenemase - Class A serine carbapenemases belong to functional group 2f include chromosomally encoded NMC(not metalloenzyme carbapenemase), IMI (Imipenem hydrolyzing β-lactamase) and SME(Serratia marscenscens enzyme) and plasmid mediated KPC (Klebsiella pneumoniae carbapenemase) and GES/IBC(integron borne cephalosporinase) (Queenan & Bush, 2007). All have the ability to hydrolyse carbapenems, cephalosporins, penicillins and aztreonem and all are inhibited by clavulanate and tazobactam. The chromosomal class A carbapenemase are infrequently found and can be induced by imipenem and cefoxitin. The KPC (Klebsiella pneumoniae carbapenemase) producing strains are found in Klebsiella pneumoniae, Enterobacter species, Salmonella species and other Enterobacteriaceae (Hossain et al, 2004; Miriagou et al, 2003).

Class D Serine carbapenemases: The OXA (Oxacillin hydrolysing) β-lactamase with carbapenemase activity was detected by Patow et al in 1993 and the enzyme was purified from Acinetobacter baumani (Queenan & Bush, 2007). They have been also found in Enterobacteriaceae and P.aeruginosa and were described as penicillinase capable of hydrolyzing oxacillin and cloxacillin (Bush & Sykes, 1987; Naas & Nordmann, 1999). They were poorly inhibited by clavulanic acid and EDTA and were designated as ARI-1 (Acinetobacter Resistant to Imipenem) and reside on large plasmid. The OXA carbopenemases have hydrolytic activity against penicillins, some cephalosporins and imipenem. The widespread use of reserved antibiotics such as β-lactam /β-lactamases inhibitor combinations, monobactams and carbapenem has caused persistent exposure of bacterial strains to a multitude of β-lactam leading to overproduction of β-lactamases (Goossens et al, 2004; Manoharan et al, 2010; Lee et al, 2003). Consequently the emergence of carbapenem resistance is a world-wide public health concern since carbabapenems are used as last resort to treat serious infections caused by ESBL producing organisms. Approximately 40% strains of P.aeruginosa are resistant to anti-pseudomonal drugs including carbapenems. Therefore, early detection of of ESBL, AmpC β-lactamase & MBL producing P. aeruginosa strains is of crucial importance for prevention of their inter and intra hospital dissemination.

1.2 Aims and objectives

The present study was undertaken with the aim to study Pseudomonas aeruginosa with special reference to β-lactamase production isolated in the Department of Microbiology, Jawaharlal Nehru Medical College, Wardha (M. S.), India.

1.2.1 To fulfill the aim the following objectives were taken

- To study the prevalence of Extended Spectrum β-lactamases (ESBL), Amp C β-lactamases, Metallobetalactamases (MBL) producing Pseudomonas aeruginosa strains, isolated from different clinical samples of patients attending the Hospital
- To study the antibiotic susceptibility profile of Extended Spectrum β-lactamases (ESBL), Amp C β-lactamases and Metallobetalactamases (MBL) producing Pseudomonas aeruginosa strains isolated.

2. Material and methods

The study was conducted from 1st September 2008 to August 2010 (2 year period). A total number of 250 P.aeruginosa strains were isolated from different clinical samples e.g. urine, pus and wound swab, blood, catheter tips, endotracheal tube secretions, different body fluids etc. received from indoor as well as outdoor patients departments (IPD &OPD) of our hospital, which is a tertiary care hospital in a rural set-up. P.aeruginosa strains were characterized according to conventional identification tests. P.aeruginosa ATCC 27853 were used as positive control for all conventional tests. All antibiotic disks and culture media used in the study were procured from HiMedia laboratories Pvt. Limited, India. Ethylene Diamine Tetraacetic acid (EDTA) and 3-amino phenylboronic acid (APB) were procured from Sigma-Alderich.

2.1 Antibiotic susceptibility testing

All 250 P.aeruginosa strains were subjected to antibiotic susceptibility testing to different antimicrobial agents using Mueller-Hinton agar plates by Kirby-Bauer disk diffusion method according to CLSI guidelines (CLSI Document M2-A9, 2006). Using sterile swab, lawn culture of the test strain (turbidity adjusted to 0.5 McFarland standard) was made on Mueller Hinton Agar plate. With all aseptic precaution, the antibiotic disks were put on that inoculated plate. Six antibiotic disks were put on a 90mm diameter plate. The antibiotic sensitivity tests were put for aminoglycosides such as amikacin (Ak-30μg), netilimicin (Nt-30μg); cephalosporin such as ceftazidime(Ca-30μg), cefepime(Cpm-30μg); fluoroquinolones i.e. ciprofloxacin(Cf-5μg); monobactams i.e. aztreonam (Ao-30 μg); carbapenems such as imipenem(I-10μg), meropenem(Mr-10μg); piperacillin/tazobactam (Pt-100/10μg), ceftazidime/clavulanic acid (Cac-30μg /10 μg) and polymyxin B (Pb-300μg) etc. (Fig. 1)

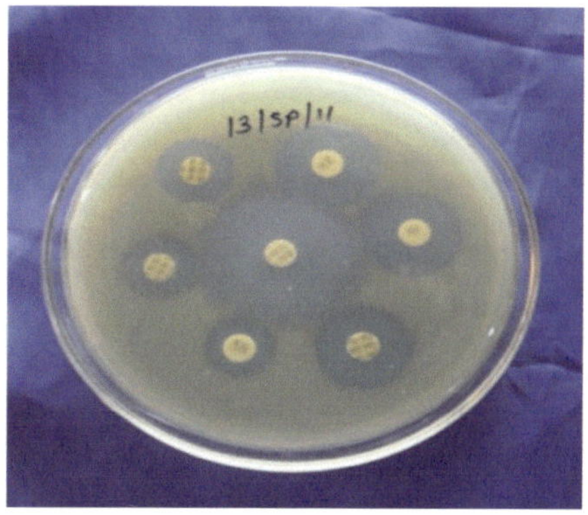

Fig. 1. Antibiotic susceptibility test.

Detection of newer β-lactamases

Though several methods both phenotypic and genotypic have been described for detection of newer β-lactamases, we restricted our study only to phenotypic methods. There is no CLSI guideline given for detection of ESBL, AmpC β-lactamases ans MBL producing P.aeruginosa.

2.1.1 Detection of extended spectrum β-lactamases (ESBL)

Screening test: ESBL production was detected by reduced susceptibility to Ceftazidime, Cefotaxime.

Confirmatory tests: As per Clinical and Laboratory Standard Institute (CLSI) guidelines for Enterobacteriaceae (Waynepa CLSI, 2008; Storenburg, 2003), we used the same combined disk method as confirmatory test for Pseudomonas aeruginosa also, as the principle remains the same.

1. **Combined Disk Method** (Carter et al, 2000)
   Broth cultures of test strains were adjusted to McFarland 0.5 standard and used to inoculate Mueller Hinton agar plates with a sterile swab. Commercialized disks containing ceftazidime (Ca) 30 μg and ceftazidime plus clavulanate (Cac) 30μg plus 10μg respectively were used in this method. An increase in diameter of ≥5mm with ceftazidime plus clavulanate (Cac) disk as compared to ceftazidime(Ca) disk alone was considered positive for ESBL detection. All 250 P. aeruginosa strains were also tested using piperacillin (Pc)100 μg & piperacillin-tazobactam (Pt) 100 μg plus 10 μg respectively in combination.
2. **E test ESBL strip** (Washington et al, 2006)
   The E-test ESBL confirmatory test strips are based on the CLSI dilution method. The strip has concentration gradients of ceftazidime (TZ) 0.5 to 32 μg/ml on one half and ceftazidime 0.064 to 4 μg/ml plus 4 μg/ml clavulanic acid (TZL) on another half . The ESBL E-test was performed and interpreted using test strains and Quality Control strains according to the manufacturerer's instructions. In this method lawn culture of test strain was done on a Mueller Hinton agar plate. With a sterile forceps the ESBL E-test strip was placed onto the inoculated plate. After overnight incubation at 37°C, the zone of inhibition was read from two halves of the strip. MIC ratio of ceftazidime/ceftazidime clavulanic acid (TZ/TZL) ≥ 8 or deformation of ellipse or phantom zone present was considered as positive for ESBL production.

2.1.2 Detection of Amp C β-lactamases

For detection of AmpC class of β-lactamases, no satisfactory technique has been established till date as per CLSI guidelines. Induction of C β-lactamase synthesis was Amp based on the disc approximation assay using several inducer substrate combinations.

Screening test: Several inducer/substrate combinations disks like Cefoxitin/Piperacillin, Imipenem/Ceftazidime,Imipenem/Cefotaxime, Imipenem/Cefoxitin, Imipenem/Piperacillin -Tazobactum were used as described by Dunne and Hardin et al. Imipenem and cefoxitin were used as inducers of AmpC β-lactamases (Dunne & Hardin, 2005).

Interpretation: Strains were considered inducible if a positive test was obtained with any of the inducer/substrate combinations. A test was considered positive if the zone of inhibition was reduced by ≥2 mm on the induced side of the substrate disc or even blunting of substrate zone of inhibition adjacent to inducer disc. Also, if the zone of inhibition produced by ceftazidime/ceftazidime-clavulanic acid (Cac) disk was ≥2mm less than the zone produced by a ceftazidime (Ca) disk, the strain was considered to be inducible Amp C positive. Similarly, same criteria was used for piperacillin & piperacillin/tazobactam (Pc/Pt) disks.

Confirmatory test: Disk potetiation(DP) test and Double disk synergy test (DDST) using 3-aminophenylboronic acid (APB) (100mg/ml dissolved in DMSO) (Yagi et al, 2005). An increase in zone size of ≥5mm around the Ceftazidime- APB disk compared to ceftazidime only disk was recorded as a positive result for disk potentiation test. In DDST, the presence of change in the shape of growth inhibitory zone around ceftazidime or cefotaxime disk through the interaction with the 3- Aminophenyl boronic acid containing disk was interpreted as positive for AmpC production.

2.1.3 Detection of metallobetalactamases (MBL)

All imipenem resistant strains were screened for Carbapenemase activity by Classical Hodge Test and Modified Hodge Test (MHT) (Lee et al, 2001a; 2003b). Pseudomonas aeruginosa strains which were positive by Classsical Hodge Test(IHT) and Modified Hodge Test (MHT) were tested for metallobetalactamase (MBL) production by Imipenem/EDTA double disk synergy test (Lee et al, 2001)and disk potentiation test or imipenem-EDTA combined disk test (Yong et al, 2002) using Di-potassium EDTA (10µl of 0.5 M).

Imipenem-EDTA double disk synergy test (DDST) (Lee et al, 2001)

The IMP-EDTA double disk synergy test was performed for detection of metallobetalactamases. Test strains i.e. Pseudomonas aeruginosa (turbidity adjusted to 0.5 McFarland standard) were inoculated on to Mueller Hinton agar plate. After drying, a 10µg Imipenem disk and a blank sterile filter paper disk (6mm in diameter, Whartman filter paper no.2) were placed 10mm apart from edge to edge. 10 µl of 50mM zinc sulfate solution was added to the 10 µg imipenem disk. Then, 10µl of 0.5 M EDTA(Sigma, USA) solution was applied to the blank filter paper disk. As disodium-EDTA is difficult to be solubilised in sterile water, we had used dipotassium-EDTA which is easily soluble in sterile water. Enhancement of the zone of inhibition towards the EDTA disk was interpreted as a positive result.

Disk Potentiation test or Imipenem-EDTA combined disk test (Young et al, 2002)

The test was performed for detection of metallobetalactamases. Test strains (turbidity adjusted to 0.5 McFarland standard) were inoculated on to Mueller Hinton agar plate. Two imipenem disk (10 μg) were placed on the plate wide apart and 10 μl of 50mM zinc sulphate solution was added to each of the imipenem disks. Then 10μl of 0.5 M EDTA solution was added to one of the disk to obtain the desired concentration. The inhibition zones of the imipenem and imipenem-EDTA disks were compared after 16-18 hours of incubation at 35°C. If the increase in inhibition zone with the Imipenem and EDTA disk was ≥7 mm than the imipenem disk alone, it was considered as MBL positive.

The MBL producing strains were further confirmed by using MBL - E test strip (AB bioMerieux) (Walsh et al, 2002).

MIC ratio of Imipenem /Imipenem-EDTA (IP/IPI) of ≥8 or deformations of ellipse or phantom zone indicate MBL production by MBL E-test.

2.2 Observations and results

Maximum 204(81.6%) P.aeruginosa strains were isolated from Indoor Patient Department (IPD). No newer β-lactamase producing strains were isolated from patients attending Out Patient Department

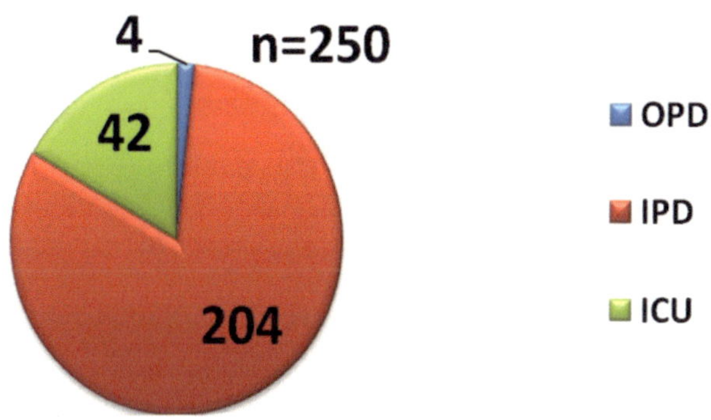

Fig. 2. Isolation of Pseudomonas aeruginosa strains from OPD, IPD and ICU patients.

Fig. 3 shows 165 (66%) P.aeruginosa strains were ESBL, AmpC β-lactamases and MBL producers.

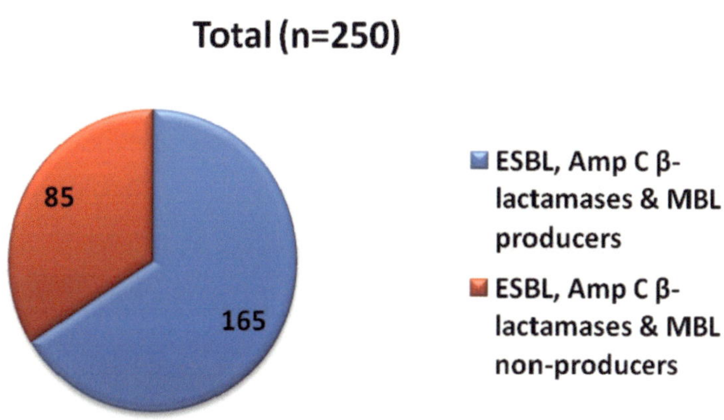

Fig. 3. Prevalence of newer β-lactamases producing P. aeruginosa strains (n=250).

P.aeruginosa	ESBL		AmpC		MBL	
	No.	Percentage	No.	Percentage	No.	Percentage
n=250	100	40	105	42	28	11.2

Table 1. Prevalence of ESBL, AmpC β-lactamase and MBL producing P. aeruginosa (n=250)

Amongst the 100 ESBL (Fig. 4) and 105 Amp C β-lactamase producers (Fig. 5 & 6), 68 (27.2%) P. aeruginosa strains had produced both ESBL as well as AmpC β-lactamases. 28 (11.2%) P. aeruginosa strains were Metallobetalactamase (MBL) producers.

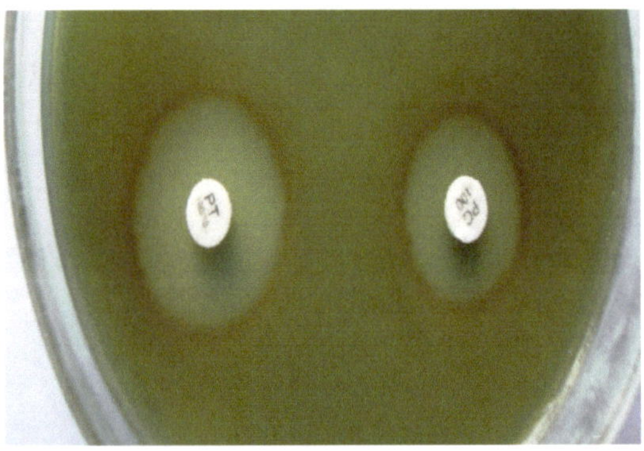

Fig. 4. Detection of ESBL(Combined disk method)

Detection of AmpC β-lactamases (Figure 5&6)

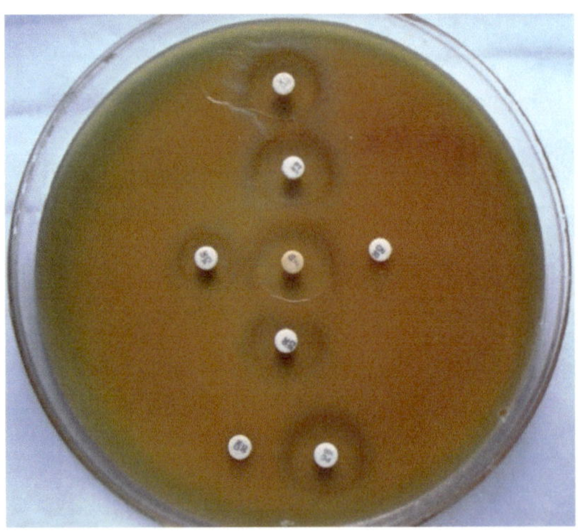

Fig. 5. Inducer-substrate combination disk test.

Fig. 7 shows amongst 100 ESBL and 105 AmpC β-lactamase producers 68 (41.2%) strains had produced both ESBL as well as AmpC β-lactamases. There was no strain which produced all the 3 types of β-lactamases. Similarly, no strain produced ESBL or AmpC β-lactamase along with MBL.

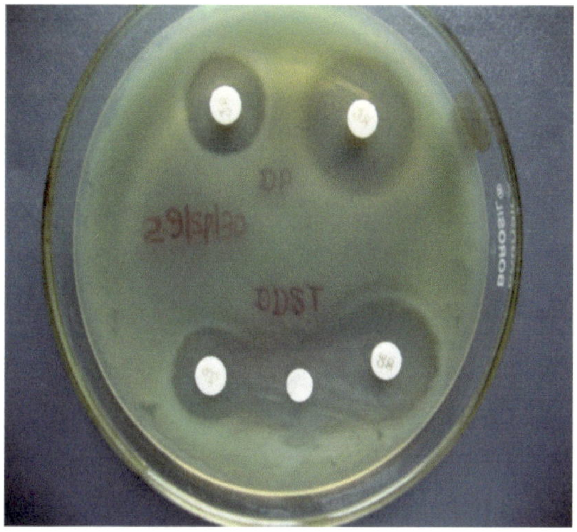

Fig. 6. DDST & DP test using 3-Aminophenyl-boronic acid (3-APB).

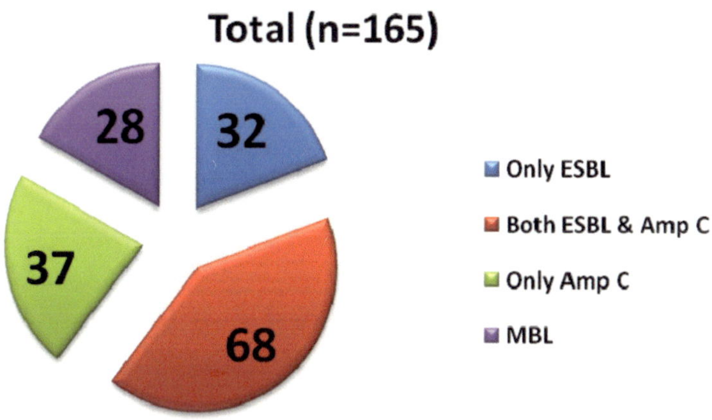

Fig. 7. Incidence of different newer β-lactamases producing P.aeruginosa strains(n=165)

Table 2 shows that out of 250 P. aeruginosa strains studied, 31 (12.4 %)were imipenem resistant and 28 (11.2 %) were metallobetalactamase (MBL) producers. 31 imipenem resistant strains were screened for carbapenem hydrolysis by Classical Hodge test (HT) & modified Hodge test (MHT). Amongst these 31 imipenem resistant P. aeruginosa strains, 28 (90.3%) were positive for Classical Hodge test (HT) & modified Hodge test (MHT) for carbapenem hydrolysis and these 28 strains were also positive for metallobetalactamase (MBL) production by Double disk synergy test (DDST) and disk potentiation test (DP).

Imipenem resistant P. aeruginosa	Screening test for carbapenem hydrolysis		Confirmatory test for MBL		
	Classical Hodge test	Modified Hodge test	Double disk synergy test	Disk potentiation test	MBL E-test
n = 31	28	28	28	28	28

Table 2. Prevalence of MBL producing P. aeruginosa (n =250)

These 28 strains were also confirmed for metallobetalactamase (MBL) production by using MBL E-test strip (AB bioMerieux). MBL E-test (Fig. 9) shows MIC ratio of imipenem IP/ imipenem-EDTA IPI for test strain P. aeruginosa as 16/1 i.e. 16 and MBL E-test positive. The phantom zone shown in Fig. 9 is another criteria for MBL E-test positivity. MBL E-tests done for those 28 P. aeruginosa strains showed that the MIC ratio of imipenem / imipenem-EDTA i.e. IP/IPI were > 8 such as 16/1 for 9 strains, 24/1.5 for 3 strains, 32/1 for 5 strains, 48/1 for 8 strains, 64/1 for 2 strains and 128/1 for 1 strain.

Confirmation of MBL by E-test : Figure 8 & 9

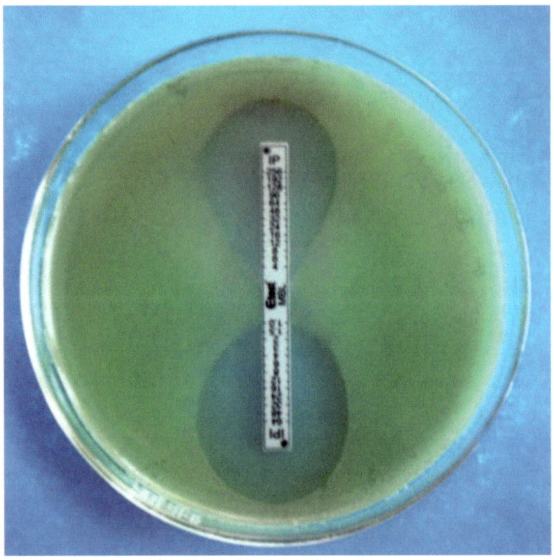

Fig. 8. Quality control: P.aeruginosa ATCC 27853 (MBL E test negative).

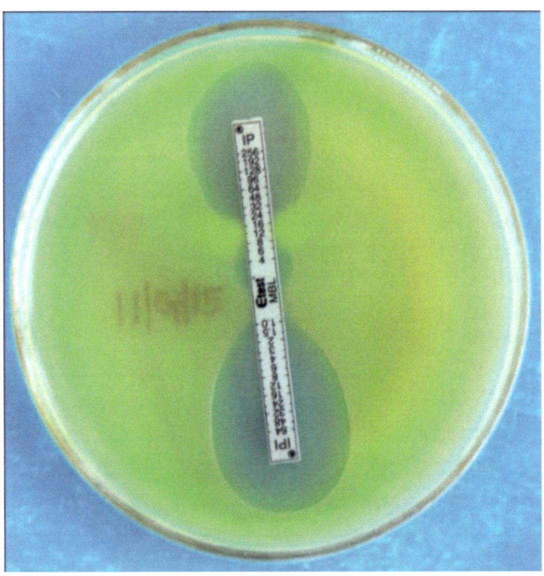

Fig. 9. MBL E-test (positive).

Fig. 10 shows from ICU 6 (14.3%) strains produced both ESBL and AmpC β-lactamases whereas 9(21.4%) strains produced MBL.

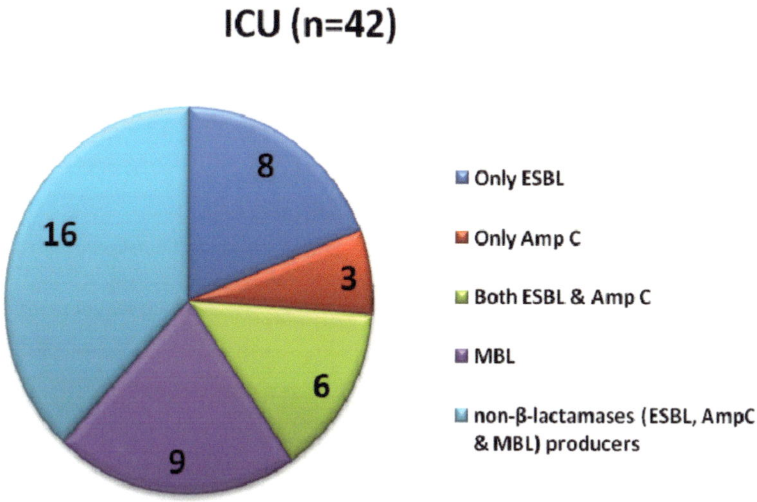

Fig. 10. Isolation of different β-lactamases producing P. aeruginosa strains from ICU.

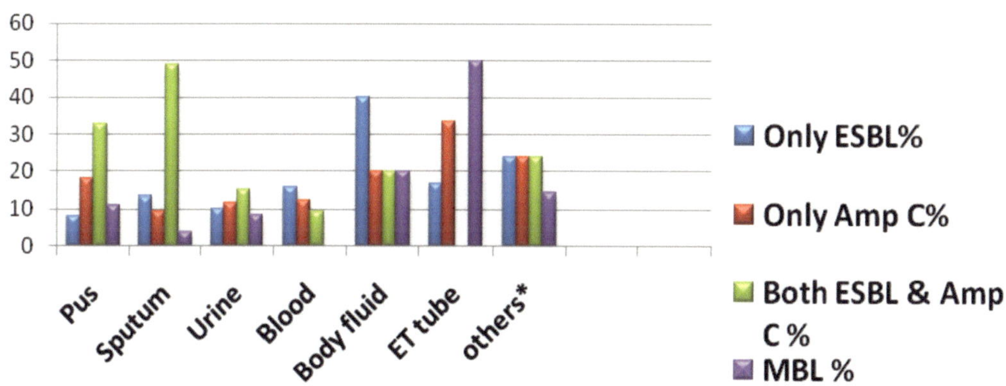

*others include throat swab, vaginal swab, ear swab, bronchial wash, tip of catheter & drain fluid.

Fig. 11. Isolation of β-lactamases producing P.aeruginosa strains from different clinical specimens.

In the present study, maximum P.aeruginosa strains isolated from pus and wound swab, 73 (29.2%) followed by 60(24%) from urine. The fig. 11 shows 26(49%) P.aeruginosa strains isolated from sputum sample were both ESBL and AmpC β-lactamase producer. 50% P.aeruginosa strains isolated from endotracheal tube secretions were MBL producers. Though no MBL producing strains were isolated from blood culture.

Fig. 12 shows maximum 36.2% strains isolated from Medicine ward produced both ESBL and AmpC β-lactamase. From surgery ward maximum 10(35.7%) strains were MBL producers. No MBL producing P.aeruginosa strains were isolated from Neonatal Intensive Care Unit(NICU) and 3(20%) strains were only ESBL producers.

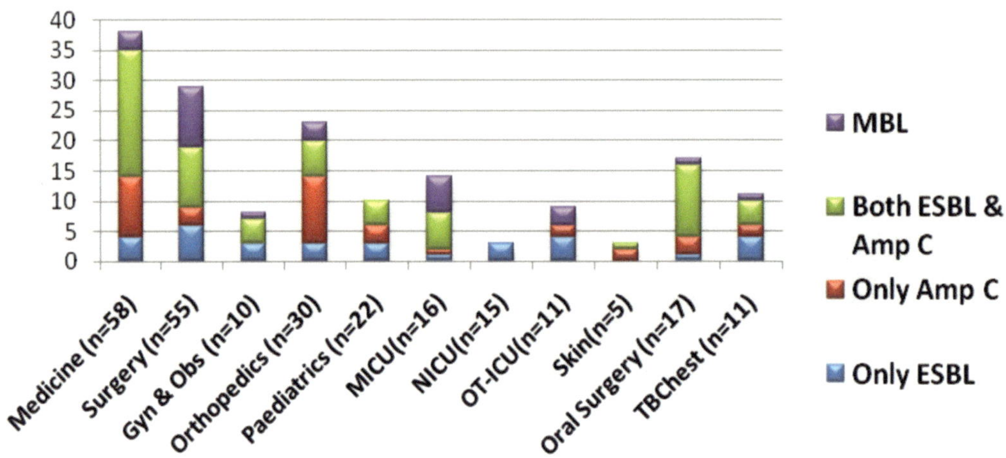

Fig. 12. Isolation of β-lactamases producing P. aeruginosa strains from different clinical specialities

Fig. 13 shows that P.aeruginosa strains showed a high degree of resistance to cefepime (90.4%), cefoxitine(91.6%) and ceftazidime(67.2%). However effective antimicrobial agents were found to be polymyxin B (100%), Imipenem(87.6%) and piperacillin-tazobactum (86%) sensitive.

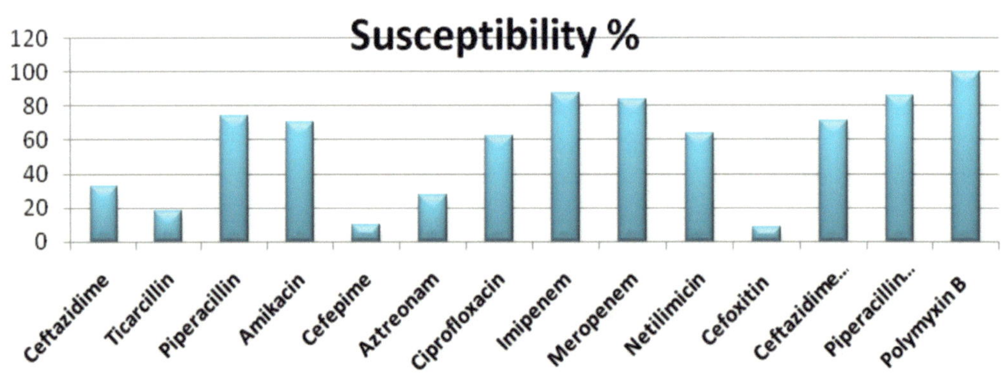

Fig. 13. Antibiotic susceptibility profile of P. aeruginosa strains (n=250)

Fig. 14 shows most effective antimicrobial agent against ESBL andAmpC β-lactamase producing P.aeruginosa strains were Imipenem(100%) and Polymyxin-B(100%). However, sensitivity of ESBL and AmpC β-lactamase producers to piperacillin-tazobactam were 100% and 82.8% respectively.

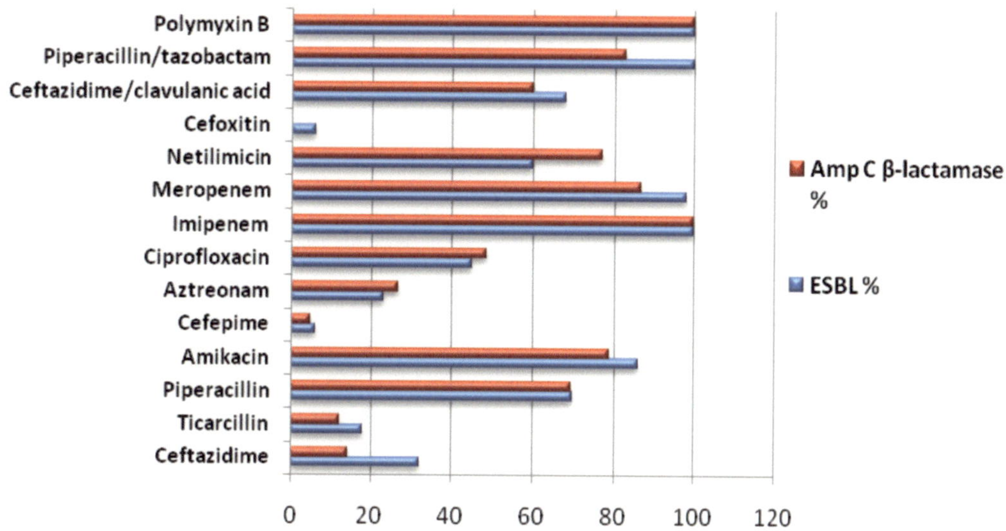

Fig. 14. Antibiotic susceptibility profile of ESBL & Amp C β-lactamases producing P.aeruginosa strains

Fig.15 shows all(100%) MBL positive isolates were sensitive to polymyxin-B. 1(3.7%) each MBL producing strain was sensitive to Amikacin and Netilmicin respectively. But no MBL producing strain was susceptible to Aztreonam.

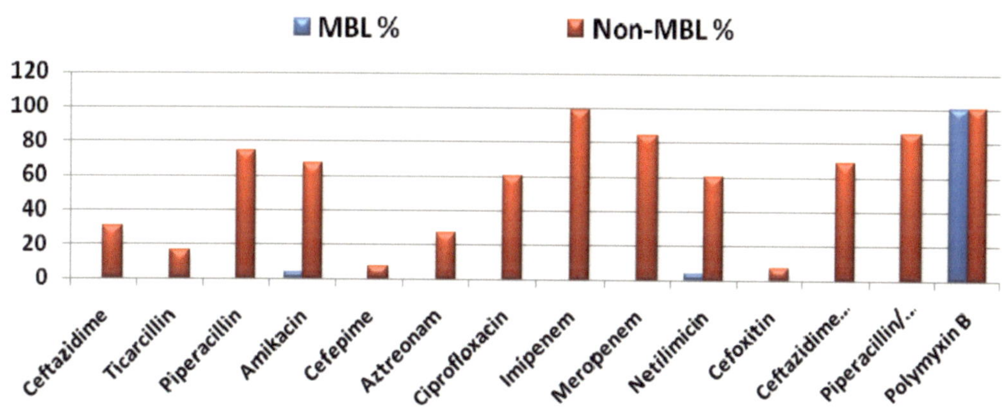

Fig. 15. Antibiotic susceptibility profile of MBL & non-MBL P. aeruginosa strains

2.3 Discussion

Pseudomonas aeruginosa is one of the most important microorganisms which causes problems clinically as a result of its high resistance to antimicrobial agents and is therfore a particularly dangerous & dreaded bug. Despite the discovery of ESBL, Amp C β-lactamases and MBL at least a decade ago, there remains a low level of awareness of their importance and many clinical laboratories have problems in detecting ESBL& Amp C β-lactamases. Failure to detect these enzymes has contributed to their uncontrolled spread and commonly to therapeutic failures.

Detection problems arise especially with organisms that produce an inducible Amp C β-lactamases, as clavulanate can induce high level production of Amp C , which may obscure recognition of ESBLs (Moland et al, 2008). According to Clinical & Laboratory Standards (CLSI) interpretive definations, ESBLs do not always increase MICs to levels characterized as resistant (Livermore, 2002). Not only that ESBL producing organisms may give false sensitive zones in routine disk diffusion test. The number of infections caused by Amp C β-lactamases producing P. aeruginosa is on rise and poses a threat to patients due to therapeutic failure if they remain undetected (Arora & Bal, 2005). Metallobetalactamase (MBL) producing P.aeruginosa is an emerging threat and a cause of concern for treating physicians as it can hydrolyze carbapenems which are given as a last resort to the patient having infection with ESBL and AmpC β-lactamase producing P.aeruginosa. The MBLs have become more notorious as therapeutically available inhibitors are not available and for their potential for rapid and generalized dissemination to different other Gram negative bacilli. Hence, accurate identification of MBL producing strains are very urgently needed. Though PCR gives specific and accurate results, it's use is limited to few laboratories because of it's high cost and different types of ESBLs, AmpCβ-lactamases and metallobetalactamases (MBLs) present worldwide (Moland et al, 2008b).

In the present study 81.6% P.aeruginosa strains were isolated from IPD patients Algun et al from Turkey in 2004 reported isolation of P. aeruginosa 61% from IPD patients. Basak et al in 2009 reported 89.3% isolation from IPD and 10.7% from ICU from our hospital.

In the present study, co-existence of MBL producing P. aeruginosa was not observed along with ESBL & Amp C producers. Saha et al in 2010 reported 86% strains producing both MBL and Amp C β-lactamases while only one strain was observed to produce both ESBL and MBL. In the present study 68(27.2%) strains were both ESBL & Amp C β-lactamases producers amongst 250 P. aeruginosa strains studied.

6(22.2%) MBL producing strains were isolated from Medicine ICU. Sarkar et al in 2006 reported 36.4% of imipenem resistance in nosocomially infected patients with P. aeruginosa. In present study, we found 15 (35.7%) P. aeruginosa from NICU and all were from blood cultures of neonates and all were imipenem sensitive. Only 3 (20%) of these were found to be positive for ESBL production. Arkawa et al, 2000 recommended testing ceftazidime-resistant isolates for MBL production because in their study some MBL producing Gram negative bacilli were inhibited by low concentration of imipenem and they were difficult to detect. But Lee et al, 2001 reported that in their study, not a single MBL-producing isolates were detected among imipenem susceptible isolates.

In Japan, Sugino et al, 2001 used only carbapenem non-susceptible isolates for screening of MBL. Hence we also used carbapenem resistant isolates for detection of MBL. Though Arkawa et al, 2000 and other authors have done DDST & Disc potentiation test with ceftazidime and EDTA, in our study we used imipenem and EDTA for DDST & Disc potentiation test. As in our study, even in non MBL producing *P.aeruginosa* strains, the ceftazidime resistance was quite high (69.8%). The MBL producing strains may also have another ceftazidime resistance mechanism (Lee et al, 2003b). With such type of strains, DDSTs using an imipenem disc can show positive results for MBL but a ceftazidime disc can not; just as a cefepime disc but not a ceftazidime disc can detect extended spectrum β-lactamase (ESBL) production in Amp-C β-lactamase producing strains.

Though Franklin et al, 2006 have reported that 87% of their MBL producing Enteobacteriaceae isolates had >30mm of zone with aztreonam, we did not find any MBL producing *P.aeruginosa* strain to be susceptible to aztreonam. This can only be explained by the fact that there are presence of some other mechanisms for aztreonam resistance in P. aeruginosa strains isolated.

Aggarwal et al in 2008 found that polymyxin B was the most effective antibiotic recording 0% resistance, similar was the finding of our study. In our study we found 67.2% resistance against ceftazidime which was quite high and corelated well with the study of Behra et al in 2008 who had reported 70% resistance to ceftazidime.

3. Conclusion

Microbial drug resistance is now a global problem due to newer β-lactamases produced by Gram-negative bacteria including Pseudomonas aeruginosa. E-test and Polymerase chain reaction (PCR) can be used for accurate detection of newer β-lactamases , but both are costly and require expertise and cannot be done routinely.

Hence to conclude, for detection of ESBL, combined disk method using piperacillin/piperacillin-tazobactam (Pc/Pt), for detection of Amp C β-lactamases confirmatorty Disk potentiation test using 3-aminophenylboronic acid and for detection of MBL producing P. aeruginosa disk potentiation test using imipenem-EDTA should be done by all clinical Microbiolgy laboratories to prevent its dissemination and also for a good therapeutic outcome as these tests are economical, easy to perform and quite specific.

4. Acknowledgment

The author highly acknowledge the Datta Meghe Institute of Medical Sciences, Deemed to be University for funding this project.

5. References

Aggarwal G., Lodhi R B., Kamalakar U P., Khadase R K., Jalgaokar S V. (2008). Study of metallobetalactamases production in clinical isolates of P. aeruginosa. *Indian J Med Microbiol.* Vol 26 No.4 pp. (349-351).

Algun U., Arisoy A., Gunduz T., Ozbakkaloglu B. (2004). The resistance of Pseudomonas aeruginosa strains to Fluoroquinolone group of antibiotics. *Indian J Med Microbiol.* Vol 22 No.2 pp. (112-114).

Ambler, R. P. (1980). The structure of β-lactamases. *Phil. Trans. R.Soc. Lond. B. Biol. Sci.* Vol 289 pp. (321-331).

Arkawa Y., Shibata N., Shibayama K., Kurokawa H., Yogi T. Fusiwara H, et al. (2000). Convenient test for screening metallobetalactamases producing gram-negative bacteria using thiol compounds. *J Clin Microbiol* Vol 38 pp. (40 - 43).

Arora S., Bal M. (2005). Amp C β-lactamases producing bacterial isolates from Kolkata hospital. *Indian J Med Res.* Vol 122 pp. (224-233).

Basak S., Khodke M., Bose S., Mallick SK. (2009). Inducible AmpC Beta-Lactamase Producing Pseudomonas Aeruginosa Isolated In a rural Hospital of Central India. *Journal of Clinical and Diagnostic Research.* Vol 3 pp. (1921-1927).

Behra B., Mathur P., Das A., Kapil A., Sharma V. (2008). An evaluation of four different phenotypic techniques for detection of metallobetalactamases producing Pseudomonas aeruginosa. *Indian J Med Microbiol* Vol 26 No.3 pp. (233-237).

Bush, K., and R. B. Sykes. (1987). Characterization and epidemiology of β-lactamases. Elsevier Science Publishers BV, Philadelphia, PA.

Bush K., Jacoby GA., Medeiros A. (1995). A functional classification scheme for beta lactamase and its correlation with molecular structure. *Antimicrob Agents Chemother.* Vol *39 pp.* (1211-1233).

Carter MW., Oakton KJ., Warner M., Livermore DM. (2000). Detection of extended spectrum beta lactamases in Klebsiellae with the Oxoid combination disk method. *J Clin Microbiol* . Vol *38* pp. (4228-4232).

Clinical and Laboratory Standards Institute. (2006). *Performance standards for antimicrobial disk tests;* Approved Standards, 9th ed. *CLSI Document M2- A9,* Vol. 26 No 1. Wayne PA.

Dunne WM. and Hardin DJ. (2005). Use of Several Inducer and substrate Antibiotic Combinations in a Disk Approximation Assay format to screen for AmpC induction in patient isolates of Pseudomonas aeruginosa, Enterobacter spp, Citrobacter spp and Serratia spp. *J Clin Microbiol* . Vol 15 pp. (5945-5949).

Franklin C., Liolios L., Peleg AY. (2006). Phenotypic Detection of carbapenem susceptible Metallobetalactamase producing Gram-negative bacilli in the clinical laboratory. *J of Clin Microbiol.* Vol 44 No.9 pp. (3139-3144).

Free J.M., Galleni M., Bush K., Didiberg O. (2005). Is it necessary to change the classification of β-lactamases? *J. Antimicrob. Chemother.* Vol 55 pp. (1051-1053).

Goossens H., Malhotra Kumar S., Eraksoy H., Unal S., Grabein B., Masterton R. *et al.* (2004). MYSTIC study group: Results of two world wide surveys into physician awareness and perceptions of extended spectrum spectrum beta lactamases. *Clin Microbiol Infect.* Vol *10 pp.* (760-762).

Hossain, A., Ferraro MJ., Pino RM., Dew III RB., Moland ES., Lockhart TJ., Thomson KS., Goering RV., Hanson ND. (2004). Plasmid mediated carbapenem-hydrolyzing enzyme KPC-2 in an *Enterobacter* sp. *Antimicrob. AgentsChemother.* Vol 48 pp. (4438–4440).

I.O.M.(1998) eds. Harrison, P.F. & Lederberg J. pp. (8-74), National Academy Press Washington, DC.

Lee K., Chong Y., Shin H B., Kim Y A., Yong D., Yum J H. (2001). Modified Hodge and EDTA disk synergy test to screen metallobetalactamases producing strains of Pseudomonas spp and Acinetobacter spp. *Clin Microbiol Infect.* Vol 7 pp. (88 - 91).

Lee K., Lim Y S., Yong D., Yum J H., Chong Y. (2003). Evaluation of Hodge test and imipenem-EDTA double disk synergy test for differentiation of metallobetalactamases producing clinical isolates of Pseudomonas spp and Acinetobacter spp. *J Clin Microbiol.* Vol 4 pp. (4623 - 4629).

Lee K., Lee WG., Uh Y., Ha GY., Cho J., Chong Y. (2003). VIM and IMP - type metallobetalactamase producing Pseudomonas spp. and Acinetobacter spp in Korean hospitals. *Emerg Infect Dis.* Vol 9 pp. (868-871).

Lim HM., Pene J.J., Shaw RW. (1988). Cloning, nucleotide sequence and expression of the Bacillus cereus 5/B/6 β-lactamase II structural gene. *J. Bacteriol.* Vol 170 pp. (2873-2878).

Livermore DM. (2002). Multicentre evaluation of the VITEK 2 Advanced Expert System for interpretive reading of antimicrobial resistance tests. *J Antimicrob Chemother.* Vol 49 pp. (289-300).

Manoharan A., Chatterjee S., Mathai D., SARI Study Group. (2010). Detection and Characterization of metallobetalactamases producing Pseudomonas aeruginosa. *Indian J Med Microbiol* . Vol 28 No.3 pp. (241-243).

Me deiros A A. (1984). β-lactamases *Br. Med Bull.* Vol 40 pp. (18-27).

Miles RS., Amyes SGB. 2008 Laboratory control of antimicrobial therapy chapter 8 In *Mackie & McCartney's Practical Medical Microbiology,* 14th ed, JG Collee, AG Fraser, BP Marmion, A Simmons, Editors, pp. (151-178) Churchil Livingston, ISBN: 978-81-312-0393-4, Indian Reprints.

Miriagou, V., Tzouvelekis L. S., Rossiter S., Tzelepi E., Angulo F.J., Whichard J.M. (2003). Imipenem resistance in a *Salmonella* clinical strain due to plasmid-mediated class A carbapenemase KPC-2. *Antimicrob.Agents Chemother.* Vol 47 pp. (1297–1300).

Moland E S., Kim S., Hong S G., Keneeth & Thomson. (2008). Newer β-lactamases: Clinical & Laboratory Implication Part 1. *Clinical Microbiology Newsletter,* Vol 30 No.10 pp. (71-78).

Naas, T., P. Nordmann. (1999). OXA-type β-lactamases. *Curr. Pharm.Des.* Vol 5 pp. (865–879).

Philippon A., Arlet G., Jacoby GA. (2002). Plasmid-determined Amp C type β-lactamases. *Antimicrob Agents Chemother.* Vol 46 pp. (1-11).

Pitt T L. (1990). Pseudomonas: vol 2 chapter 2.12. *Topley & Wilson Principles of Bacteriology, Virology and Immunity,* 8th ed, MT Parker & BI Duerden, Eds., pp. (256-269). Edward Arnold, ISBN : 0 340 88565 3., London, UK.

Queenan AM., Bush K. (2007). Carbapenemases : the versatile β-lactamases. *Clinical Microbiology Review,* Vol 20 No.3 pp. (440-458).

Saha R., Jain S., Kaur IR. (2010). Metallobetalactamase producing Pseudomonas species - a major cause of concern among hospital associated urinary tract infection. *J Indian Med Assoc.* Vol 108 No.6 pp. (344-348).

Sarkar B., Biswas D., Prasad R. (2006). A clinicomicrobiological study on the importance of Pseudomonas in nosocomially infected ICU patients with special reference to metallobetalactamases production. *Indian J Pathol Microbiol.* Vol 49 pp. (44-48).

Soughakoff W., Goussard S., Courvalin P. (1988) TEM-3-β-lactamases which hydrolyzes broad spectrum cephalosporins, is derived from the TEM-2 penicillinases by two amino acid substitutions. *FEMS Microbiol Lett.* Vol.56 pp. (343-348).

Stórenburg E., Mack D. (2003). Extended-spectrum beta-lactamases: Implications for the clinical microbiology laboratory, therapy, and infection control. *J Infect* Vol 47 pp. (273-295).

Sugino Y., Iinuma Y., Nada T., Tawada Y., Amano H., Nakamura T., Hasegawa Y., Shimokata K., Shibata N., Arkawa Y. (2001). Antimicrobiol activities and mechanism of carbapenem resistance in clinical isolates of carbapenem resistant P. aeruginosa and Acinetobacter spp. *J Jpn. Assoc. Infect. Dis.* Vol 75 pp. (662–670).

Thomson K. S. (2001). Controversies about Extended-Spectrum and AmpC Beta-Lactamases. *Emerging Infectious Diseases* Vol 7 No.2 pp. (333-336).

Toleman MA., Vinodh H., Sekar U., Kamat V., Walsh TR. (2007). blaVIM-2 harboring integrons isolated in India, Russia, and the United States arise from an Ancestral

Class 1 integron predating the formation of the 3′ conserved sequence. *Antimicrob Agents & Chemother* Vol 51 No.7 pp. (2636-2638).

Tzouvelekis L S., Bonomo R A. (1999). SHV-type beta-lactamases. *Curr. Pharm Des.* Vol 5 pp. (847-864).

Walsh, T. R., Bolmstrom A., Qwarnstrom A., GalesA. (2002). Evaluation of a new Etest for detecting metall-lactamases in routine clinical testing. *J. Clin. Microbiol.* Vol 40 pp. (2755–2759).

Washington CW Jr., Stephen DA., Williams MJ., Elmer WK., Gary WP., Paul CS., Gail LW. (2006). Antimicrobial Susceptibility Testing chapter 17 In *Koneman's Colour Atlas and Textbook of Diagnostic Microbiology*, 6th ed, pp. (945-1021) Lippincott Williams & Wilkins, ISBN : 10: 0-7817-3014-7., Philadelphia PA, USA.

Watanabe M., Iyobe S., Inove M., Mitsuhashi S. (1991) Transferable imipenem resistance in P. aeruginosa. *Antimicrob Agent Chemother* . Vol 35 pp. (147-151).

Wayne PA. (2008). Performance standards for antimicrobial susceptibility testing; 18th informational supplement. *Clin Lab Standards Inst.* M100-S18.

Yagi T., Wachino J., Kurokawa H., Suzuki S., et al. (2005). Practical methods using boronic acid compounds for identification of class C β-lactamase producing Klebsiella pneumoniae and Escherichia coli. *J of Clin Microbiol.* Vol 43 No.6 pp. (2551-2558).

Yong D., Lee K., Yum J H.., Shin H B., Rossolinism, Chong Y. (2002) Imipenem - EDTA disk method for differentiation of metallobetalactamases producing clinical isolates of Pseudomonas spp and Acinetobacter spp. *J Clin Microbiol* . Vol 40 pp. (3798 -3801).